NURSING
RESEARCH

AN EXPERIENTIAL APPROACH

BARBARA SCHALK THOMAS, Ph.D.

Professor
College of Nursing
University of Iowa
Iowa City, Iowa

with 50 illustrations

THE C. V. MOSBY COMPANY

ST. LOUIS • BALTIMORE • PHILADELPHIA • TORONTO   1990

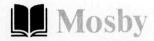

Editor: N. Darlene Como
Developmental editor: Laurie Sparks
Project manager: Patricia Tannian
Cover designer: Elise A. Stimac

Printed in the United States of America

The C.V. Mosby Company
11830 Westline Industrial Drive, St. Louis, Missouri 63146

Library of Congress Cataloging in Publication Data

Thomas, Barbara, 1930-
    Nursing research: an experiential approach / Barbara Schalk
  Thomas.
        p.   cm.
    Includes bibliographical references.
    ISBN 0-8016-6061-0
    1. Nursing—Research. I. Title.
    [DNLM: 1. Nursing Research. WY 20.5 T454n]
  RT81.5.T49   1990
  610.73'072—dc20
  DNLM/DLC
  for Library of Congress   89-14551
                                                        CIP

GW/GW/D 9 8 7 6 5 4 3 2 1

TO MY FAMILY

Preface

The philosophy of this book rests on the premises that nursing is both a science and an art and that the role of research in nursing is to strengthen its scientific base. Nursing science has made tremendous strides in the past decade, including adoption of research preparation in all nursing education programs, expansion of nursing's leadership base from vastly increased numbers of nurses holding master's degrees, dramatic increases in the number of doctorally prepared nurse scientists, greatly expanded support for nursing research, and the resulting steady growth of respect for research-based nursing knowledge. Recognition of nursing as a profession has steadily improved as the role of nursing research has expanded.

There are different expectations regarding research skills needed by nursing students at different levels. The aim of this book is to provide undergraduate and master's level nursing students with a solid understanding of nursing research and its role in contemporary nursing practice. The discriminating use of nursing research findings depends on knowledge of the research process, nursing knowledge, and positive attitudes toward nursing research. Active involvement in the learning process is the hallmark of this book.

Students develop more positive attitudes toward research if instruction is geared to depth rather than breadth. To facilitate the growth of nursing science, all nurses must have positive attitudes toward research as a source of nursing knowledge. Such attitudes stimulate nurses to approach nursing practice with skills of critical thinking and to develop lifelong habits of learning.

My background in the hard sciences and science education convinced me that a research methods course (or an integrated approach) must not sacrifice depth to achieve breadth. Students' understanding of science and scientific methods is most effectively promoted when they experience the complete research process, no matter how limited or elementary the topic or methodology of the research may be. However, the trend in nursing research textbooks has been toward breadth. Through years of teaching research methods at both the undergraduate and graduate levels, I have become increasingly dismayed at the appearance of longer and longer research textbooks. Students are given more to *read about* research, but little in the way of *experience in* research. Over the past 15 years my use of textbooks has decreased while the course syllabus containing experiential exercises and problems has grown. Students' performance from this problem-oriented approach was the stimulus for writing this book.

I am grateful to the Literary Executor of the late Sir Ronald A. Fisher, F.R.S., to Dr. Frank Yates, F.R.S., and to the Longman Group Ltd., London, for permission to reprint Tables III and VII from their book *Statistical Tables for Biological, Agricultural and Medical Research* (6th Edition, 1974).

I am grateful for the encouragement and support of my family in helping me to put forth the sustained effort that writing a manuscript requires. My thanks also go to Professor Nancy Jordison and Leigh Moore for their assistance in reviewing the chapters of the textbook and instructor's manual. I would like to thank the reviewers for their blind reviews of each chapter of the textbook. Their comments and suggestions were extremely helpful. My thanks also to Darlene Como, Barbara Carroll, Laurie Sparks, Patricia Tannian, Liz Fett, and others behind the scenes at Mosby for turning the manuscript into a finished product.

BARBARA SCHALK THOMAS

Contents

NURSING
RESEARCH

AN EXPERIENTIAL APPROACH

CHAPTER 1

Introduction to nursing research

Objectives

After completing this unit of study, students will be able to:

1. List milestones in the development of nursing research
2. Discuss contributions to nursing research by such leaders as Nightingale, Nutting, Johnson, Goodrich, Stewart, Abdellah, and Johnson
3. Describe the relationship between progress in nursing education and development of nursing research
4. Identify barriers to the growth of nursing research
5. Identify facilitators for the growth of nursing research
6. Describe studies that have had the most impact on nursing practice as identified by contemporary nursing leaders
7. Identify the process of dissemination and utilization of research findings

A BRIEF LOOK AT BEGINNINGS
Florence Nightingale's legacy

Florence Nightingale (1850-1910) was the first nurse to be described as a researcher. She demonstrated great independence in her thinking and in her nursing practice even though she was a Victorian (Simmons and Henderson, 1964). She had an insatiable curiosity and an analytical mind that led her to reject "the prevalent standards of divine revelation, authority and majority opinion and substitute as her criteria conscience, feeling, sense of justice, and experience" (Palmer, 1977, p. 85). Her greatest contributions to nursing as a science were her outstanding work as a statistician, her notes on nursing, her work during the Crimean War, and her establishment of St. Thomas, an independent school of nursing. Nightingale was a statistician who presented her work carefully and clearly, and through this work she became known as a change agent and reformer. She made notes about relationships between environmental factors and patients' welfare and about the factors associated with soldiers' morbidity and mortality during the Crimean War. She discovered that the military hospitals' record keeping was chaotic; for example, they had no way of identifying British soldiers who could not identify themselves. An able administrator, she established new systems that enhanced both administrative practices and nursing care.

Nightingale was interested in increasing educational opportunities for women and lauded Queen's College for opening its doors to women in 1878, but she did not envision college-based education for nurses. However, in establishing St. Thomas as a nursing program independent of hospital services, she obviously considered the importance of separating nursing education and nursing services.

In Florence Nightingale's time, what were the sources of nursing knowledge and skills for novices?

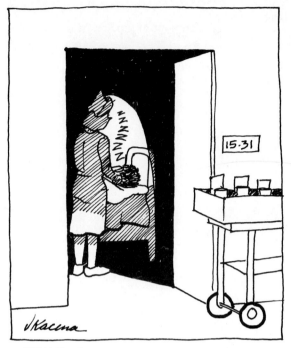

TIME FOR YOUR SLEEPING PILL
MR. WILSON . . . MR. WILSON . . .

Fig. 1-1 Tradition in action.

Hospital-based nurses' "training"

Although Florence Nightingale is generally credited with beginning nursing research, her work did not stimulate nurses to pursue research in the early twentieth century. Nurses were concerned primarily with the rapidly increasing need for nursing services as new health care agencies emerged and existing ones expanded. It should be noted also that nursing educators in the United States did not follow Nightingale's leadership in establishing independent nursing education programs. Instead the programs were operated and controlled by hospitals (Simmons and Henderson, 1964). Nursing students were required to spend long hours learning about and giving patient care. Tradition and authority were the primary sources of nursing knowledge that formed the basis for practice (Fig. 1-1). Experienced nurses passed on their knowledge and skills to student nurses as a means of ensuring safe patient care. Physicians were the instructors, and they selected topics for nursing students that would perpetuate nurses' roles as "handmaidens" to physicians. From Nightingale's time through the early 1900s, nurses had few incentives to question the traditions of nursing practice; conformity was expected and rewarded. Research activity was scattered and sparse. The first nursing study was M. Adelaide Nutting's survey of nursing education in 1906 (Simmons and Henderson, 1964).

What factors hindered the development of nursing as a science?

Nursing started as a women's occupation. How did the status of women affect the development of nursing as a profession?

Exceptions to hospital-based training

There were two exceptions to the prevailing state of hospital-based nurses' training programs in the early twentieth century. In 1909 an undergraduate school of nursing opened at the University of Minnesota, largely through the efforts of a physician, Richard Beard. That same year a department of nursing education was established at Teachers College, Columbia University (Simmons and Henderson, 1964). These were the first nursing programs to offer systematic study of the basic sciences and foundations of nursing, as well as clinical learning activities.

Hospital-based programs dominated nursing education for many years. Their near monopoly was not maintained without protest, however. Such leaders as Annie Goodrich, M. Adelaide Nutting, and Isabel M. Stewart objected strongly to the lack of quality in training and to the exploitation of student labor in hospital programs, and they called for nursing education to be moved to colleges and universities (Simmons and Henderson, 1964). A formal survey of conditions in nurse training programs, the Goldmark Report, was completed in 1920, and another by the Committee for the Study of Nursing Education, completed in 1923, recommended separating the educational and service functions of hospitals. Additional university-based nursing programs were established, notably at Yale University and Western Reserve University. There were 138 collegiate nursing schools by 1946.

Why do you think hospitals had such a firm grip on nursing education?

Move to colleges and universities

The transfer of nursing education to colleges and universities was important in the development of nursing research because in those settings nursing was studied as a science as well as an art. Before collegiate and university programs in nursing began, studies about nurses (that is, their characteristics, staffing, and turnover) and especially about nursing education dominated reseach activity. In the academic environment, however, research on nursing interventions was initiated, although studies of occupational and educational concerns constituted the major part of nursing research for some years.

Research: a growing tradition

The year 1952 saw the first publication of *Nursing Research,* a journal devoted entirely to nursing studies. In a much later publication about gerontology and nursing, Gunter and Miller (1977) noted that an article on nursing gerontology was published in the first issue of *Nursing Research.* This article, by Mack (1952), discussed the urgent need for nursing research on gerontology because of rapidly increasing numbers of elderly people. However, there were no additional nursing gerontology studies by Mack or anyone else for nearly a decade (de Tornyay, 1977). As avenues opened for the publication of research findings, the studies published revealed a shotgun approach to nursing research. There was an amazing breadth and diversity of topics, but there were no discernible bodies of focused research. Specialty journals and the venerable *American Journal of Nursing* also began to publish the results of nursing research. In 1959 the first abstracting service for periodicals concerning nursing research was established (Simmons and Henderson, 1964).

Dorothy Johnson (1959) was one of several nursing leaders to note that, if nursing is to be regarded as a profession, there must be a theoretical body of knowledge upon which practice rests. This message has been repeated in various terms for the last 30 years and is no longer regarded as controversial. As late as 1965, however, a highly respected textbook on nursing research called "nursing as a science . . . one of the most controversial concepts today" (Abdellah and Levine, 1965, p. 13). Most nurses today see research as a principal (but not sole) way of obtaining knowledge to determine their practice.

In 1962 the American Nurses' Association published a national plan for nursing research. Because there were widespread feelings that occupational and educational research should move aside for research on nursing practice, it was no surprise that clinical nursing studies headed the list (ANA, 1962). Since the mid-1950s, clinical research has been more valued than research on nursing administration, education, or history, although there is general agreement that all types of research are needed. As Gortner stated, "nurses . . . are urged to move on all fronts vigorously and not allow one to fall behind the other" (Gortner, 1975, p. 193). Recent years have seen a renewed interest in research on nursing administration in particular. Nursing administration has far-reaching effects on the environment in which care is given, and its components are being studied for ways to improve the environment for patients, their families, and caregivers. In 1980 the American Nurses' Association defined its three priorities for clinical research: health promotion and the prevention of illness, development of efficient health care delivery systems for nursing care, and improved nursing interventions for the nursing care of high-risk groups. The statement of these priorities reflected the growing cadre of nurse scientists who were prepared to take the initiative and provide the leadership needed to establish stimulating research programs.

Another major stimulus for developing nursing science was, as mentioned previously, the move of education to colleges and universities. Attention to rigor in the nursing curriculum came from several sources and included research preparation as a goal for every nurse (Carnegie, 1974). Expectations for research and publication by nursing faculty began to resemble those held for faculty in other disciplines. The number of master's degree programs in nursing increased dramatically, and doctoral programs began to appear.

Better-prepared faculty led to improvements in both research and research preparation in colleges and universities. As advanced levels of nursing education were established, more realistic expectations about nurses' involvement in research were established. Whereas in the early 1970s it was believed that every nurse should be an independent investigator, more recently it was realized that the prime function of basic nursing education is to prepare nurses who can evaluate nursing studies for implementation in their practice, that is, who can be consumers of research (Thomas and Price, 1980). Preparing students for the consumer role is a difficult task in today's crowded nursing curricula, and there are serious disagreements about how it should be done. Some programs focus on critiquing research reports, primarily those in nursing journals. Others include study about research practices as an abstract topic, with little or no hands-on experience. The development of a research proposal is a common requirement, an apparent contradiction to consumer-oriented objectives. Involvement of nursing students in faculty research is considered desirable, but far too few opportunities exist for this sort of experience. There appears to be a consensus, however, that basic nursing education programs should focus on preparing nurses to be consumers of research, reserving the role of generating research for nurses with advanced academic preparation.

With the growth of doctoral programs in nursing, and with increasing numbers of nurses earning doctorates in other disciplines, the research role of the master's-prepared nurse has also been redefined. In the past, nurses with master's degrees were expected to fulfill leadership roles as independent nurse scientists. Today's master's-prepared nurse is expected to function in a collaborative role or as a beginning investigator. The doctorate is now the research degree in nursing as it is is other academic disciplines. The three types of doctorates held by most nurse scientists are doctor of philosophy (Ph.D.), the traditional research degree; doctor of nursing science (D.N.S.), the degree that recognizes clinical expertise at an advanced level; and doctor of education (Ed.D.), which represents preparation as an educator at an advanced level. All of these doctoral degrees are regarded as research degrees, but their focuses differ. The earned doctorate is now merely the beginning of a research career, and continuing education regarding research skills is needed at all stages of nurse investigators' careers (Hinshaw, 1988).

Funding

An overview of the beginnings of nursing research would not be complete without attention to the development of funding for nursing research. An early source of support was Sigma Theta Tau International, the national honor society of nursing, which has been funding nursing research since 1936 (Kreuger, Nelson, and Wolanin, 1978). Chapters of Sigma Theta Tau International at colleges and universities have sponsored research conferences and symposia for many years. Locally sponsored "research days" have brought clinicians, nursing faculty, and nursing students together. What a marvelous way to demonstrate and further the interdependence of nursing practice, administration, research, and education! Although the gap between the generation of information and its use in practice and education remains a problem, efforts are being devoted to narrowing this gap. Both the funding and the prestige attached to conducting nursing studies have been important stimuli for research.

The American Nurses' Foundation, established in 1952, has sponsored a small grants program, which in turn has supported a wide variety of nursing studies. The application procedures have remained relatively simple, and the funds are made available in only a few months. The American Nurses' Association also has encouraged research by sponsoring widely publicized research conferences.

The Public Health Service Act of 1944 created a federal Division of Nursing to support research and research training; however, there was little activity until 1955 (Kreuger, Nelson, and Wolanin, 1978). Remarkable growth of federal funding for nursing research occurred while the Division of Nursing was part of the Bureau of Health Professions, until 1985 when the National Center for Nursing Research became one of the institutes in the National Institutes of Health. Clinical research proposals received the most funding, but all kinds of research were supported. In 1955, $500,000 was appropriated (de Tornyay, 1977); 30 years later, $9.7 million was made available (Solomon, 1986).

The expenditures for nursing research included funds set aside for special projects grants and fellowships in nursing. Many of the special projects grants had research components, and some were designed specifically for faculty development in research. Moreover, funds for nursing fellowships were substantial. In 1985, $52.3 million was allocated to nursing education and another $550,000 was dedicated to faculty fellowships (Solomon, 1986). In addition, nurses were highly successful in competing with other scientists for funds from the National Institutes of Health, such as those from the National Center for Maternal and Child Health, and from other government agencies, such as the National Center for Health Services Research and the National Institute for Mental Health. Funds were also provided by private organizations such as the Robert Wood Johnson Foundation and the March of Dimes Foundation.

The creation of the National Center for Nursing Research in the National Institutes of Health was approved by Congress in November 1985. Its first director, Dr. Ada Hinshaw, identified the challenges facing the new staff and advisory council as delineation of research priorities, development of more depth in nursing research, and more systematic implementation of research findings in practice (Hinshaw, 1988). She asserted that priorities are needed to focus on society's greatest needs and to increase the rigor of nursing studies. She suggested that greater depth in nursing studies could be accomplished by assisting individuals and groups to develop *programs* of research, not isolated studies. She cited the need for a "critical mass" of nurse investigators studying the same general area, who would attract doctoral candidates to their school because of shared research interests.

Milestones

Some milestones in the development of nursing research are summarized in the box on p. 9. These milestones show that the growth of nursing research has been faltering and difficult. It is through the tireless work of certain nurses and enlightened physicians that nursing has taken its place among the professions in universities. Social and behavioral scientists also contributed to the growth in nursing research, especially through their support and mentoring of nurse fellows and their collaboration with nurses in faculty development projects.

FROM FINDINGS TO PRACTICE
Selecting research findings for implementation

Professional responsibilities. Nurses and nursing students are continually urged to base nursing practice on firm foundations of knowledge gleaned

Milestones In the Development of Nursing Research

1859	Nightingale's *Notes on Nursing* was published.
1899	International Council of Nurses was organized.
1900	*American Journal of Nursing* began publication.
1909	Nursing program was established at the University of Minnesota.
1909	Department of Nursing Education was established at Teachers College, Columbia University.
1909	Waters' study, *Visiting Nursing in the United States,* was completed.
1912	American Nurses' Association was established from the Nurses Associated Alumnae (founded in 1897).
1920	Goldmark Report was published.
1925	First *Facts about Nursing* was published.
1927	First clinical study was published (Broadhurst, 1927).
1934	Nightingale International Foundation was established.
1952	National League for Nursing was established from the National League for Nursing Education.
1952	*Nursing Research* began publication.
1953	*Nursing Outlook* began publication.
1955	Public Health Service nursing grants were implemented.
1955	American Nurses' Foundation was chartered.
1957	Department of Nursing Research was established at Walter Reed Army Hospital.
1962	American Nurses' Association set priorities for nursing research, emphasizing clinical research.
1962	*Nursing Forum* began publication.
1963	*International Journal of Nursing Studies* began publication.
1967	*Image* began publication.
1970s	Interest in computing in nursing emerged.
1971	ANA Council of Nurse Researchers organized.
1978	*Research in Nursing & Health* began publication.
1978	*Advances in Nursing Science* began publication.
1980s	Use of computers in nursing research became commonplace.
1982	Conduct and Utilization of Research in Nursing (CURN) project's 11 volumes were published.
1983	Three computer grants were awarded by the Division of Nursing.
1985	Congress allocated funding for the National Center for Nursing Research.
1986	Ada Sue Hinshaw was named first director of the National Center for Nursing Research.
1988	Research priorities were set by the National Center for Nursing Research.

through research. Although the value of other ways of knowing, such as experience and even intuition, is fully recognized, the growth of nursing as a science depends on generating new knowledge through research and implementing these findings in practice. Before research findings are implemented, however, they should be subjected to sufficient study to remove questions about the credibility of the results. We cannot depend on the findings of a single study to develop protocols for use in clinical settings. Replications are needed to provide a consistent body of new knowledge on which innovations in nursing practice can be based.

Oberst (1981) defined four persons or groups who bear responsibility for implementing research when appropriate and ignoring studies that should not be implemented. First is the investigator. The investigator should report the procedures used, the assumptions made, and the limitations of the study, as well as giving readers an objective report of findings. Second, the reviewers or editorial boards who serve the scholarly journals should be responsible for seeing that misleading conclusions or outright misinformation does not find its way into print. Third, nurse scientists who read the report should, through letters and commentary, question methods, results, or conclusions that appear unsound. Equally important, they should point out strengths of research reports and should note when findings are well established enough to warrant implementation. Finally, the consumers of nursing research (clinicians, administrators, and educators) must decide whether findings should be implemented in practice and taught in curricula. All potential consumers of nursing research should develop the habit of reading current nursing research articles—and also the scholarly dialogue and letters to the editor that commend or question reported studies.

Criteria for evaluating research for practice. In Chapter 10 the critical evaluation of a research report as part of the literature review is discussed. At this point our concern is with the general criteria for evaluating the potential of research findings for practice. Haller, Reynolds, and Horsley (1979) developed three categories of such criteria: existence of a research base for practice, relevance of the findings for utilization in practice, and potential for evaluation of the innovation in the clinical setting.

When evaluating the research base, nurses should look for multiple studies of a phenomenon to avoid inferring that an improved outcome is a consequence of a new intervention, when in fact such an association is false. This is termed a type I error (see Chapter 4). In many areas of study, exact replications will not be found, but several studies demonstrating the same outcomes from similar interventions are often available, and these complementary studies help to establish the credibility of the findings. For example, a number of investigators (such as Leininger, 1980; Larson, 1986; and Rieman, 1986) examined differences in patients' and nurses' perceptions of nurses' caring behavior. The studies varied in the designs and methods used, but their overall findings were clear: patients look for positive interactions in communication and when nurses perform routine or special procedures. The nurses studied had insufficient understanding of patients' perspectives and were often seen as hurried and uncaring.

Such consistent findings should cause nurses to seek an awareness of patients' needs and perceptions during the assessment process. These studies represent one of the easiest research bases to implement in practice. In this case implementation requires no organizational change and no consensus among the nurses that the indicated changes should be made!

Scientific merit, another facet of the research base, refers to the quality of the study design and its implementation. The nurse should ask whether the study builds on prior work and whether the design, sampling procedures, and methods of data collection and analysis selected enhance the credibility of the findings. Key issues include adequacy and representativeness of the sample; validity, reliability, and sensitivity of the data collected; and appropriateness of the data analysis procedures. The results and conclusions should be based firmly on the data and not go beyond them.

Risk, the third dimension of the research base, is a mediator in relation to replication and scientific merit (Haller, Reynolds, and Horsley, 1979). The greater the risk to human subjects, the greater the number of rigorous replications needed before implementation. Research findings are more readily implemented in practice settings when risk is small than when it is great. Early implementation of a finding should be conducted as field research, commonly called clinical trials, so the innovation's value can be assessed further.

Criteria concerning the relevance of research findings to practice are the degree of clinical merit (its clinical significance and usefulness), extent of clinical control over the variables (control over outcomes and over the instrumentation needed to measure outcomes), feasibility or ease of implementation (which varies from setting to setting), and cost benefit considerations.

The final set of criteria described by Haller et al. is related to potential for clinical evaluation. A study must have outcome measures that can be used in clinical settings. Clinicians' evaluations do not merely replicate the research but go beyond it to judge whether the outcomes justify continuing use of a new protocol once it has been implemented. Data collected before and after implementation should be compared to determine the impact of the innovation on resources and environment, as well as outcomes.

Utilization and nonutilization of research findings

In 1982, 11 volumes of work resulting from the Conduct and Utilization of Research in Nursing (CURN) project were published. These booklets should be required reading in all nursing curricula. Horsley was the principal investigator for the project, which was a 5-year effort by the Michigan Nurses' Association to identify research findings that should without doubt be implemented, to develop protocols for implementing the findings, and to define the essential components of planned change, using Havelock's knowledge utilization model. The areas of research whose merit was deemed sufficient for implementation were as follows:

1. Structured preoperative teaching
2. Reduction of diarrhea in tube-fed patients
3. Preoperative sensory preparation to promote recovery

4. Prevention of decubitus ulcers
5. Intravenous cannula change
6. Closed urinary drainage systems
7. Distress reduction through sensory preparation
8. Mutual goal setting in patient care
9. Clean, intermittent catheterization
10. Specific nursing interventions for pain

There is evidence that research findings have been implemented when the criteria for implementation have not been met (Oberst, 1981) and that findings have not been implemented when the criteria have been met (Brett, 1987; Ketefian, 1975; Kirchoff, 1982). Oberst (1981) noted that topical insulin is recommended as an appropriate treatment for decubitus ulcers in several nursing textbooks, even though two investigators, Gerber and Van Ort (1979, 1981), reported no significant improvement of ulcers in their tests of topical insulin and in fact warned that a safe dosage had not been determined even for further trials.

An interest in continuing education of nurses led Ketefian (1975) to examine knowledge about temperature taking and practices based on that knowledge. She tested several hypotheses about which groups of nurses would be better informed regarding recent research in oral temperature determination. She discovered no differences in knowledge or use of correct procedures based on level of basic nursing education, recency of basic nursing education, or participation in continuing nursing education. In short, she found little impact from a set of solid research findings regarding correct oral temperature determination.

Kirchoff's study (1982) focused on the discontinuation of coronary care precautions, such as ice water restrictions and rectal temperature restrictions, in intensive care units (ICUs). She found that only 24% and 35% of nurses in ICUs had stopped using these restrictions, respectively, even though the nursing literature contained ample evidence for discontinuing them.

Brett's study (1987) of the utilization of research findings is an excellent overview of some contributions made by nurse scientists and of the problems of reaching consumers of research. Her first step was to identify research findings that should be implemented and had been published at least 2 years before her study. Using the criteria developed by Haller, Reynolds, and Horsley (1979), she selected nine studies published in five nursing journals between 1978 and 1983. She added five studies from the CURN project, creating a list of 14 sets of research findings that should be implemented. She surveyed 216 nurses to determine their knowledge about and use of these research findings.

Brett used Rogers' model (1983) in which the diffusion of an innovation occurs in five stages. In the first stage, *knowledge*, a potential adopter is exposed to a research finding and understands how and when it applies. Next comes the *persuasion* stage, in which an attitude toward the research finding is formed. The nurse considers, evaluates, and either accepts or rejects the finding in the *decision* stage. If the finding is not rejected (which it may be at any stage), the nurse moves to the *implementation* stage when use of the research finding begins. If the innovation can be accepted and accommodated readily in the practice setting, its implementation will continue and spread. If use of the innovation runs counter to agency policy and practices, the implementor will be forced to recognize this resistance to change and either abandon it or take appropriate actions to become a change agent. A change agent generally tries to reduce the barriers to the innovation rather than increase the forces propelling it toward implementation. The final stage, *confirmation,* occurs when the decision to implement the finding is reinforced by positive feedback from colleagues and further adoption of the innovation.

Brett (1987) questioned nurses about the 14 sets of research findings to learn the stages of their implementation. She split the implementation stage into "use sometimes" and "use always"; there was no focus on the confirmation stage in her questionnaire. She determined that one item was at the knowledge stage, seven were at the persuasion stage, four were at the "use sometimes" stage, and the remaining two were at the "use always" stage. These last two interventions were the use of closed sterile urinary drainage to maintain the sterility of urine in patients who have been catheterized less than 2 weeks, with a closed drainage system maintained at all times, and the use of skilled verbal interaction by a nurse to improve patients' relief from pain and decrease pain medications.

Thomas and McKeighen (1989) attempted to identify and describe nursing research that has had the most substantial impact on nursing practice. The question posed was, "What comes to your mind first as the study or body of research which has had the most impact on nursing practice?" Participants, all Fellows in the American Academy of Nursing, were asked to identify studies or bodies of work and then rate each according to its importance and the extent of its utilization. Twenty-nine bodies of work were identified, with most receiving high ratings on importance but decidedly lower ones on utilization. In relation to importance, the studies were rated as to how well they met the following criterion: the importance of the work is exceptional both in significance and in scientific merit; the work represents the best of scholarly productivity in nursing. With regard to utilization, the criterion for the highest rating was as follows: the work has been thoroughly disseminated in all settings; it has been incorporated into nursing practice, and the information is part of forward-looking nursing curricula (Thomas and McKeighen, 1989).

Study participants selected the five most important and five most used studies from the list of 29 works. Ranked first was Abdellah's work (1954, 1955, 1957, 1961, 1965, 1967) on job satisfaction of nurses and its relationship to patient welfare, staffing, other aspects of nursing administration, and research methods, including attention to ethical concerns. The book on research methods that she wrote with Levine (1965) set high standards for research preparation of nurses at a critical point in the development of nursing research. Ranked second was Esther Brown (1948); her work, a continuation of the Goldmark Report, was a major impetus in moving nursing education from hospitals to colleges and universities. Jean Johnson's work (1978, 1984, 1985) on strategies to facilitate patients' recovery, comfort, and early mobility after surgery was uniformly viewed as a strong record of research. This work (with others such as Fuller, Endress, Rice, Christman, and Stitt) came at the critical time when ambulation of patients soon after surgery was being introduced. Fourth, Barnard's work (1975, 1980) on infant development, particularly her studies of the effects of stimulation on premature babies, was highly valued. She examined three outcome measures: sleep-wake patterns, weight gain, and general maturational development. The fifth choice of study participants was Burgess' work (with Holmstrom and Laszlo; 1973, 1974, 1975, 1976, 1977, 1978, 1979), which defined a "rape trauma syndrome" and discussed the needs of rape victims, effective counseling approaches, factors associated with recovery from rape trauma, and the delivery of appropriate care to rape victims.

In the rating of utilization, an obvious choice of Brown's work (1948) was made; the changes in nursing education she recommended have been carried out. The three other bodies of work that received high ratings for utilization were those of Johnson, Abdellah, and Barnard in that order. The fifth area selected was Carol Lindeman's work (with Stetzer and Van Aernman; 1971, 1973) on preoperative nursing activities, especially structured teaching, in speeding the recovery and increasing the comfort of surgical patients. Lindeman's work stimulated additional studies on preoperative teaching and provided the foundation for including this important nursing intervention in basic nursing programs.

Participants noted that selecting five from the list of 29 was difficult for both categories. Dissemination and utilization of new information take time, and a study's importance is often misjudged in the period immediately after its completion. Thus, when the choice was limited to five most utilized studies, older works were more likely to be selected.

The goal of implementing research findings that should be included in practice is far from realized. Information from the CURN project has not been disseminated as widely as it should be, and too few nurses read research reports regularly. On the brighter side, nurse scientists are assuming the responsibility of writing for a practice audience as well as a research audience. Their articles bridge the gap between research and practice by identifying what should be implemented and describing protocols that can be applied practically in clinical settings. Journals are publishing more articles about implementing research findings, and there is even a new journal, *Applied Nursing Research*, that is devoted entirely to this task.

REFERENCES

Abdellah F (1957). Methods of identifying covert aspects of nursing problems. *Nursing Research* 6:4.

Abdellah F (1961). Criterion measures in nursing. *Nursing Research* 10:21-26.

Abdellah F (1967). Approaches to protecting the rights of human subjects. *Nursing Research* 16:316-320.

Abdellah F and Levine E (1954). Work sampling applied to the study of nursing personnel. *Nursing Research* 3:11-16.

Abdellah F and Levine E (1955). Effects of nurse staffing on satisfaction with nursing care. *Hospital Monograph, Number 4*, Chicago: American Hospital Association.

Abdellah F and Levine E (1965). *Better patient care through nursing research*. New York: Macmillan Publishing Co.

American Nurse's Association (1962). Committee on Research, ANA blueprint for research in nursing. *American Journal of Nursing* 62:69.

Barnard K (1975). Trends in the care and prevention of developmental disabilities. *American Journal of Nursing* 75:1700-1704.

Barnard K (1980). Knowledge for practice: directions for the future. *Nursing Research* 29:208-212.

Brett J (1987). Use of nursing practice research findings. *Nursing Research* 36:344-349.

Broadhurst J (1927). Hand-brush suggestions for visiting nurses. *Public Health Nursing* 19:487.

Brown E (1948). *Nursing for the future.* New York: Russell Sage.

Burgess AW and Holmstrom LL (1973). The rape victim in the emergency ward. *American Journal of Nursing* 10:1741.

Burgess AW and Holmstrom LL (1974). Crisis and counseling requests of rape victims. *Nursing Reseach* 23:196.

Burgess AW and Holmstrom LL (1975). Accountability: a right of the rape victim. *Journal of Psychiatric Nursing* 13:11.

Burgess AW and Holmstrom LL (1976). Coping behavior of the rape victim. *American Journal of Psychology* 133:413.

Burgess AW and Holmstrom LL (1978). Recovery from rape and prior life stress. *Research in Nursing and Health* 1:165.

Burgess AW and Holmstrom LL (1979). Rape: sexual description and recovery. *American Journal of Orthopsychiatry* 49:648.

Burgess AW and Laszlo AT (1977). Courtroom use of hospital records in sexual assault cases. *American Journal of Nursing* 1:64.

Carnegie E (1974). The research attitude begins on the undergraduate level (Editorial). *Nursing Research* 23:99.

de Tornyay R (1977). Nursing research: the road ahead. *Nursing Research* 26:404-407.

Gerber R and Van Ort S (1979). Topical application of insulin in decubitus ulcers. *Nursing Research* 28:16-19.

Gerber R and Van Ort S (1981). Topical application of insulin to pressure sores: a questionable therapy. *American Journal of Nursing* 81:1159.

Gortner S (1972). Research for a practice profession. *Nursing Research* 24:193-197.

Gunter L and Miller J (1977). Research in the practice areas: toward a nursing gerontology, Part 5. *Nursing Research* 26:208-230.

Haller D, Reynolds M, and Horsley J (1979). Developing research-based innovation protocols: process, criteria and issues. *Research in Nursing and Health* 2:45-51.

Hinshaw A (1988). The National Center for Nursing Research: challenges and initiatives. *Nursing Outlook* 36:54-56.

Horsely J, Crane J, Crabtree M, and Wood D (1978). *Using research to improve nursing practice: a guide.* CURN Project. New York: Grune & Stratton Inc.

Johnson D (1959). The nature of a science of nursing. *Nursing Outlook* 7:291-296.

Johnson J (1984). Coping with surgery. In Werley HH and Fitzpatrick JJ (Editors). *Annual Review of Nursing Research. Vol II.* New York: Springer Publishing Co Inc, pp 107-132.

Johnson J, Christman N, and Stitt C (1985). Personal control interventions: short- and long-term effects on surgical patients. *Research in Nursing and Health* 8:131-145.

Johnson J, Fuller S, Endress M, and Rice V (1978). Altering patients' responses to surgery: an extension and a replication. *Research in Nursing and Health* 1:111-121.

Johnson J, Rice V, Fuller S, and Endress M (1978). Sensory information, instruction in a coping strategy and recovery from surgery. *Research in Nursing and Health* 1:4-17.

Ketefian S (1975). Application of selected nursing research findings into nursing practice. *Nursing Research* 24:89-92.

Kirchoff K (1982). A diffusion survey of coronary precautions. *Nursing Research* 31:196-201.

Kreuger J, Nelson A, and Wolanin M (1978). *Nursing research: development, collaboration and utilization.* Germantown, Md: Aspen Publishers Inc.

Larson P (1986). Cancer nurses' perceptions of caring. *Cancer Nursing* 9:86-91.

Leininger M (1980). Caring: a central focus of nursing and health care services. *Nursing and Health Care* 1:135-143.

Lindeman C and Stetzer S (1973). Effects of preoperative visits by operating room nurses. *Nursing Research* 22:4-6.

Lindeman C and Van Aernman B (1971). Nursing interventions with the presurgical patient— the effects of structured and unstructured preoperative teaching. *Nursing Research* 20:319-332.

Mack M (1952). Personal adjustment of chronically ill old people under home care. *Nursing Research* 1:9-30.

Oberst M (1981). Responsibility and the research consumer. *Cancer Nursing* 4:407-408.

Palmer I (1977). Florence Nightingale: reformer, reactionary, researcher. *Nursing Research* 26:84-89.

Rieman D (1986). Noncaring and caring in the clinical setting: patients' descriptions. *Topics in Clinical Nursing* 8:30-36.

Rogers E (1983). *Diffusion of innovations.* 3rd ed. New York: Free Press.

Simmons L and Henderson V (1964). *Nursing research: a survey and assessment.* New York: Appleton & Lange.

Solomon S (1986). Congress overrides presidential veto: nurses triumph. *Nursing and Health Care* 7:14-15.

Thomas B and McKeighen R (1989). An analysis of the importance and utilization of selected research findings. In press.

Thomas B and Price M (1980). A survey of research preparation in nursing education. *Nursing Research* 29:259-261.

Watson J (1981). Nursing's scientific quest. *Nursing Outlook* 29:413-416.

REFERENCES FOR FURTHER STUDY

Abdellah F (1972). Evolution of nursing as a profession. *International Nursing Review* 19:219-235.

Amos L (1985). Influencing the future of nursing research through power and politics. *Western Journal of Nursing Research* 7:460-470.

Blomquist K (1986). Replication of research. *Research in Nursing and Health* 9:193-194.

Cook E (1913). *The life of Florence Nightingale.* Vol I. London: Macmillan Publishing Co, Inc.

Diers D (1988). On clinical scholarship (again). *Image* 20:2.

Feldman H (1981). A science of nursing—to be or not to be? *Image* 13:63-66.

Gortner S (1983). The history and philosophy of nursing science and research. *Advances in Nursing Science* 5:1-8.

Haller K (1986). The value of replication research. *Maternal Child Nursing Journal* 11:364.

Horsley J, Crane J, and Bingle J (1978). Research utilization as an organizational process. *Journal of Nursing Administration* 8:4-6.

Lawson L (1988). Building research credibility. *Journal of Nursing Administration* 18:7, 24

Meleis A (1987). International nursing research for knowledge development. *Western Journal of Nursing Research* 9:285-287.

Nightingale F (1859). *Notes on nursing.* Philadelphia: JB Lippincott Co.

See E (1977). The ANA and research in nursing. *Nursing Research* 26:165-171.

Stevenson J (1987). Forging a research discipline. *Nursing Research* 36:60-64.

Werley H (1977). Nursing research in perspective. *International Nursing Review* 24:75-83.

Woods N (1986). The winds of change . . . dramatic changes in nursing research. *Nursing Research* 19:1-14.

CHAPTER 2

Research process

Objectives

After completing this unit of study, students will be able to:

1. Define research
2. Define replication and describe the steps in completing a replication
3. Describe scientific methods
4. Describe ways of acquiring knowledge
5. Identify and describe kinds of articles in nursing journals
6. Explain the steps of the research process
7. Compare and contrast the research process with the nursing process and with ordinary problem solving
8. List at least five ways of classifying nursing research

Nursing leaders and most nurses recognize research as vitally needed if nursing is to be regarded as a profession. By definition, a profession is an occupation requiring advanced education and involving intellectual skills that rest on a body of tested knowledge.

Compare nursing based on apprenticeship training in hospitals (for example, from 1900 to 1930) with contemporary nursing in relation to its status as a profession.

Did early nurses have intellectual skills that rested on a body of tested knowledge? On what did they rely?

Contemporary nursing requires advanced education and bases its practice on foundations of tested knowledge from all health professions, the basic sciences, the social sciences, and the behavioral sciences. There has been a phenomenal growth of research-based knowledge in nursing during the past three decades. The proliferation of graduate programs alone accounts for an enormous body of new knowledge. Master's and doctoral degree graduates in nursing have produced studies that have been widely published. Nursing faculties have accepted the challenge to "publish or perish." It is not uncommon for nursing faculty members to average five or more publications per year. In addition to research generated in academic settings, many hospitals encourage research activities for nurses and some have even established research departments. Moreover, theories have been borrowed and adapted from other disciplines, and nursing theories have been developed. Nursing is firmly established as a profession.

WAYS OF GENERATING KNOWLEDGE

Before turning to ways that scientific methods generate knowledge and sometimes produce theories, we should consider other sources of knowledge nurses use in determining their practice.

Common sense

Common sense is an important source of knowledge that can be acquired in various ways: reasoning from experiences, observation, using other senses, and trial and error. Reasoning from experiences includes both personal and educational experience. Thus common sense tells us that a baby's bath water should be comfortably warm and that precautions should be taken to prevent chilling of the baby during the bath. Common sense dictates that nurses remind new mothers never to leave infants or toddlers alone in a bath for even a moment. Commonsense knowledge, which often has origins that are only vaguely recognized, guides nursing practice in all areas.

That common sense is an important source of nursing knowledge can be demonstrated by looking at the origin of the word "nurse"—the Latin *nutricia*, nourishing. Most people perform or receive nursing or nursinglike acts in their daily lives. The teenage babysitter may not be able to describe the causes and manifestations of separation anxiety, but he or she knows that something needs to be done if an infant starts to cry when the mother leaves. The babysitter may have commonsense knowledge from observation, from caring for other young children, or from a course, book, or pamphlet on child care. Through experience, then, people develop ways of dealing with situations, needs, or problems— with varying degrees of success or predictability. Herein lies the problem with common sense. It may or may not be successful. Individuals and situations are unique; the outcomes of a given intervention based on common sense may not be predictable.

Identify some examples of commonsense knowledge in nursing.

Trial and error

A young mother may use another method of acquiring knowledge—trial and error—to soothe a fussy baby. She may try many things to comfort the child before she succeeds in stopping the crying. The next time the baby is fussy, she is likely to use those measures her experience has shown to be effective—she uses knowledge gained from trial and error. Will she be successful? Not necessarily! Through trial and error, people build repertoires of behaviors for dealing with certain situations. Some are effective; some are not.

Should nursing knowledge be built on knowledge of questionable authenticity? How much nursing practice do you think is based on common sense? On trial and error?

Intuition

In many cases, when faced with a need to make a decision and with no ready solution from either education or experience, the nurse may use intuition—a hunch or idea that has no foundation for predicting what the consequences of implementing it will be. The word "intuition" refers to a grasp of knowledge as a whole, immediate possession of knowledge, or acquisition of knowledge without reasoning. Although intuition has sometimes been the basis of nursing practice in the past, descriptions of its use have been strangely absent from the nursing literature until recent years. Rew and Barrow (1987) examined 14,971 article titles from the *American Journal of Nursing* for the years 1900, when the journal originated, until 1970. Only one of these titles contained the word "intuition," and that article was advocating the use of systematic assessment rather than intuition in making clinical nursing decisions (McCain, 1965). The problems with intuition are obvious and stem from its failure to be based on facts, experience, or any known foundation. The outcomes of actions based on intuition are unpredictable.

The role of intuition has received more attention recently, which has enhanced its credibility somewhat. Loye (1983) asserted that ethical dilemmas, expert nursing care, and the ability to predict behavior based on inadequate or ambiguous data all require the nurse's intuitive thinking. Intuition probably does not operate in a vacuum. It is likely that nursing actions based on intuition are really responses dictated by verbal and nonverbal cues and relationships the nurse has experienced only subliminally. The real source of the intuitive behavior remains obscure, even to the caregiver.

Authority

A fourth basis for nursing actions is expert knowledge in nursing, often called *authority*. When learning about nursing, a student is usually exposed to a wide body of knowledge in the sciences and the humanities, as well as nursing course work. Here knowledge is accumulated through synthesis of that which the student brings to the program, that which is acquired in formal courses, that which is learned through independent study or informal experiences, and finally that which is acquired through laboratory work, field trips, or clinical experiences. The underlying sources of knowledge may not be readily apparent. They may be common sense, trial and error, intuition, or unknown; all we can say is that they are traditional. In nursing programs, as in most other disciplines, a considerable body of knowledge is conveyed to students as authoritative evidence. The expert nurse clinician has synthesized knowledge from various sources over years of experience and ultimately acquires the voice of authority. All disciplines are based largely on authoritative evidence so that information and skills can be transmitted effectively and efficiently. The obvious advantages are efficiency and growth of the discipline as its body of knowledge grows. The disadvantage is that traditional "truths" may be accepted without challenge, when in fact research is needed to validate or refute them.

The voice of authority need not come from a teacher. It may come from the printed page. We tend to think that anything that appears in textbooks, monographs, periodicals—anything in writing—has a basis in fact. However, the transmission of conventional wisdom via the printed page does not make common sense, trial and error, intuition, or even the voice of authority any more reliable than if the information were transmitted orally.

Research reports

Nursing research can be defined simply as a scientific activity designed to reveal new nursing knowledge. The key words are *scientific* and *new knowledge*. Scientific means that a question or problem has been identified and a systematic study has been designed and conducted to determine the answer. *New knowledge* reminds us that research must extend current frontiers of knowledge; the mere collection of existing information is not research. Sometimes the word "research" is used rather loosely. For example, research is sometimes used to refer to looking up existing information: "I am going to the library to do some research for my paper." This is not research. Research is systematic, scientific inquiry directed toward producing *new* information.

Research reports are fairly easy to distinguish from other types of journal articles. The research author describes reasons for the study and the background information on which it builds. Research reports refer to data gathered for a systematic study of the phenomena of interest. The methodology is described in enough detail to allow other investigators to duplicate the study with another sample in another setting—that is, to replicate the study. The results, conclusions, and discussion are precise and objective. Implications for nursing research and practice should be suggested. It is especially important that investigators identify the limitations of their studies. Such information allows readers to decide for themselves whether the findings can be extrapolated to other populations or whether further study is needed.

Judge whether each of the following is research (R) or not research (NR):

A nursing student gathered information about funding for nursing research from 1960 to 1980 from records of the American Nurses' Association.

Two nurses interviewed parents of children with leukemia to determine what nursing actions were most and least helpful during hospitalization of the children.

A team of nursing faculty members compiled information from editors of journals that publish nursing articles about the manuscript selection and publication process. _____

A community health nurse used questionnaires, interviews, and pharmacy records to examine compliance with therapeutic regimens among hypertensive clients. _____

A nurse historian studied the papers of Isabelle Maitland Stewart to learn about the philosophy of nursing education in Stewart's time. _____

Rarely does a single study provide sufficient evidence to change nursing practice, because the study of human beings is so complex and difficult. The holistic approach needed is virtually impossible to implement. Difficulties faced in nursing research and ways of resolving them or making the best possible compromises are discussed in subsequent chapters.

Other types of journal articles

Descriptive and prescriptive narrations. Many of the nursing journals publish several kinds of articles. Among the most common are descriptive and prescriptive narrations. The former describe the outcomes of a nursing intervention, new ways of approaching problems in nursing administration, or perhaps teaching strategies used in nursing education or continuing education. These articles convey the authors' experiences, ideas, and opinions. In prescriptive narrations the authors tell nurses (or nurse administrators or nurse educators) what to do, to whom, and when. Again, prescriptive narrations usually consist of recommendations based on the authors' experiences, ideas, and opinions, but an increasing number of these articles are syntheses of research written especially for nurses in practice settings. Nurse investigators are taking greater responsibility for dissemination of research findings to practicing nurses. The basis for the recommendations in descriptive or prescriptive narrations should be examined carefully. In many cases the articles pool recommendations from various sources, including common sense, trial and error, intuition, authority, and research. The information is only sometimes based on scientific studies; in other cases there has been no scientific test on which to base the conclusions and recommendations.

Position papers. Many journals publish another kind of article, which might be termed a position paper. These articles advocate certain positions or changes of position based on logic, identification of trends, new ideas, opinions, and possibly research. The primary purposes of such papers are to inform readers about new developments and to persuade them to adopt the author's point of view. The impact of the article depends on the soundness of the reasoning, the factual basis for the ideas and conclusions presented, and the persuasiveness of the presentation.

Literature reviews. In another kind of journal article, research findings are cited and summarized; research results constitute the sole basis for the article. Such an article is termed a review of the research literature. The usefulness of a literature review article depends on several factors: a focus on an important topic, a comprehensive summary of all of the truly relevant literature on the topic, a scope that is carefully delimited (by years or topic), a critical appraisal of the summarized research, and an organized, synthesized presentation. A well-written review article does more than summarize studies; it points out areas of consensus and areas of disagreement, solid discoveries and tentative findings, and methodological strengths and weaknesses. A literature review can be a gold mine for nurses and nursing students, since it summarizes the literature on a topic and analyzes the summarized studies. Literature reviews often recommend changes in nursing practice or improvements in the research base.

In the figure below, draw lines from the sources of knowledge to the proper spot on the continuum that represents weak and strong bases for knowledge.

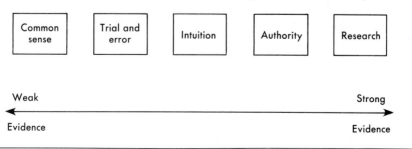

CHARACTERISTICS OF RESEARCH
Use of scientific methods

Research has several characteristics that make it a desirable source of knowledge for nursing. Researchers use scientific methods, not guesswork, to arrive at results and conclusions. Scientific methods allow investigators to evaluate their work; their conclusions are regarded as tentative until a substantial body of evidence has been gathered for verification of their findings.

Evaluate the statement, "Facts are regarded as truth only as long as there is general consensus about them."

Cumulative nature

Research is cumulative; it builds on the work of others. Scientists today are better informed than those in the past because of an ever-increasing knowledge base and because of new technology that has enhanced methods and capabilities of study. Science and technology are inextricably linked. For example, imagine the work made possible by the invention of thermometers, sphygmomanometers, microscopes, neutron accelerators, and computers.

We can assert that science today is better than it was in the 1800s. Is this true? Is it true of art? Music? Literature? Nursing?

Empirical nature

Research is empirical. The word "empirical" refers to knowledge based on factual information derived from observation or direct sensory experience. Empirical knowledge is not speculative, nor is it deduced from theories. Rather, it is based on observations and measurements of phenomena under study. It is open and encourages additional study of a topic. A scientist describes the methodology in a research report in enough detail for other scientists to repeat (replicate) the study. Subsequent work may support or challenge the original research. Thus research is self-correcting.

Which of the following are characteristics of research? Write a Y for yes or an N for no.

Scientific methods employed _____

Subject to evaluation _____

Cumulative _____

Self-correcting _____

Empirical _____

Interdependent with technology _____

STEPS IN THE RESEARCH PROCESS

Research is a series of activities moving from the formulation of a problem through the scientific investigation of the problem to findings and dissemination of study conclusions. In real life the flow of activities is neither in such discrete steps nor as straightforward as the following description suggests. For example, it is necessary at the problem formulation stage to think about the methodology that will be employed. The limits placed on a study by such problems as access to research subjects, the rights of human subjects, or measurement error in data collection must be considered from the earliest planning stages. Thus it is useful to think of the steps of the research process as dynamic, sometimes overlapping and sometimes moving back and forth. Fig. 2-1 shows the cyclical nature of the knowledge base and research activities. Through a literature search, questions about nursing or health lead to formulation of a precise problem. The investigator identifies the context of the problem, indicating who should be studied and how they should be studied. Once the design has been determined, relevant variables must be identified and data concerning these variables must be gathered. These data may be analyzed and summarized in various ways. The data may be used to describe phenomena. Relationships may be examined or groups of subjects may be compared with each other. The results must be interpreted carefully and objectively to reach valid conclusions that address the problem statement. This information raises questions for further study.

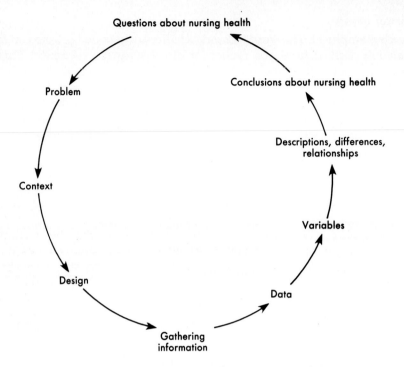

Fig. 2-1 Cyclical nature of nursing research.

Identifying the purpose of the study

The purpose of a study is first stated broadly and reflects the investigator's interest in a topic. This interest may be derived from such sources as observations made in the course of providing nursing care, discussions with colleagues or patients, and reading about a topic or from existing research on a topic. As explained in Chapter 1, some of the most important research by nurses has been developed from their clinical practice. Discussions with other nurses, with physicians, or even with patients may elicit questions important enough to warrant study. Often a research report published in a journal or delivered at a conference raises more questions than it answers. Such reports often evoke additional ideas or stimulate better ways of approaching the phenomena under study. Another reason for reading research reports to identify problems for study is that the report contains at least a brief overview of the relevant literature, and the reader is given leads to additional information and can decide early whether the topic truly interests him or her.

The research purpose must identify the study concepts, which are the ideas or topics of interest—for example, anxiety, pain, wellness, or self-care agency. At this point the investigator may have little knowledge about prior work in the topic area and may even be fuzzy about the nature of some of the concepts of interest. Before formulating a research question or hypothesis (an educated guess about the concepts' effects or relationships), the investigator must determine what is known about the topic and where gaps in information are.

Reviewing the literature

Once a problem area has been identified, the investigator must review the literature as thoroughly as possible. The objective is to learn more about relevant concepts and possible relationships among them so that the study will extend knowledge in the field rather than cover old ground. At this stage students often fear that their topics will have already been studied. Not to worry! Most areas of nursing research are wide open, with many questions remaining unanswered.

Another consideration is the possible need for a replication or a partial replication. A replication is a repeat of an existing study, keeping all factors the same (for example, data collection instruments) except the study sample. A partial replication is similar to an existing study, but with some changes in hopes of improving the study's design and credibility. The perfect study has yet to be conducted. Instruments used to collect data for the study may be flawed, a sample may be too small or too unrepresentative to provide credible findings, or the study samples may be quite different from the population of current interest.

Formulating a conceptual or theoretical framework

Information from the review of the literature must be organized to reveal where there is consensus about the nature of selected variables or about relationships among them. Variables are simply concepts, such as anxiety or pain, that take on different values from situation to situation, time to time, or person to person. The review of the literature might indicate a cause-and-effect relationship between two variables. The causal variable is formally known as the independent variable; the outcome (effect) variable is called the dependent variable. The nature of the study determines whether a concept is a dependent or an independent variable. For example, a research problem may focus on the effects of anxiety on postsurgical pain. In this problem, anxiety is the independent variable and pain is the dependent variable. In another study the research problem might involve an investigation of the antecedents of anxiety among surgical patients. In such a study, anxiety is the dependent variable and the antecedent variables (to be identified) are the independent variables.

Information about relevant variables can be summarized and explained to show what is known and what remains to be studied. Such a discussion is called a conceptual framework. It forms the basis for transforming a broad purpose for a study into a more precise and limited statement, question, or hypothesis.

Draw a single line under the independent variable(s) and double lines under the dependent variable(s) in each of the research problems that follow:

What are the effects of relaxation training on patients' anxiety in relation to cardiac catheterization?

Will there be significant dissimilarity in the oral and rectal temperature differences between normal persons (less than or equal to 20 respirations per minute) and patients with tachypnea (more than 20 respirations per minute)?

How is the anxiety of wives whose husbands have had a first myocardial infarction affected by their perceptions of their support roles?

Do overweight adults differ from normal weight adults in their perception of their health status or their self-care agency?

What is the impact of social support, self-esteem, and autonomy on adolescents' health practices?

A conceptual framework can be illustrated briefly by reporting the nature of a variable, self-esteem, and its relationships with other concepts. Assume that adolescents are the population of interest. First, there are several views of self-esteem. A single definition must be selected. Suppose that the definition of self-esteem as merely a person's view of himself or herself is chosen. However, self-esteem is also a reflection of the ways others treat the person, and it is directly related to gregariousness and academic achievement and inversely related to depression and dependence. The literature reveals that low self-esteem among adolescents is associated with substance abuse. There may be no evidence of a cause-and-effect relationship, but the conceptual framework formulated from these and other findings might indicate several research paths. Can adolescents' self-esteem be enhanced with interventions designed to reduce dependence and depression while improving social and academic skills? Will such a program affect adolescents' attitudes toward the use of mood-altering drugs? Or better, will the program make a difference in the actual behavior of adolescents in relation to substance abuse? Nurses have a vital stake in learning more about health promotion strategies such as these. The study questions are derived from a conceptual framework consisting of the variables self-esteem, sociability, gregariousness, academic achievement, depression, dependence, and risk of substance abuse.

In some cases the review of the literature contains sufficient information about the concepts that have been studied to generate a theory. A theory is a systematic statement about apparent relationships or underlying principles of certain observed phenomena that has been verified to some degree. If the relationships among certain variables have been consistently demonstrated, a theory may have been devised to describe, explain, and predict relevant phenomena. To survive, however, a theory must be continually verified. One theory about aging asserts that people withdraw from business and social interactions as they grow older. This withdrawal, termed disengagement (Cummings, Dean, and Newell, 1960), is viewed as beneficial to both the elderly and society; it is thought to be desired by older people. Disengagement theory has been both supported and challenged, and an alternative theory, activity theory, has been proposed (Havighurst, 1968). Activity theory posits that older people want to remain active in all phases of their lives and that any withdrawal is against their desires and in fact is an outcome of discrimination toward the elderly. Although research to test disengagement theory is still conducted, many of its supporters now agree that it applies only to some people, primarily those in poor health or with passive personalities. More recent research on healthy older adults provides support for activity theory.

Formulating the problem statement

Formulating a research problem involves moving from the general purpose of the research as originally perceived to specific statements, questions, or hypotheses suggested by the review of the literature. Information about relevant variables and prior work in the area points to gaps, and one or more of these lead to the problem statement. In an area where little is known about the concepts, the research problem may be stated as a declarative sentence: "The purpose of this research is to explore factors that impinge on . . . ." Such a problem statement indicates that the research will be an exploratory study. In an exploratory study the investigator attempts to identify relevant variables and perhaps relationships among them. Hypotheses are often generated from exploratory studies. A hypothesis is simply an educated guess.

If a topic has received enough study to suggest tentative relationships among relevant, known variables, the research problem is usually stated as a question or series of questions. These questions focus on gaps identified in the literature review—but not necessarily *all* of the gaps. It is common for two or more investigators to start out with similar research purposes, read the same body of literature, and derive very different problem statements. Similarly, if the literature indicates that certain relationships or differences in groups need to be substantiated, the investigator may wish to test hypotheses about the variables in question to challenge or verify existing findings or to extend understanding of these findings.

Delimiting and delineating the research problem are important parts of stating it. Delimiting refers to defining boundaries—determining which phenomena will be included in the study and which will be excluded. Delineation refers to describing all of the questions and subquestions to be addressed in the study. The problem statement should be sharply focused. Relevant variables must be defined, both conceptually and operationally. A conceptual definition is like one obtained from a dictionary, although it may be derived from books or articles about the concept. A conceptual definition may be abstract. By comparison, an operational definition of a variable must be concrete. The investigator explicitly states how variation in the concept will be empirically indicated. A conceptual definition of pain may include a range of feeling from dull distress to acute, sometimes unbearable agony. It may refer to illness or injury. By contrast, an operational definition specifies how higher levels of pain are to be distinguished from lower levels. Overt physical signs of pain may be combined with verbal expressions of pain on a checklist, producing a pain score. Or physiological measures, such as pulse rate or use of pain medications, may suffice as the operational definition of pain.

Label each of these definitions as conceptual (C) or operational (O):	**Anxiety**—the score on Spielberger's State Anxiety Scale (Spielberger, 1983) _____
	Social support—"a characteristic of the social situation that buffers the effects of stress on the health of the individual" (Northouse, 1988) _____
	Psychosocial adjustment to illness—score on the Psychosocial Adjustment to Illness Scale (PAIS) (Derogatis, 1975) _____
	Stroke—a focal brain disorder resulting in continued neurologic deficits of 12 hours or more because of interruptions in the blood supply to the brain (Sahs and Hartman, 1976) _____
	Self-concept—score on the Piers-Harris Scale (1967)
	Primipara—a woman bearing a child for the first time
	Apical pulse—the rate of beat obtained by placing the stethoscope over the apical area of the heart (Brown and Murphy, 1977) _____
	Elderly—a person aged 65 or older _____

Determining the research methodology

The first aspect of methodology that must be decided is the general approach. Fig. 2-2 summarizes some of investigators' options. It is apparent from this diagram that research can be regarded as a series of decisions, each of which limits subsequent choices. Most components of this diagram are self-explanatory. The main differences between basic and applied research lie in the purposes of the study. If the study is pursued to satisfy the investigator's curiosity, it is probably basic research. Basic research usually leads eventually to practical applications, that is, to solving problems, but the time between the discovery and the application of findings may be long. Problem solving is not the stimulus for the study as it is in applied research.

The review of the literature suggests the level of study appropriate to a topic. If little is known about the topic, it would be premature to develop an experimental study, one that attempts to establish cause and effect among phenomena. First, variables must be identified and studied. On the other hand, if there has been substantial study of an area and one or more independent variables can be manipulated in an effort to determine cause and effect, an investigator may well proceed with an experimental approach. Experimental approaches involve

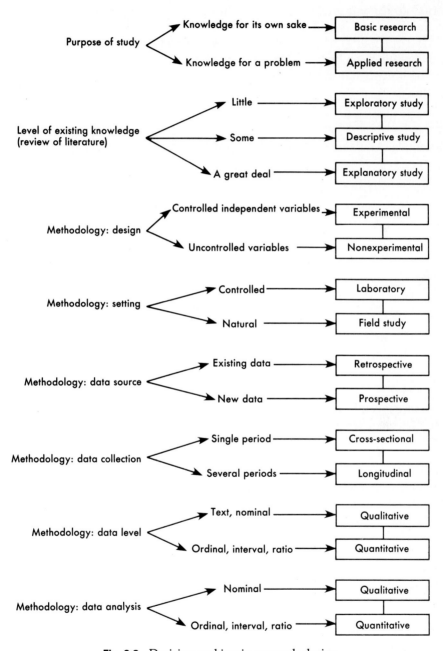

Fig. 2-2 Decision making in research design.

comparisons of experimental and control groups with the investigator determining the treatment that each receives. Giving one treatment to the experimental group and another to the control group is referred to as manipulating
the independent variable.

Most nursing studies focus on the real world of nursing care, education,
administration, or history. Thus most are field studies, and variables are examined in their natural context, in contrast to studies conducted in laboratory
settings.

What kinds of nursing studies might be carried out in a laboratory setting?

A retrospective study concerns research on data from the past. Chart audits
or studies of an organization's minutes or a nursing leader's papers are examples
of data collection for retrospective studies. The data were recorded for purposes
other than the study at hand. In prospective studies, data collection follows
formulation of the problem and the data are collected specifically for the research.
(Differences in these approaches, as well as their advantages and disadvantages,
are discussed in Chapter 4.)

The last two methodological items in Fig. 2-2 contain terms that may be
unfamiliar. Briefly, there are four levels of data. Nominal data are in the lowest
level and consist merely of narrative materials that can be placed in different
categories or classes. Religion and ethnicity are examples of nominal data. One
category is not more or less in any way than another category. There is no logical
way of putting the categories in descending or ascending order.

The next higher step is ordinal data. Ordinal data go beyond mere categories.
The data can be ranked on some attribute so that a hierarchy may be established.
If a nursing instructor were to rank six students in order of their demonstrated
clinical competence, the resulting set of ranks would constitute ordinal data.
The differences between the ranks need not be equal; that is, if the rankings
were placed in the descending order B, D, A, E, C, and F, the difference between

the clinical skills of B and D need not be the same as between E and C. It is known, though, that B is ranked better than D who is ranked better than A. In a horse race, horse A that wins the race is first and horse B that finishes next is second, regardless of whether it is by a length or a nose!

If six nursing students are arranged in descending order according to height, the situation is quite different. Each student's height can be recorded in scale values such as inches or centimeters, and the difference between any two pairs is measurable. A difference of 3 inches between two pairs is the same as another difference of 3 inches between two other pairs. Such measures are referred to as interval data. If the data have a real zero, they are called ratio data. The levels of data are discussed further when measurement is studied in Chapter 4.

Conducting the research

Nursing research methodology is dictated by the research problem(s). After a thorough review of the literature and a formulation of statements, questions, or hypotheses, the investigator has a fairly firm grasp of what has been done and what needs to be done. The methodological decisions that need to be made are the general approach, the population and sample, data collection procedures and instruments, ethical considerations for protection of the rights of human subjects, and techniques of data analysis to be used. The decisions about general approach are illustrated in Fig. 2-3.

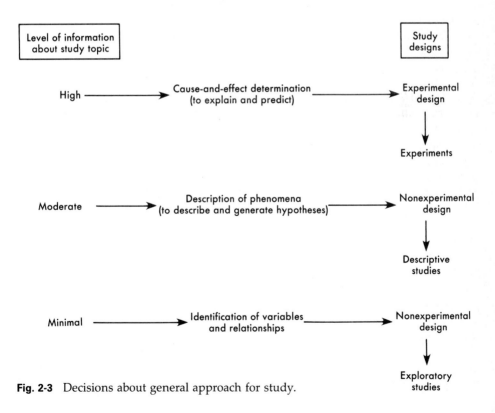

Fig. 2-3 Decisions about general approach for study.

The first decision is whether there is sufficient background information to warrant an experimental study. If not, a choice of nonexperimental approaches must be made. Next is the selection of the target population. The target population is the large group or *study population* from which the sample will be selected. The investigator must specify the nature of the research subjects that will be studied and the geographical and temporal limitations placed on the study population. The target population constitutes the frame from which a sample is selected. The sample must be both adequate and representative so that generalization of study findings from the sample to the target population is reasonable. Sampling is a broad and complex subject; entire textbooks are devoted to the methods and statistics of sampling.

The data collection instruments will have been selected in the problem formulation stage if operational definitions for all variables were developed. Attention must also be given to procedures for data collection. Will interviews be used? Will they be combined with questionnaires or perhaps with chart audits? Ethical considerations must be taken into account. Is the subject placed at risk, either physiologically or psychosocially? Do the potential benefits of the research clearly outweigh the potential risks? Have research subjects been given a clear *option* to participate? The methodology of a research project should not place research subjects at risk for physical or psychosocial harm or distress. The procedures followed must protect human subjects and ensure confidentiality of data. In many cases anonymity should be maintained to prevent possible negative repercussions from responses given.

The variables and their operational definitions, along with the research problem, usually give the investigator some leeway in selecting methods of data analysis. Although the primary focus of data analysis is to answer the specified research problem, it is usual also to collect information to describe the sample. For quantitative studies, both descriptive and inferential statistics are generally used. Descriptive statistics are those used to describe the investigator's data and some of the findings. Inferential statistics allow investigators to reach conclusions about differences among groups or relationships among variables in the sample. In a well-designed study the inferences about the sample can be generalized to the target population. Several techniques of data analysis may need to be employed. Some studies benefit from additional analyses to strengthen the findings by eliminating potential sources of bias.

Reporting the research

The final step in the research process is the dissemination of research findings and a report of the approach used. Research is not complete until this step has been taken. Many nurse investigators believe that findings in which statistically significant results are reported have a better chance of being published than reports in which the results were not statistically significant. If this is true, it is unfortunate. The study's worth rests on its focus on an important topic and its scientific merit, not on the statistical significance or nonsignificance of its findings.

Investigators often report their research informally at a research conference or symposium before publishing it. Thus reports at conferences usually contain the most up-to-date information on a subject. Students of nursing research should take all opportunities to attend research conferences. The meetings are helpful to the investigators as well as the audience. Generally there is a question-and-answer period after each presentation. The questions posed and the ensuing discussion often provide clues to the investigator about areas in the report that need clarification. Aspects of the results or methodology the investigator had not viewed as questionable may be challenged. Thus discussion at a conference may help the investigator identify additional limitations and perhaps new assumptions.

Often, only abstracts of the studies presented at professional meetings are published. However, if the entire report is published in the proceedings of the conference, the investigator should ask the conference organizers for permission to publish an adapted version of the paper in a journal to reach a wider audience.

RESEARCH PROCESS COMPARED WITH NURSING PROCESS AND ORDINARY PROBLEM SOLVING

Steps in the research process are similar to those in the nursing process. Furthermore, there are strong parallels between both of these and ordinary problem solving. Fig. 2-4 illustrates these similarities and explains which parts parallel each other.

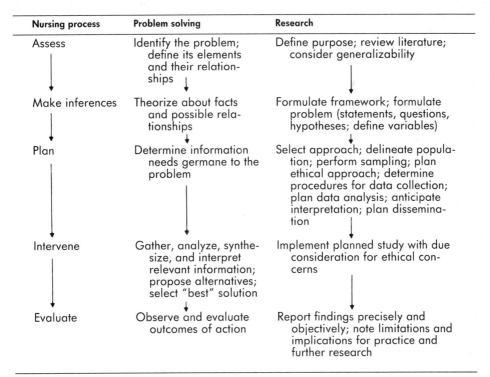

Nursing process	Problem solving	Research
Assess	Identify the problem; define its elements and their relationships	Define purpose; review literature; consider generalizability
Make inferences	Theorize about facts and possible relationships	Formulate framework; formulate problem (statements, questions, hypotheses; define variables)
Plan	Determine information needs germane to the problem	Select approach; delineate population; perform sampling; plan ethical approach; determine procedures for data collection; plan data analysis; anticipate interpretation; plan dissemination
Intervene	Gather, analyze, synthesize, and interpret relevant information; propose alternatives; select "best" solution	Implement planned study with due consideration for ethical concerns
Evaluate	Observe and evaluate outcomes of action	Report findings precisely and objectively; note limitations and implications for practice and further research

Fig. 2-4 Comparison of research with nursing process and ordinary problem solving.

The assessment phase of the nursing process corresponds to identifying the problem in problem solving and to defining the purpose, reviewing the literature, and considering the generalizability of potential results in the research process. In problem solving, the problem must be systematically identified and clarified with its elements specified before information can be gathered for the problem's solution. The review of the literature takes place in the assessment stage because it must precede planning. The problem(s) for study cannot be identified until the literature review is complete.

The stage of the nursing process at which inferences are made corresponds in problem solving to theorizing about facts and possible relationships among them. This theorizing is aimed at identifying needed data. In the research process this phase includes formulation of the conceptual or theoretical framework and the problem statement. When the problem is formulated, variables are identified and defined both conceptually and operationally. Explication of study variables is one vital reason for the literature review.

The planning phase of the nursing process corresponds to the determination of data needs for solving problems and to planning the entire study for the research process. For research, a general approach must be selected (Fig. 2-2) and decisions must be made about the population and its sampling, employment of ethical procedures, data collection, and data analysis. At this point the investigator should anticipate the kinds of results the study will produce. Dummy tables should be prepared for displaying the quantitative findings if the study is quantitative. A means of completing the research process by dissemination of findings should also be planned at this time.

The intervention phase of the nursing process is straightforward if the planning phase has been completed properly. This is also true of both problem solving and the research process. If there are flaws in the plan, there will be difficulties in the intervention, problem solving, or implementation of the research plan.

The final step of the nursing process is evaluation. Its parallel in problem solving is observation of the selected solution's outcomes. If the outcomes are unsatisfactory, the problem solver must return to one of the alternative solutions identified earlier or perhaps must identify a new solution. In the research process the investigator evaluates the findings by objectively discussing them along with the limitations of the study and in the context of prior work on the topic. Thus readers of the research report are given enough facts to make their own judgments about the credibility and generalizability of the findings.

Parallels between the research process, the nursing process, and problem solving should not be surprising. After all, nursing science requires that all three processes be used in professional practice.

REFERENCES

Brown M and Murphy M (1977). *Ambulatory pediatrics for nurses*. New York: McGraw-Hill Inc.

Cummings E, Dean R, and Newell D (1960). Disengagement: a tentative theory of aging. *Sociometry* 23:23-35.

Derogatis L (1975). *Psychosocial adjustment to illness scale*. Baltimore: Clinical Psychometric Research.

Havighurst R (1968). Personality and patterns of aging. *The Gerontologist* 8:20-23.

Loye D (1983). *The Sphinx and the Rainbow*. London: New Science Library.

McCain RF (1965). Nursing by assessment, not intuition. *American Journal of Nursing* 65:82-84.

Northouse L (1988). Social support in patients' and husbands' adjustment to breast cancer. *Nursing Research* 37:91-95.

Piers E and Harris D (1967). *Manual for the Piers-Harris children's self-concept scale*. Nashville, Tenn: Counselor Recordings and Tests.

Rew L and Barrow E (1987). Intuition: a neglected hallmark of nursing knowledge. *Advances in Nursing Science* 10:49-62.

Sahs A and Hartman E (1976). *Fundamentals of stroke care*. DHEW Pub No 76-14016, Health Resources Administration, Washington, DC: US Government Printing Office.

Spielberger C (1983). *Manual for the state-trait anxiety inventory*. Palo Alto, Calif: Consulting Psychologists Press.

REFERENCES FOR FURTHER STUDY

Aggleston P and Chalmers H (1986). Nursing research, nursing theory and the research process. *Journal of Advanced Nursing* 11:197-202.

Derdiarnen A (1988). A valid profession needs valid diagnoses. *Nursing and Health Care* 9:136-140.

Huckstadt A (1986). In search of a scientific base for nursing practice. *Kansas Nurse* 61:4-5.

King I (1987). Keynote address: translating research into practice. *Journal of Neuroscience and Nursing* 19:44-48.

Newman M and O'Brien R (1978). Experiencing the research process via computer simulation. *Image* 10:5-9.

Norbeck J (1987). In defense of empiricism in nursing research. *Image* 19:28-30.

Schmitt M (1986). The research process versus related processes. *Oncology Nursing Forum* 13:125-126.

Solberg L (1987). Is library work research? *Family Practice Research Journal* 6:117-119.

Visitainer M (1986). The nature of knowledge and theory in nursing. *Image* 18:32-38.

Wise P (1987). The research responsibility: spreading the word. *Journal of Continuing Education in Nursing* 18:105.

Wright P (1986). Review of the research process. *Journal of the Association of Pediatric Oncology Nurses* 3:26-27.

CHAPTER 3

Formulating research problems

Objectives

After completing this unit of study, students will be able to:

1. Identify the most important step in the research process

2. Describe four sources of researchable problems and illustrate each source

3. List three barriers to formulating researchable problems

4. Give reasons for acquiring research skills if one's aim is to be a consumer of research rather than an investigator

5. Identify efficient ways of locating published nursing studies

6. Describe the five major aims of the literature review

7. Describe the process of completing a literature review

8. Identify a systematic approach to evaluating research studies critically

9. Describe the process of developing a researchable problem

10. Identify criteria for evaluating research problems

11. Describe the dual role of the nurse investigator and the difficulties the duality raises

12. Describe practices for ensuring that nursing research is ethical

WHAT IS A RESEARCHABLE PROBLEM?

A research project begins with a specific research aim. The aim might be to identify relevant variables in a little studied area; to describe the current status of phenomena related to nursing practice, administration, education, or history; or to investigate person- or situation-based variables in order to explain differences in outcomes from specific interventions with different people or under different circumstances. The statement of purpose generally indicates what is being studied and why. The statement of purpose is frequently modified and refined several times. As the investigator gains familiarity with the problem area through study of the literature, discussions with colleagues, and reflection, the problem becomes more focused and the choices about the study population and the methodology narrow.

Problem formulation is the single most important step in the research process. A person who wishes to undertake a nursing research project should take the time to devise a problem that is interesting to himself or herself, as well as important to nursing. Since the many phases of the research process require attention to detail and sessions of tedious work, as well as exciting stages, the topic should be one that holds the investigator's attention. Where do ideas for research originate? Nurses and nursing students often feel overwhelmed when asked to develop a researchable problem. The usual first effort is simply to find a problem. As information about the problem area is gathered, the second task is to choose among the many problems that emerge!

Before we turn to sources of research problems, three types of questions that are *not* researchable should be noted. Value-oriented or "should" questions may require philosophical analysis and study, not research. For example:

Should the school of nursing operate a home health care agency?
Should additional clinical experiences be included in the nursing curriculum?
Should nursing faculty maintain practice roles?

The word "should" is a clue that we are asking about the desirability of the phenomena—which may require a value judgment. Questions such as these can be revised to focus on beliefs, perceptions, or impact of the proposed actions, and the revised question may then be researchable. For example, the first of the preceding questions might be restated as follows:

How favorably do faculty view the operation of a home health care agency by the school of nursing as a way of enriching clinical experiences for students and maintaining practice skills among faculty?

Devise researchable questions from the second and third questions above.

A second type of nonresearchable question is one that can be answered by a simple yes or no. For example:

Do nurses experience greater satisfaction with primary care nursing than with team care?

Do male nursing students experience discrimination regarding clinical rotations?

Are school nurses' skills used efficiently?

These questions may require collection of data to answer the question posed, but they do not contribute to an overall conceptual or theoretical framework of *new* knowledge. The first question might be restated as follows:

How does job satisfaction of primary care nurses compare with that of functional care nurses?

Restate the other two questions in researchable forms.

Finally, questions that require only the collection and manipulation of existing information do not constitute a research problem. For example:

What proportion of registered nurses in New Jersey maintain their licenses but remain inactive?

How many grants did the Center for Research in Nursing award in the period 1985 to 1990?

What proportion of nursing students who enrolled in graduate study at university X during 1985 completed their work for the master's degree within 2 years?

Choose one of the preceding questions and revise it so that it will be researchable.

In the discussion that follows, four sources of research problems are identified and explained. Most research problems evolve from the use of two or more of these overlapping and complementary sources.

SOURCES OF RESEARCH IDEAS
Experience

Everyday experiences of nurses and nursing students are a prime source of research problems. A nurse who has a spirit of inquiry will question traditional ways of doing things. What is the basis for a certain recommendation in a textbook? What are the possibilities for improving nursing care in a particular situation? Many nursing care practices are based on unscientific ways of knowing; such traditional practices should be examined in a systematic way.

It may seem unrealistic to ask students who are just learning about nursing to identify a problem that will generate new knowledge for nursing. However, finding a worthwhile problem is not as difficult as it may sound. Students simply need to be alert to discrepancies between authoritative evidence about what should be done (for example, from textbooks) and what is actually done in practice. For example, Williamson (1978) questioned the effects of reconditioning on bladder dysfunction caused by prolonged catheterization. She noted that nursing textbooks advocated reconditioning by clamping and unclamping the drainage tubing to simulate normal filling and emptying of the bladder, but that there had been no systematic study of the basis for this practice. Moreover, reconditioning was not being used in her hospital. Since bladder dysfunction can lead to problems such as discomfort from mucosal irritation, bladder distention, retention of residual urine, and bacteriuria necessitating reinsertion of the catheter and prolonging hospitalization, the problem was deemed valuable for nursing. Williamson's study (1978, 1982) provided support for reconditioning as did later study of the same phenomena by Oberst, Graham, Geller, Stearns, and Tiernan (1981). Nursing literature contains numerous examples of studies gleaned from clinical experience or from questioning tradition.

Problem 3-1

A research problem based on experience

Review an issue or two of *Nursing Research, Research in Nursing and Health,* or the *Western Journal of Nursing Research* and find an article that you judge to be based on the investigator's experience. List the citation and the research problem from the study you find.

Citation (author, year, title, journal, volume, pages):

Research problem(s):

Does this study need to be replicated?

What additional ideas for research does it suggest?

Theory

A second source of researchable problems is theory—both nursing theory and theory from related disciplines. The investigator becomes thoroughly versed in the theory and devises a way to test one or more of its abstract components in practical, concrete terms. Nursing theories have been tested in a variety of ways and settings. For example, Heidt (1981) and Quinn (1983) tested Rogers' energy field premise (1970) that "all changes in the human field occur via a rhythmic flow of energy waves as the field engages in interaction with the environmental energy field" (Quinn, 1983, p. 44). State anxiety was the dependent variable in both studies. Heidt used actual physical contact, whereas Quinn tested non-contact therapeutic touch. Both studies provided support for Rogers' theory.

Another nursing theory that has found wide use is Orem's theory of self-care (1980, 1985). Although Orem refers to her model as "concepts of practice," it is generally regarded as a nursing theory for two reasons: it is logical, and it interrelates concepts of wholly compensatory, partly compensatory, and supportive-educative as ways of looking at nursing. Fig. 3-1 illustrates both the nurse's and the patient's actions in these three systems. Nursing actions focus on activities that help patients perform self-care to maintain life, health, and a sense of well-being. People have self-care needs that require minimal nursing interventions in the supportive-educative system, but as their needs exceed their ability to meet those needs, a self-care deficit becomes evident. Such deficits are related to attitudes and beliefs about the value of self-care, physical or mental ability to perform self-care, and knowledge, that is, having the information to make correct decisions, solve problems, or perform self-care activities requiring specific skills.

Nursing care, termed "helping actions" by Orem, plays more active roles in the partly and wholly compensatory systems than in the supportive-educative system. Nursing is defined in terms of its role in providing care to persons with deficits in self-care ability and excessive needs. The helping actions include acting or doing for another, guiding, supporting, providing for a developmental environment, and teaching. In all three systems the characteristics and beliefs of the patient or layperson and of the nurse affect self-care practices and thus influence patient outcomes.

Orem's theory can be generalized to a number of settings, and nursing research literature is replete with ideas for testing hypotheses based on this theory. Orem's theory is consistent with other validated theories; in fact, she used role theory and force field theory to support her premises. A glance at three published studies based on Orem's theory indicates its wide applicability.

Sirles A (1988). Self-care education, parent knowledge and children's health care visits. *Journal of Pediatric Health Care* 2:135-140.

Lakin J (1988). Self-care, health locus of control and health value among faculty women. *Public Health Nursing* 5:37-44.

Nakagawa T and Kogan H (1988). Self-management of hypertension: predictors of success in diastolic blood pressure reduction. *Research in Nursing and Health* 11:105-115.

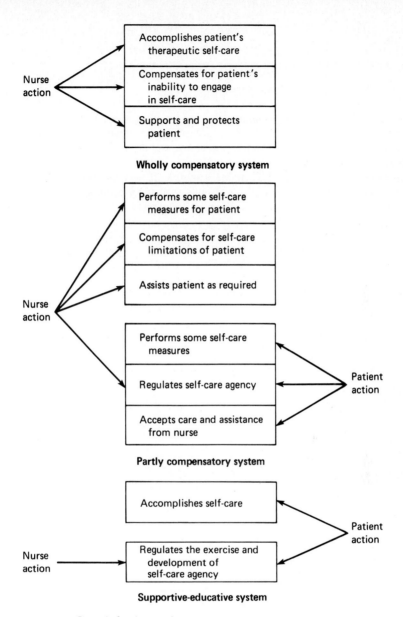

Fig. 3-1 Orem's basic nursing systems.

From Orem D (1985). *Nursing: concepts of practice.* 2nd ed. New York: McGraw-Hill Inc.

A further example of a hypothesis that might be formulated to test Orem's theory is the assertion that a hospitalized patient's involvement in his own care will improve his well-being in a tangible way, such as shortening his hospital stay.

Problem 3-2

Testing Orem's theory of self-care

Study Fig. 3-1 with a view to testing Orem's theory among different populations. Devise a research problem (exploratory statement, research question, or hypothesis—do not be too concerned about the form of your problems!) for each system:
1. *Supportive-educative system.* Focus on a sample of new mothers. State a research problem that would test Orem's theory concerning some aspect of the mothers' (not the infants' or families') wellness.

2. *Partly compensatory system.* For this research statement, question, or hypothesis, assume that you are working with a sample of healthy elderly people. Choose any area of self-care that would be relevant for this sample.

3. *Wholly compensatory system.* In formulating this research problem, imagine that you are concerned about a patient in an acute care setting. Specify the element(s) of self-care involved and the expected benefit(s) in your research problem.

Orem's theory in its entirety is not tested in any of your answers to Problem 3-2; that is not possible. Theory testing really involves evaluating how well the explanations and predictions that evolve from the theory hold up.

Theories from psychology, sociology, education, and anthropology form the basis for many nursing studies. For example, theories of learning have been frequently tested in patient care situations, and sociological theories about role conflict, turnover, and job satisfaction have been tested on samples of nurses in various settings.

Problem 3-3

A research problem based on theory

Locate a study on role conflict and list the full citation of the journal article you find. State the theoretical premise being tested.
Citation:

Theoretical premise tested:

State a related problem for further research.

Research reports

Ideas for researchable problems often come from research reports, both published studies and those presented at research conferences. A proper research report provides readers with background information in the study area, a precisely stated problem, defined variables, a comprehensive explanation of the methodology employed, results and conclusions, and finally recommendations for nursing practice and further research.

In many cases it is obvious that a replication is needed. Definitive studies that answer a research question once and for all are rare in nursing—as they are in any discipline. Additional study of the same topic is needed to verify or challenge the reported results. Replicating a study is one way to get started in research. Replications are simply studies that apply the same approach and data collection instruments from a reported study to a new sample. Thus a beginning researcher has ready-made guidance for conducting a replication.

Reports often stimulate readers or listeners to think of different ways of approaching the problem. The new problem statement may be identical to that reported, but the methodology and data collection tools are changed. Perhaps a slight modification of the problem comes to mind as an interesting question. Another common variation is to focus the general problem on a different population. In addition, most investigators include recommendations for further study in their reports.

The more exposure an investigator has to research reports, the easier it is to formulate researchable problems. One of the best habits a nursing student can develop is to adopt a journal for regular reading. The choice may be made from research journals, such as *Nursing Research, Research in Nursing or Health*, and the *Western Journal of Nursing Research*, or from one of the specialty journals, such as *Heart and Lung, Pediatric Nursing*, and the *Journal of Gerontological Nursing*, or the student may choose to read a variety of journals. The main thing is to read. Information useful for nursing practice will be gathered, and ideas for researchable problems will be stimulated.

Problem 3-4

Ideas from a research report

Locate a research report in a journal of your choice and complete the following information:
Citation (author, year, title, journal, volume, pages):

Research problem studied:

Results:

Problem 3-4, cont'd

Ideas from a research report

Additional research problems identified by the investigator:

Additional research problems formulated by you:

Technology

Technology is a technical means for achieving a practical purpose. Health care is becoming more technologically sophisticated, and nurses as primary caregivers must stay abreast of these changes. Moreover, nurses are often in a position to note adverse effects or foresee problems that accompany technological changes, such as new measuring, monitoring, or treatment devices. An obvious question is whether a technological advance depersonalizes patient care or adversely affects patient welfare or delivery of care. To improve patient care or maintain patient-caregiver interactions, nurses may need to develop new procedures — based not on trial and error or hunches but on scientific evidence. The best way to evaluate potential solutions to practical problems is through a controlled study. In such a study the new practice is used for one group while the traditional practice is maintained for a comparable group. The new practice is evaluated on the basis of observed outcomes in each group.

Technological changes are occurring in almost every area of health care. A relatively simple change illustrates this source of research problems. Enteral feedings have been made more comfortable for patients through the adoption of soft, small-bore feeding tubes, but mechanical problems, particularly clogging, occur with their use. Metheny, Eisenberg, and McSweeney (1988) noted that clogging and failure to clear a clogged tube result in patient discomfort, risk of trauma, interruption of feeding, and additional costs. The expense factor is included because the tubes cost $10 to $20 each and replacing one requires radiological confirmation of correct positioning before feeding can be resumed. Metheny and her co-workers conducted a laboratory experiment to examine the effects on clogging of the physical properties of the tubes and three irrigant fluids. They found that polyurethane tubes were consistently superior to silicone tubes and that either water or Coca-Cola was superior to cranberry juice as an irrigant. Tube diameter made no difference in the incidence of clogging (Metheny, Eisenberg, and McSweeny, 1988).

Problem 3-5

A technological advance in need of research

Ultrasonography is a part of many prenatal management regimens. Formulate a research problem to address the potential improvements in monitoring fetal health that this technology is designed to deliver.

Formulate another research problem that focuses on potential adverse effects of using ultrasound equipment.

Identify another technological advance whose effects should be evaluated. Formulate a researchable statement, question, or hypothesis to study this problem.

FACTORS INHIBITING PROBLEM FORMULATION

Development of important nursing research problems depends largely on the investigator's grasp of the subject area. Lack of in-depth knowledge about specialties in nursing practice prevents many nursing students and some practicing nurses from identifying important, researchable problems. Education as a generalist simply prevents a student from synthesizing fundamental and state-of-the-art knowledge about specific nursing problems. Thus expectations for graduates of basic programs focus generally on using research findings appropriately in practice. As mentioned previously, the role of research consumer is now generally considered most appropriate for basic nursing graduates, and the "doer" role in research is reserved for graduate students of nursing.

Even with sufficient substantive knowledge about a problem area, inadequate understanding of the research process can cause difficulties in problem formulation. The research process is dynamic and interactive. For example, at the same time as problem formulation proceeds, the investigator needs to think ahead to ways of approaching the study of the topic. The investigator must have some knowledge of methodology to visualize a useful, feasible topic. Thus learning about the research process is a preliminary step to formulating researchable problems.

The third major barrier to problem formulation is ignorance of the state of the art in nursing research. In the best of all possible worlds, all nursing students would have opportunities to work with faculty members on professors' research studies, and the students would learn research skills by involvement in actual research. Although faculty members in schools of nursing are becoming more active in research programs, the ideal of sufficient faculty research activities for all students' involvement is not yet possible in most schools. Furthermore, students in basic nursing education programs have few opportunities to attend research conferences; many become registered nurses without ever attending a conference or symposium. Some schools of nursing, especially those that have graduate programs, have begun to sponsor research days or seminars at which graduate students and faculty share their studies. All students in the program are encouraged to attend, and the presentation and discussion are both informative and stimulating.

Few nursing students are required to read research literature regularly, and therefore nursing students often have difficulty distinguishing published research reports from other kinds of journal articles. In today's crowded nursing curricula, students have few opportunities to read research studies on a single topic intensely enough to uncover inconsistencies in the literature and thereby identify researchable problems. They also lack the time to read research reports systematically and somewhat leisurely so that the research problem, background information, methodology, or results can stimulate their imaginations to identify practice implications and new problems.

LOCATING NURSING STUDIES
Preliminary steps

After identifying a broad purpose for a study, the researcher must review the literature to develop a researchable problem. From the statement of purpose, the investigator lists the different components (variables) and identifies synonyms or related concepts for each one. New sources of information, as well as textbooks or lecture notes, may be consulted to produce a useful list. This list serves as a tool in locating information about the topic area. For example, the topic may be burnout of nurses in intensive care units (ICUs). In addition to "burnout," words and phrases the researcher should look for include stress, stress management, distress, coping, and job satisfaction and turnover. Besides special information about ICUs, articles about burnout in other settings or in other occupations might be valuable.

Once the key words for locating relevant information have been identified, there are several sources to consult. In general, it is wise to start with the most recent publications and work backwards. The exception to this rule is classic work; landmark studies or descriptions of theory development should be part of the literature review regardless of date of publication.

Before going to library resources to find relevant information, the researcher should think about how the information that is gathered will be recorded. Frequently students simply list sources on a piece of paper, either as complete citations or more briefly by the journal title and volume and page numbers. The search begins and continues in a rather disorganized way. The student takes notes on some articles and photocopies others.

A more efficient approach is recommended: Decide first which style of listing references and citing them will be used in the text. Suppose a widely used citation system such as the guidelines of the American Psychological Association (1983) is selected. Study these guidelines and make brief notes about referencing books, articles, monographs, and other sources. Using this system, record each source on a different index card; be careful to record the complete citation. Underline the names of books and periodicals. Put your cards in several alphabetized sets: one for books, one for periodicals, one for government publications, and so on. Alphabetize them by the way they are organized in the library. Books may be alphabetized either by author or by title. Periodicals should be alphabetized by name of the journal. In this way you will move systematically from one location in the library to another instead of running back and forth among the stacks.

As materials are found, the index cards can be used for recording the most important points in the selection. Although inexpensive photocopying machines encourage copying articles or book excerpts instead of taking notes about them, there is a greater price to pay for this approach than the mere deposit of coins into the machine. If the material is not read when it is located, irrelevant information may be copied, resulting in a waste of time and money. More important, photocopying delays the critical processes of reflection and synthesis. Reading and summarizing important points contribute to new insights, clarify concepts and possible relationships, and lead to a search for new kinds of information. These processes must occur sometime, and it is more efficient to approach the literature review as a continual learning process than as separate steps of gathering and then thinking. Of course, if travel to a library is difficult, library time should be used for data gathering, leaving the reading for home.

College and university libraries often have computers that can be used effectively during a literature search. First, computers can be used to locate materials, as discussed in the following sections on sources of information. Computer word processing or database systems can also be used to record information and store it in readily retrievable forms. Students can enter their notes directly into files and add labels such as problem ideas, definitions, theory, data collection tools, results, and ethical concerns as the information is entered. As the collection grows, the information can be retrieved, studied, and summarized. Conflicts and consistencies show up quickly, and the computer does most of the tedious, time-consuming organizational work. Computer software for this purpose is inexpensive and easy to use, but of course the hardware must be available where it can be used efficiently.

Books

The subject card catalog can be used to locate books that focus on key concepts. If a study based on theory is planned, accurate, comprehensive information about the theory is necessary, and this means that the primary source, usually a book, should be consulted. A primary source is simply one that reports original work. For full understanding of the theorist's model, additional work concerning the theory should be sought in author card catalogs and indexes.

If your interest is in self-care theory, where should you start?

Secondary sources focus on other people's work. Research reports are generally both primary and secondary sources. They report the investigator's work, which is primary source material, and they include a review of the literature, sometimes under the heading "Background for the Study," which consists of secondary source material. Articles that review the literature on a topic consist solely of secondary sources.

Even if a study is based on a conceptual framework instead of theory, material from books may provide in-depth information and explanations that can improve an investigator's understanding of the potential variables for a study. In addition, information in books may help the researcher focus on the most interesting aspects of a problem. Since usually it takes more than a year to write a book and possibly another year to publish it, the most up-to-date information on a topic cannot be found in books.

Bibliographies

Most students are familiar with bibliographies provided by instructors on selected topics in nursing courses. These lists of references have been compiled to serve as a guide to the literature on the topic. Finding a bibliography on a specific research topic saves time. Examples of two types of bibliographies are Taylor's *Bibliography on Nursing Research: 1950-1974* (1975), which includes more than a thousand citations, and Riggar's *Stress Burnout: An Annotated Bibliography* (1985), which is indexed according to "Signs and Symptoms," "Causes and Sources," and "Coping Strategies."

The researcher should not rely wholly on bibliographies because they may not be comprehensive and because the list of sources ends at least several months before the publication of the bibliography.

An annotated bibliography provides a list of references on a topic with brief summaries of important points. These bibliographies can be helpful in distinguishing pertinent references from those with little relevance to a topic. However, they should be used as starting points for locating relevant literature rather than as complete sources of information. In choosing the points in the summaries, the bibliographer may have omitted information that is highly germane to the researcher's study purposes. Information in annotated bibliographies may even have been distorted.

Abstracts

Summaries of articles that have appeared in journals are compiled in books of abstracts, such as *Psychological Abstracts* and *Abstracts of Health Care Management Studies*. Each volume contains an index that can be used to locate abstracts of articles on the topic by number. The complete citation of the article is given so that those of special interest can be located and studied in their entirety.

Dissertation Abstracts deserves special mention. Research completed by nurses for doctoral study often appears in *Dissertation Abstracts* before it is published in a journal. If the abstract seems particularly helpful, the entire dissertation can be ordered either as a photocopied document or on microfiche. The dissertation generally contains a thorough review of the literature and copies of data collection tools, as well as detailed information about the study.

Another abstract, *Nursing Studies Index*, includes summaries of nursing reports, studies, and historical materials in periodicals, books, and pamphlets. However, the abstracts cover only the years 1900 to 1959, which limits their usefulness.

Indexes

The researcher should always read the directions for using an index because they provide important information about abbreviations, the scope and subject headings of the index, format of the citations, and journals covered. The indexes most useful for nursing students and nurses are the *Cumulative Index to Nursing and Allied Health Literature* (CINAHL), *International Nursing Index, Hospital Literature Index, Index Medicus*, and *Medoc*. Fig. 3-2 illustrates a typical CINAHL item.

Some libraries have special collections they have acquired and indexed. For example, the University of Iowa's health sciences library has the Adelaide Nutting Historical Nursing Collection and the Archives of the Department of Nursing Education of the Teachers College of Columbia University. These materials are in microfiche form and have been indexed according to both subject and author. The reference librarian can be consulted about any special collections that might contain useful sources of information.

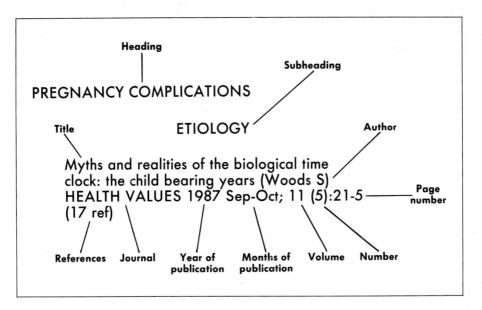

Fig. 3-2 CINAHL entry.

The *Cumulative Index to Nursing and Allied Health Literature* (CINAHL) has been published in five bimonthly issues and an annual cumulation since 1956. Its coverage is wider and it is published more frequently than the *International Nursing Index*. CINAHL indexes about 250 English-language journals, including nursing journals, biomedical journals, allied health journals, and even popular periodicals when they contain articles of interest to nurses. Publications from such organizations as the American Nurses' Association and the National League for Nursing are also indexed, as are publications from the U.S. Department of Health and Human Services. Until 1978 CINAHL contained an appendix that was valuable for locating audiovisual materials, book reviews, and pamphlets.

CINAHL can be searched by computer in some libraries. The researcher should work with a librarian to identify key words and decide what and how many years to include in the search. In some cases a search can be performed immediately. Such a search, called an on-line search, retrieves citations and abstracts for display on the cathode ray tube (CRT) of the computer. If inappropriate or inadequate materials are found, the search strategy can be modified with more or different key words and a new search can be initiated immediately. When the list of sources is adequate, it can be printed out as a document. Computer searches cost very little considering the work they perform. Costs vary according to the topic, key words used, restrictions, and years searched. Most librarians can provide an estimate of costs or will start with a less expensive restricted search to see whether it is adequate.

The *International Nursing Index* includes citations from both foreign and American journals. The foreign citations are placed at the end of each subject section. This index has been published quarterly with an annual cumulation since 1966. It includes approximately 200 nursing journals in all languages and nursing articles from more than 2600 nonnursing journals indexed by *Index Medicus*. The focus is on journals, but the appendixes also index publications of nursing organizations, nursing books, and doctoral dissertations. Computer searches of this index are available in most large libraries.

The *Hospital Literature Index* has been published quarterly with each fourth issue an annual cumulation since 1945. It indexes more than 600 journals concerning the literature on the administration and delivery of health care in both acute care and long-term care facilities. Such topics as personnel, financial management, equipment, education, legislation, and utilization are included. Most large libraries can perform computer searches of the literature indexed in the *Hospital Literature Review Index*.

Index Medicus has been published monthly and cumulated annually since 1879. It is probably the best-known index in the health sciences and covers more than 2600 journals worldwide. Foreign language entries are listed in brackets at the end of each subject section. *Index Medicus* can be accessed by subject or author. Volume 2 of each annual cumulation includes a "Bibliography of Medical Reviews," an index to current medical review articles. Computer searches are generally available in large libraries.

Medoc has been published quarterly with an annual cumulation since 1978. It focuses on U.S. government publications in the health sciences and also

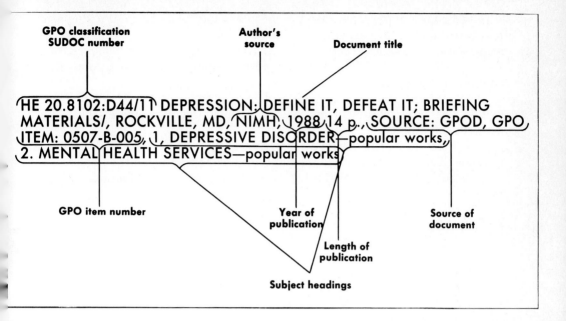

GPO classification
SUDOC number

Author's
source

Document title

HE 20.8102:D44/11 DEPRESSION: DEFINE IT, DEFEAT IT; BRIEFING
MATERIALS/, ROCKVILLE, MD, NIMH, 1988, 14 p., SOURCE: GPOD, GPO,
ITEM: 0507-B-005, 1, DEPRESSIVE DISORDER—popular works,
2. MENTAL HEALTH SERVICES—popular works

GPO item number

Year of
publication

Source of
document

Length of
publication

Subject headings

indexes pamphlets and monographs. Sources are indexed by title, author, report number, and subject/keyword. Computer searches are not available. Fig. 3-3 illustrates a typical *Medoc* listing.

PURPOSES SERVED BY THE LITERATURE REVIEW
Identifying a problem
The overall purpose of reviewing the literature is to identify and delimit a researchable problem from a broad statement of purpose. This involves gaining an understanding about the importance of the study area, major concepts of interest, the theoretical underpinnings of the research topic if applicable, the state of the art regarding research on the selected topic, and methodological issues. Information from the literature review must be synthesized to identify explanatory or predictive products of theories or gaps or inconsistencies in conceptual frameworks that merit study.

Researchers tend to focus on too large a problem. Most investigators must be aware of the need to narrow the scope of a research topic and to search for hierarchical relationships that can produce research problems and related subproblems.

Establishing the significance of the study
After identifying a general problem, the investigator should try to determine whether it is truly valuable for nursing research. The evaluation of nursing interventions that are in use based on trial and error or tradition is always an important topic for study.

Other topics' importance may not be so obvious. A search of the literature may reveal that the problem involves intense suffering or loss for a certain group of patients or families; research that would lead to interventions to ameliorate these conditions would be valuable, even if the proportion of the population concerned is not great.

Another topic's importance might rest on the number of individuals affected. In this case small improvements that would affect many people establish the subject's importance.

The literature search may reveal that the problem area has been understudied in terms of either condition outlined above. In such a situation the importance of the topic area is ensured and further work on problem development is warranted.

Identifying and defining relevant variables

Reviewing the literature should provide an investigator with a rationale for doing a study. Students may develop a general research purpose and go to the literature to find out more about the topic's relevant variables, or they may study the literature in a general area in search of a topic. In the latter case, study of basic references such as textbooks and reference books should probably precede study of the research literature. These books help the student focus on problems of greatest interest and identify variables that must be considered.

For example, our neophyte investigator might be interested in nursing care of infants admitted to neonatal intensive care units, particularly very low birth weight (VLBW) infants. Textbooks and reference books define VLBW infants as weighing less than 1500 grams (Butnarescu, Tillotson, and Villarreal, 1980). Our investigator decides that this population is of greatest interest. One decision that narrows the study topic has been made.

Further perusal of the literature reveals that study is needed in several areas: prevention of very low birth weights, intrapartum risks for VLBW infants, practices for successful resuscitation measures, practices for successful nursing management of VLBW infants, parental support, and practices for discharge planning and follow-up. The investigator selects prevention of VLBW infants. Another decision that narrows the study topic has been made. An opportunity to read a minireview of the literature on VLBW infants and to formulate a problem based on this information is provided later in the chapter.

Defining the conceptual or theoretical framework

Another reason for the literature review is to ascertain whether there are theoretical underpinnings for the emerging study topic. Any theories that touch on the study topic should be carefully studied to identify real-life questions that will test the explanatory or predictive functions of the theory. The researcher must become very familiar with the theory and any modifications and tests it has undergone. The search includes information about the status of the theory. What studies have been done to support it? What findings challenge or even refute it? This sort of information must be synthesized to develop a theoretical framework that reveals what is known about the theory and how existing information justifies or suggests further work. At this point the investigator may or may not have narrowed the topic to a single problem.

In the absence of theory on a study topic, the investigator searches the literature for studies on the topic and synthesizes the findings to reveal research needs. There may be studies that need to be replicated. There may be areas of consensus and areas of dispute. Generally a review of existing studies suggests untapped areas—gaps or disputed points that merit study. Results of existing work must be synthesized in such a way that research needs are identified. This is the conceptual framework for the proposed study. The review of the literature points clearly to research problem(s) that merit study.

Exploring methodological issues

Exploration of methodological issues is an important function of the literature review. The approaches used by others and the limitations imposed on their studies by these approaches can be instructive. A particularly helpful aspect to examine is the sampling plan used in each prior study reviewed. Random samples are generally desirable for reasons discussed in Chapter 4, but they are difficult to come by. Should existing studies be replicated with improved sampling plans, or with a larger sample?

Another useful focus is data collection. What instruments were used as operational definitions of the study variables? Instrument development is a demanding project in itself, and investigators who can find acceptable tools in the literature have made tremendous progress toward their study goals. Data collection procedures furnish more clues. Why did an investigator choose a certain mode? What alternatives are there? Would alternative procedures produce different results? Would they be better?

Provisions for ensuring that ethical research practices were maintained is another area to be covered in the literature search. Ethics review committees look for provisions that benefit research subjects rather than those that are merely harmless. Innovative ways of helping research subjects are sometimes reported and can be useful in planning further research.

Finally, data analysis techniques that have been used in prior studies should be examined for possible usefulness to the proposed study. Usually an investigator has several choices for analyzing data, and an informed choice is facilitated through study of others' methods.

Delineating and delimiting the problem

The problem identified from the literature review is the one that emerges as most interesting or important from the theoretical or conceptual framework. As noted earlier, it is common for beginning investigators to address problems that are too large. There is no magic way to delineate what a problem will address and delimit it to a feasible level of inquiry. However, the scope of problems chosen by other investigators provides clues.

Developing a researchable problem statement requires diligent study of the literature review, and a thinking through of the project itself. A tentative problem statement should be written. Does it contain subproblems? Should it? Are the variables of greatest interest contained in the problem statement? Are there clear indications of the nature of the independent variable(s), the dependent variable(s), and intervening variable(s)? Is the study focus clear and limited to a practical scope?

PROCESS OF DEVELOPING A RESEARCHABLE PROBLEM
Types of research problems

A statement of a problem may take three forms: a simple declarative sentence, a question, or a special declarative sentence (a hypothesis). Although each of these forms is generally associated with a different type of study, the dividing lines among them are not always distinct. Fig. 3-4 illustrates the relationship between the level of the study and the type of the research problem statement that is generally appropriate for each.

In general, simple declarative sentences focus on identifying variables in a study setting, identifying relationships among discovered variables, or generating hypotheses about discovered variables. All of these study purposes relate to *exploratory* studies. For example:

The purpose of this study is to explore . . .

the factors associated with resumption of smoking after completion of a smoking cessation program.

actions performed by world-class athletes to maintain optimum health and fitness during competition.

changes in body image after childbirth when postpartum depression occurs.

For better-known areas, one or more questions may be posed about the topic or situation to describe them or learn more about variables or relationships among them. In such studies there is not enough information available to make

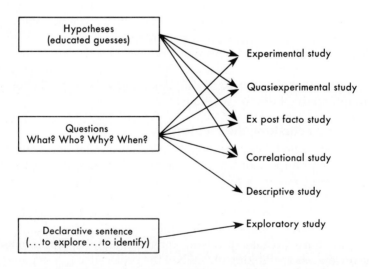

Fig. 3-4 Forms of research problems and levels of study.

educated guesses (hypotheses) about differences in populations or relationships among variables, but the study may enable investigators to develop such hypotheses. Thus questions are generally associated with *descriptive* studies. For example:

> What coping strategies do adolescent patients with diabetes employ in relation to dietary limitations associated with socialization activities?
>
> What is the relationship between seizure control of children with epilepsy and (1) their self-concept, (2) their mother's adjustment to the disease state and (3) their father's adjustment to the disease state?

Sometimes the review of the literature or a theory allows the investigator to make educated guesses about phenomena to be studied. In such cases one or more hypotheses can be formulated as the problem statement(s). The research hypotheses state the predictions in a positive manner. Fig. 3-1 illustrates the major components of Orem's self-care theory. Any number of research hypotheses can be generated from it because there are many manifestations of self-care and there are numerous populations and situations to test. For example:

> Health teaching geared to self-care practices focused on imagery and progressive relaxation will improve patients' adjustment to chronic hemodialysis.

What other populations could replace hemodialysis patients in this hypotheses?

What other aspects of self-care could replace imagery and progressive relaxation in this hypothesis?

Problem 3-6

Prevention of very low birth weights

Return now to the subject of VLBW infants. Suppose that your interest is in the prevention of VLBW births. Further reading is necessary to identify the state of the art regarding prevention of VLBW infants. Is this an important area for study? What is known about the etiology of the VLBW phenomenon? What variables have been linked with VLBW infants? What methods have been used to study the problem? Where are the important gaps in our knowledge of this phenomenon? What do you want to study? Selected information is described in the following abstracts of a few published studies. In an actual literature review

Problem 3-6, cont'd

Prevention of very low birth weights

many more sources would be consulted. Your task is to study the abstracts that follow as if they were a complete literature review, and do the following: (1) write a paragraph about the importance of the area for study and (2) devise one or more research problems. Your problems may be stated as simple declarative sentences, research questions, or hypotheses.

Reeder S and Martin L (1987). *Maternity nursing,* 16th ed. Philadelphia: JB Lippincott Co.
    A number of factors have been associated with VLBW births. Age at conception (under 15 or over 35), weight before conception (20% underweight or overweight), use of alcohol and other drugs, low socioeconomic status, emotional illness, and heavy smoking have been identified in retrospective studies. The nurse should take a careful health history to determine whether any of the following risk factors exist: hypertension, renal disease, diabetes, cardiovascular disease, endocrine disorders, sickle cell trait or disease, neurological disease, major psychoses, anemia, tuberculosis, cancer, or lupus erythematosus.

Naeye R and Blanc W (1974). Influences of pregnancy risk factors on fetal and newborn disorders. *Clinical Perinatology* 1:187.
    Fetal and newborn mortality rates, which are associated with low birth weight infants, are substantially higher in the United States than in other developed countries. There has been a drop in infant mortality rates, but this is due largely to great improvements in saving VLBW infants; the incidence of VLBW has not decreased. Women in the following groups have a tendency to have low birth weight infants: poor, nonwhite, unmarried, older, and receiving insufficient prenatal care.

Butnarescu G, Tillotson D, and Villarreal P (1980). *Perinatal nursing.* Vol 2. New York: John Wiley & Sons, pp 257-274.
    Three types of small for gestational age (SGA) infants are described, and SGA infants are distinguished from preterm and postterm infants. SGA infants are at particular risk for hypoglycemia, thymic atrophy, late anemia, temperature instability, pulmonary hemorrhage, congenital infections, congenital anomalies, large gastric capacities, and future retarded growth.
    Hypertensive disease in pregnancy, birth of other SGA babies, and parents' low birth weights have been associated with the incidence of low birth weights.

Andrews B, Lorhirachoonkul V, and Schott R (1970). Small-for-date babies. *Pediatric Clinics of North America* 17:185-198.
    This paper summarizes the conclusions of the group about maternal, placental, and fetal influences on the VLBW phenomenon, which are illustrated in Fig. 3-5.

Problem 3-6, cont'd

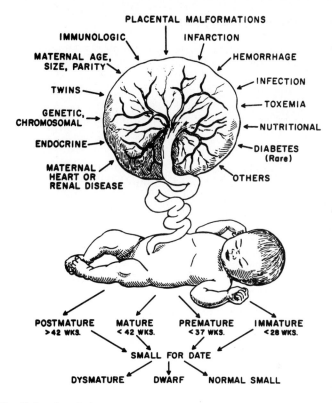

PLACENTAL MALFORMATIONS

IMMUNOLOGIC   INFARCTION

MATERNAL AGE,   HEMORRHAGE
SIZE, PARITY

                                    INFECTION
TWINS

                                    TOXEMIA
GENETIC,
CHROMOSOMAL   NUTRITIONAL

ENDOCRINE   DIABETES
                                    (Rare)
MATERNAL
HEART OR   OTHERS
RENAL DISEASE

POSTMATURE   MATURE   PREMATURE   IMMATURE
>42 WKS.   <42 WKS.   <37 WKS.   <28 WKS.

            SMALL FOR DATE

DYSMATURE   DWARF   NORMAL SMALL

Fig. 3-5 Small-for-date baby.

From Andrews B, Lorhirachoonkul V, and Schott R (1970). Small-for-date babies. *Pediatric Clinics of North America* 17:186.

Schraeder B (1986). Developmental progress in very low birth weight infants during the first year of life. *Nursing Research* 35:237-242.

Forty-one VLBW infants who were free from congenital anomalies and appropriate for gestational age were studied via chart audits and home visits. Developmental progress was studied as it related to medical and biological status (operationalized as incidence of intraventricular hemorrhage, days infant was supported by mechanical ventilation, and birth weight) and environmental factors (operationalized as length of time in NICU, characteristics of the childrearing environment, and socioeconomic status). VLBW infants are subject to canalization, meaning that natural self-righting tendencies are active in bringing the infant back into the appropriate maturational trajectory. (Maturational trajectory refers to the graph of growth with the passage of time.) The author noted the need for additional follow-up of VLBW infants,

Problem 3-6, cont'd

Prevention of very low birth weights

since 29% of the sample were in single-parent homes and another 24% were in low socioeconomic status homes.

Committee to Study the Prevention of Low Birth Weight (1985). *Preventing low birth weight.* Washington, DC: National Academy Press.
   [An investigator who wishes to study this area would find this reference invaluable—all 278 pages of it!]
   Most infant deaths occur in the first 4 weeks of life, and VLBW infants are at greatest risk. Risk assessment instruments should be used to identify high-risk pregnancies and target them for early intervention. Although no single approach reduces VLBW, initiation of prenatal care during the first trimester and continuation of regular visits throughout the pregnancy is anticipated to reduce VLBW births. Other promising preventive measures include prepregnancy health education, especially for low-income women and adolescents, and prepregnancy interventions to correct poor nutritional status, inadequate weight for height, smoking, use of alcohol and other drugs, susceptibility to rubella and other infectious agents, inadequate time between pregnancies, and high parity. Research is needed on ways to influence the behavior of individuals, especially teenagers.
   Health education about reproduction must be improved to focus on preconception counseling, early pregnancy diagnosis and prenatal care, the importance of immunizing against rubella, and the effects of an unhealthy life-style. Such education should be provided in schools, family planning clinics, and the private sector. The current inadequacy of family planning clinics is reflected by the high number of unintended pregnancies and abortions. The unmet needs are greatest among the poor and the young. Both access to and content of prenatal care must be improved. Research should focus on "(1) description and analysis of the current composition of prenatal care; (2) assessment of the efficacy and safety of numerous individual components of prenatal care; and (3) evaluation of certain well-defined combinations of prenatal care interventions" (Committee Report, 1985, p. 15).

Importance of preventing VLBW infants as a study topic?

Research problem(s):

Evaluating nursing studies critically

All nurses should have the ability to review research reports critically. This important topic is addressed in detail in Chapter 10. It is a professional responsibility for consumers of nursing research, as well as for active investigators. The aim is to complete an appraisal that will judge study findings in relation to the study's significance, scientific merits, and implications for nursing practice.

The critical review of published nursing studies should seek to identify the strengths and weaknesses of the study on a systematic basis. Too often critiques focus only on weaknesses. Each phase of the research process should be evaluated so that particular strengths or flaws in one section will not influence the overall critique. Reading widely improves an investigator's ability to appraise research reports. Critiquing also helps readers develop a sense of the scope of a reasonable problem and various ways of approaching researchable problems.

Criteria for judging the feasibility of research problems

After formulating a research problem that is interesting to the investigator and reasonable in terms of the literature review, the investigator should judge the study's feasibility before proceeding to the design stage. The major considerations are researchability, significance, ethical considerations, and practicality.

Researchability refers to whether the problem can be answered by research. A researchable problem can always be placed in the context of a theoretical or conceptual framework. The wording of problems that pass this test should be checked to be certain that they do not require value judgments, yes or no answers, or merely compilation of information from existing sources.

Another criterion for judging the feasibility of a research problem is its importance to nursing. The rationale for the study derived from the literature review and personal experience does much to establish the value of a study.

Still, more questions need to be asked. Is the problem important to nurses, patients, health care agencies, other health care professionals, or society as a whole? What benefits will the study results provide? Who will use the study results? Will information from the study build on a foundation of information for further insights and knowledge? Does the problem serve to test theories? Assumptions? Untested traditions? To meet the criterion of importance, a research problem should provide favorable answers to at least some of these questions.

Analyzing problems for importance eliminates the study of self-evident or trivial questions. However, researchers sometimes fail to focus on a problem because they feel that a more meaningful problem is just around the corner. Students and graduate nurses alike should be reminded that a small, well-conceived study may be valuable, reasonable, and appropriate. Thesis students sometimes need to be told that the purpose of the thesis study is to provide evidence of a student's ability to conduct an independent investigation, not to answer the big questions in nursing research definitively. A perfect study can never be developed.

Ethical considerations should receive attention early in the study, at the problem formulation stage. Nurses in clinical settings often have difficulty performing the roles of both nurse and investigator. Oleson and Whittaker (1967) describe four stages in the development of the research role between the investigator and the research subjects:

1. Surface encounter
2. Proffering and inviting
3. Selecting and modifying
4. Stabilizing and sustaining

Although Oleson and Whittaker are sociologists who focused on participant observation and interviewing of nursing students, the four stages can be applied in nurse-patient situations.

The surface encounter is the mutual exchange that occurs when a nurse explains a study to patients and points out that he or she will also be acting as an investigator. The study is explained in general terms, and patients are asked if they will participate. In this encounter the nurse makes it clear that the nursing care the patient will receive is entirely separate from the role the patient will assume as a research subject. In this way the nurse seeks to overcome patients' natural predisposition to identify the nurse only with the nursing role, which is of course more familiar to them.

In the proffering and inviting stage the nurse and patient offer and seek definitions of themselves for each other. As the study begins, the nurse might invite a patient to ask questions about the research role each will play, in an effort to define the dual roles of nurse/investigator and patient/subject. Patients must be told that they can limit their participation in a study or withdraw altogether at any time.

Selecting and modifying refer to choosing some role definitions and changing or rejecting others. As the study progresses, the dual roles played by the investigator and the subjects become clearer. The nurse investigator must facilitate this stage by being alert to confusion the patients may feel about the study. Patients may be reluctant to ask questions.

Stabilizing and sustaining are the final stage of the role-making process. In this stage both nurse and subjects have a balanced view of their dual roles and understand that research involvement of patients involves experiences beyond receiving nursing care. Oleson and Whittaker (1967) use the term "balanced instability" to indicate that changes in the situation necessarily cause changes in roles even though duality in roles is recognized. Even with change, the priority of patient welfare over research needs must be clear. Sometimes, as a project develops, it is apparent that a patient is experiencing physical or psychological discomfort or is at risk for discomfort. In this case the project must be modified or even abandoned in the interests of patient welfare.

In defining the research role, the nurse must remember that patients should be the ends of nursing research, not the means to the end of developing a scientific base for nursing. Fowler (1986) called attention to this premise in questioning a change in the American Nurses' Association *Code for Nurses*. The 1968 code stated: "The nurse participates in research activities when assured that the rights of individual subjects are protected" (ANA, 1968). However, this revised statement appeared in 1976 and again in 1985: "The nurse participates in activities that contribute to the ongoing development of the profession's body of knowledge" (ANA, 1976, 1985).

Which statement is preferable? Why?

Nursing investigators have the responsibility of being well versed in the rights of human subjects, the concept and requirements of informed consent, and procedures for ensuring that ethical principles are not violated. Protection of human rights requires that nurses be sensitive and responsible in their actions in relation to inalienable rights of people. First and foremost, research subjects have a right not to be harmed. Research protocols generally differ from routine nursing care and should be carefully screened for potential physical, psychological, or social risks. All risks involved in the study must be spelled out precisely in both the research proposal and the informed consent document.

In a research project a new intervention is evaluated and a control group receives routine (traditional) treatment. Very early in the experiment, it is apparent that the new intervention is far superior to the routine treatment. Are there any circumstances in which it is ethical to withhold the superior intervention from the control group? If yes, what are they?

Every person has a right to refuse to participate in research. Moreover, potential research subjects should be told that they can withdraw from participation in a study at any time. The decision to participate or continue should be based on full knowledge of the research purpose and procedures. This includes the identity and credentials of the investigator(s), the purpose, duration, and expected benefits of the research, the procedures that will involve the subjects, potential inconveniences and risks, potential long-term effects of participation, projected use of the study findings, and sponsorship, if any, of the research. Subjects also need to know about provisions for confidentiality and anonymity in collecting, coding, and analyzing data and in reporting results.

Although the preceding requirements are essential, research should be explained in ways that illuminate possible risks but minimize changes in normal behavior that information about the research might stimulate. For example, information about nonparticipant observation of staff meetings in a health maintenance organization (HMO) may well result in atypical behavior by staff, defeating the purpose of the research. Similarly, explanations about research on compliance with therapeutic regimens of hypertensive patients may cause subjects to give a more favorable picture of their compliant behavior than actually exists. These problems are no excuse for being secretive about research. Subjects must know that they are being studied! Sometimes an explanation can be quite general and yet adequately informative, which reduces the problem of producing atypical or socially acceptable but untrue responses. In observation research, it has been found that the presence of an observer makes the most difference at the beginning of the study. As the research progresses, subjects return to more typical behavior and activities. The problem is solved by delaying data collection until the novelty has worn off.

Investigators must obtain informed consent from research subjects before a study begins. The Code of Federal Regulations (1981) prohibits undue inducements or any elements of fraud or deceit and defines informed consent as

> the knowing consent of an individual or his/her authorized representative, under circumstances that provide the prospective subject or representative sufficient opportunity to consider whether or not to participate.*

---

*From Department of Health and Human Services (1981). Final rule. *Federal Register* 46:8366-8391.

Informed consent need not always be in writing. If the effects of a study on subjects' well-being are nonexistent, formal consent procedures and written forms are unnecessary. For example, a retrospective, anonymous study of hospital charts to obtain information about patient falls would not require the subjects' consent, although the hospital personnel would spell out the conditions of confidentiality and anonymity for the chart audit.

In survey studies a cover letter may explain the necessary information for potential participants, and a preaddressed, stamped envelope may be enclosed for return of a completed questionnaire. If the investigator's letter makes it clear that participation is voluntary, the mere return of the questionnaire is usually regarded as sufficient evidence of informed consent. In tape-recorded interview studies, the consent to be interviewed is sometimes collected as the first part of the tape recording. Fig. 3-6 illustrates a continuum of risks and indicates when the need for informed consent is unnecessary, necessary, and not applicable.

Practicality is an important consideration in terms of time, cost, access to research subjects, cooperation of agency personnel, personal expertise, and availability of adequate data collection instruments and procedures. Time for the study should be planned, realistically thinking through each step of the research process. Often more time than anticipated is needed for obtaining the cooperation of agency staff, gaining access to research subjects, reviewing ethical considerations, and collecting data. Time should also be allocated for reflecting on and interpreting results and for disseminating findings.

At an early stage the investigator should consider the *timing* of the study. Data collection for survey studies should be timed for the most convenient responses of the research subjects. For example, it would be unwise to send questionnaires to farmers during the planting or harvest seasons or to students during final examination week. If a specific hospital patient population is to be studied, the investigator should check the census data about such patients at different times of the year and focus on the time of greatest availability.

Cost is an important consideration. Before launching a study, the investigator should prepare a budget, allowing for expenses such as library searches, pho-

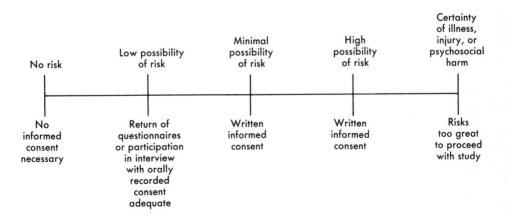

Fig. 3-6 Risks and need for informed consent.

tocopying, postage, travel, recordings, transcriptions, and computer costs. Although a budget may indicate that a study cannot be pursued without external funding, cost is often overrated as a deterrent to research. Many nurses have had the experience of developing a grant proposal and then discovering that what was needed was the exercise of developing the plan, not external funds.

Access to research subjects is obviously indispensable, and mere access is not enough. Will there be sufficient numbers of subjects during the planned data collection period? Is there a good chance that those who are asked will participate in the study? How can participation rates be enhanced? What benefits can be offered to participants? Potential subjects have little interest in contributing to the degree requirements of students. Thus improvements in nursing care or welfare of patients should be the focus of the participation request. Tangible benefits should not be overlooked. Random samples are hard to come by, and reimbursing participants for their time and effort is a good use of external funding.

Consultation with agency staff and review of admission data should be done early. To gain cooperation of agency staff, the investigator should make requests far in advance and provide sufficient rationale for the staff to be interested. Steps should be taken to minimize the effort or time staff members will have to commit to the project and to limit ways the project will change agency policies and practices.

Investigators must judge their expertise objectively. An investigator should be sufficiently expert in the substantive area to work knowledgeably with subjects and cooperating staff. For many nursing studies, clinical experience and familiarity with the nursing literature on the topic are essential. Data collection should not require experience or skills that are beyond the investigator's capabilities, such as using sophisticated technical devices or conducting interviews on sensitive topics. If the data require statistical analysis, the investigator should have a basic grasp of the necessary analytical procedures, although statisticians can be consulted. Deficiencies in any of these areas should give the investigator reason to reconsider the study.

A final aspect of practicality to consider is availability of data collection instruments and procedures. When the operational definitions of the study variables are formulated, the investigator should consider whether the limitations of the empirical indicators in representing the variables are serious enough to warrant abandoning the study. For example, attitude measures are often so transparent that respondents answer the items favorably whether the response represents their true attitudes or not. In such a situation the invesigator must qualify the results with the limitation that participants undoubtedly made socially acceptable rather than accurate responses. If this is the case, why do the study?

REFERENCES

American Nurses Association (1968). *Code for nurses.* Kansas City, Mo: The Association.
American Nurses Association (1976). *Code for nurses.* Kansas City, Mo: The Association.
American Nurses Association (1985). *Code for nurses.* Kansas City, Mo: The Association.
American Psychological Association (1983). *Publication manual of the American Psychological Association.* Washington, DC: The Association.

Butnarescu G, Tillotson D, and Villarreal P (1980). *Perinatal nursing.* Vol 2. New York: John Wiley & Sons Inc, pp 257-274.

Fowler M (1986). Ethical issues in nursing research: a shorter catechism for nursing. *Western Journal of Nursing Research* 8:461-463.

Fowler M (1988). Ethical issues in nursing research: issues in qualitative research. *Western Journal of Nursing Research* 10:109-111.

Heidt P (1981). Effect of therapeutic touch on anxiety level of hospitalized patients. *Nursing Research* 30:32-37.

Oberst MT, Graham D, Geller NL, Stearns MW, and Tiernan E (1981). Catheter management programs and post-op urinary dysfunction. *Research in Nursing and Health* 4:175-179.

Oleson V and Whittaker E (1967). Role-making in participant observation: processes in the researcher-actor relationship. *Human Organization* 26:273-281.

Orem D (1980). *Nursing: concepts of practice.* 2nd ed. New York: McGraw-Hill Inc.

Orem D (1985). *Nursing: concepts of practice.* 2nd ed. New York: McGraw-Hill Inc.

Quinn J (1984). Therapeutic touch as energy exchange: testing the theory. *Advances in Nursing Science* 6:42-49.

Riggar T (1985). *Stress burnout: an annotated bibliography.* Carbondale: Southern Illinois University Press.

Rogers M (1970). *Introduction to the theoretical basis of nursing.* Philadelphia: FA Davis Co.

Taylor S (1975). Bibliography on nursing research: 1950-1974. *Nursing Research* 24:207-225.

Williamson M (1978). *Reducing post catheterization bladder dysfunction by reconditioning.* Unpublished master's thesis. University of Kentucky.

Williamson M (1982). Reducing post catheterization bladder dysfunction by reconditioning. *Nursing Research* 31:28-30.

REFERENCES FOR FURTHER STUDY

Cassidy V (1986). Legal and ethical aspects of informed consent. *Journal of Professional Nursing* 2:343-349.

Chance K (1987). How to formulate a research question. *American Urological Association Allied Journal* 7:4-7.

Coleman D, Cooper B, Gadsberry J, Hedrick E, Larson E, and Terry B (1988). How to conduct a review of the literature. *American Journal of Infection Control* 16:45A-46A.

Damrosch S (1986). Ensuring anonymity by use of subject-generated identification codes. *Research in Nursing and Health* 9:61-63.

de Tornyay R (1987). Integrity in scientific research. *Journal of Nursing Education* 26:353.

Downs FS and Newman MA (1977). *A source book of nursing research.* Philadelphia: FA Davis Co.

Downs F (1986). Off with their heads. *Nursing Research* 35:195.

Fields WE (1983). Clinical nursing research: a proposal for standards. *Nursing Leadership* 6:117-120.

Floyd J (1988). Research and informed consent: the dilemma of the cognitively impaired client. *Journal of Psychosocial Nursing and Mental Health Services* 26:13-14, 17, 21-23.

Haller K (1988). Conducting a literature review. *Maternal Child Nursing* 13:148.

Hinshaw A (1988). Practitioners and researchers are natural partners. *American Nurse* 20:4.

Klein K (1988). Building theory through clinical practice. *Nursing Connections* 1:47-51.

Knaff K and Howard J (1984). Interpreting and reporting qualitative research. *Research in Nursing and Health* 7:17-24.

Lenz E (1987). Developing a focused research effort. *Nursing Outlook* 35:60-64.

Marchette L (1985). Research: the literature review process. *Perioperating Nurse Quarterly* 1:69-76.

Mooney N (1987). Nursing research in the clinical area: getting started. *Orthopaedic Nursing* 6:11-14, 46.

Munro B (1988). Research priorities. *Clinical Nurse Specialist* 2:44.

Rogers B (1987). Is the research project feasible? *American Association of Occupational Health Nurses Journal* 35:327-328.

Shaffer M and Pfeiffer I (1986). Nursing research and patients' rights. *American Journal of Nursing* 86:23-24.

Siantz M (1988). Defining informed consent. *Maternal Child Nursing* 13:94.

Thompson P (1987). Protection of the rights of children as subjects for research. *Journal of Pediatric Nursing* 2:392-399.

Whitney F and Roncoli M (1986). Turning clinical problems into research. *Heart and Lung* 15:57-59.

CHAPTER 4

Methodology

Objectives

After completing this unit of study, students will be able to:

1. Describe designs commonly used in nursing research and the appropriate situations for using each type of design

2. Define population

3. Define sample

4. Describe techniques of sampling and appropriate situations for the use of different techniques

5. Draw different kinds of probability and nonprobability samples

6. Describe the advantages and limitations of random samples

7. Distinguish between random sampling and random assignment

8. Describe guidelines for determining sample size

9. Distinguish between type I and type II errors

10. Identify basic concepts of measurement

11. Define internal and external validity and threats to each

12. Define instrument validity and describe content, criterion-related, and construct validity

13. Define reliability and describe four ways of establishing an instrument's reliability

14. Identify and describe at least six criteria for judging data collection instruments

15. Identify and describe at least six ways of collecting data and the advantages and disadvantages of each

GENERAL APPROACH: DESIGNS FOR NURSING STUDIES

In this chapter the elements of methodology are presented in the same order as that used in a research proposal. Research proposals must be prepared by nursing students who plan to perform studies for independent credit or for thesis work. Faculty members must review proposals to determine whether the planned work has scientific merit and to judge its practicality in terms of time and resources needed. Nurses must prepare research proposals for funding agencies and for health care agencies where research is planned. Before starting a proposal, the investigator needs to ascertain whether a special format is to be followed and whether there are limitations on the length of sections or the proposal itself. For example, proposals directed to the National Center for Nursing Research must follow scientific guidelines in format and length. A thesis chairperson may expect a more comprehensive review of the literature with less detail about budgets and time plans. Still, the table of contents for a research proposal generally follows the order used in this chapter.

The first factor to be identified is the general approach or design of the study. Designs are based on two primary considerations: the research problem and the state of knowledge about the topic area of the research problem. As shown in Figs. 2-2 and 2-3, exploratory studies and descriptive studies are both nonexperimental approaches; they are appropriate for study questions when too little is known to formulate hypotheses or perhaps even to identify variables. Some descriptive studies are undertaken to describe phenomena of interest and may also examine relationships. The final type of nonexperimental design that is discussed involves cases in which comparisons are made and hypotheses may be tested on the basis of some inherent characteristic of the population (for example, age, gender, or some personality trait) rather than on the basis of a manipulated independent variable. Such a study uses an ex post facto ("after the fact") design. In ex post facto studies comparisons are based on characteristics determined after data collection, such as age or gender. Such characteristics cannot be manipulated by the investigator.

Explanatory studies include only experimental and quasiexperimental approaches. A true experiment is one in which the investigator manipulates an independent variable and randomly assigns research subjects to comparison groups, often called experimental and control groups. In a quasiexperimental approach the investigator manipulates an independent variable but cannot assign subjects randomly to groups. Such studies can be used with varying degrees of accuracy to explain cause and effect; they are *explanatory* studies.

Selecting a design is the first major decision that must be made after delineating the problem. This occurs after a review of the literature. Before the literature review a problem statement is often so general that it could be studied at any level—exploratory, descriptive, or explanatory. The literature review spells out what is known about the subject, suggests gaps in knowledge, and ultimately points to areas where research is needed. Once a research topic has been chosen, several options are available concerning the general approach to be employed, but a preferred design can generally be identified.

Nonexperimental designs

Exploratory designs. Exploratory research designs should be employed for topics about which little is known, for example, when a foundation to formulate research questions or hypotheses is too vague or when the most relevant variables are not always apparent. Although research activities in nursing have grown exponentially in the last decade, the many questions remaining about the relationship between nursing activities and the quality of patient welfare outcomes should be studied at the exploratory stage. Experimental research about these problems would be premature because there is an insufficient foundation for designing meaningful experiments. The exploratory approach can be clarified with an example.

Several exploratory studies have looked at the use of physical restraints in acute care settings. Physical restraint of elderly patients is commonly used to prevent harm to self or others and to control behavior during treatment. However, negative effects, such as falls precipitated by wheelchair patients' removal of physical restraints and even accidental strangulation (Dube and Mitchell, 1986), have been reported. Yarmesch and Sheafor (1984) used an exploratory design in which they presented four vignettes focused on the use of physical restraints to 23 nurses and asked them what nursing actions they would take in relation to these hypothetical situations. Of the 91 decisions reported, only 10 involved alternatives to the use of physical restraints. Protection of the patient or others and control of behavior were cited as reasons for the 81 decisions to use physical restraints. In subsequent research Strumpf and Evans (1988) studied 20 elderly patients and their 18 primary nurses to answer three questions:

1. What reasons are offered by patients and their nurses for use of physical restraints?
2. What are the differences between patients' and primary nurses' perceptions of responses, effects, coping strategies, and alternatives to physical restraints?
3. What characterizes the decision-making process in the application of a physical restraint?*

Data were gathered from patients' records to validate the interview data obtained from patients and nurses. Patients were asked about their perceptions of reasons for the restraint, effects of the restraint, coping behaviors used, and alternatives they could identify. Two interview guides were used for the primary nurses. One was a Likert-type scale (1 = least important to 3 = most important) regarding reasons for using physical restraint, such as the patient's wandering off or falling out of bed. The second interview elicited nurses' perceptions of specific reasons why they had used restraints, effects of restraint use, knowledge of alternatives, personal feelings, and decision-making processes used. In this sample the periods of restraint ranged from 1 to 121 days, with a mean (arithmetic average) of 23.3 days; vests were the most frequently used restraint. Reasons stated by the patients, given by the nurses, and recorded in the charts differed widely. Most patients saw the restraints as something used for safety and spe-

---

*From Strumpf N and Evans L (1988). Physical restraint of the hospitalized elderly: perceptions of patients and nurses. *Nursing Research* 37:132.

cifically to prevent falls, whereas nurses' and charted reasons focused more on altered mental status.

Punishment and noncompliance were recorded in all three sources of data for two cases. Overall effects included anger, fear, humiliation, resistance, demoralization, discomfort, resignation, and denial. Agreement with the use of restraint was recorded in only four cases. The patients suggested a number of alternatives, almost none of which were identified by the nurses. These alternatives included increased staffing, more explanations, better access to the toilet, more comfortable restraints, and even discharge from the hospital. Nurses reported ambivalence and guilty feelings about the use of restraints, but few nurses realized how angry and humiliated the restraints made the patients feel.

Both the Yarmesch-Sheafor (1984) and Strumpf-Evans (1988) studies were appropriate exploratory level studies because they addressed an area that had been little studied. The 1984 study established that nurses chose to use physical restraints overwhelmingly in response to the situations described in the vignettes. Given this foundation the 1988 study sought to extend nursing knowledge by describing the use of physical restraints in actual situations from both the patients' and the nurses' perspectives.

Strumpf and Evans (1988) recommended that restraints be used as a special treatment requiring diagnosis, subsequent assessment, and intensive monitoring. Consultation with other members of the health team was urged. Thus the practice implications of the research tend to grow and be more specific as the body of information about an area is extended. Moreover, the research focus can turn to experimental studies as nursing knowledge is expanded. The research team identified testing of alternatives as important needed research.

The medical patients in this study were from 60 to 81 years of age, had been admitted to the hospital from the community, and were judged mentally alert enough to be interviewed. Suppose you wish to replicate this study. What criteria would you place on the sample? On the nurses? Would you collect data beyond the information gathered in this study? Would you study the problem in an acute care setting or a long-term care facility?

Simple survey designs. A simple survey study is intended merely to describe a phenomenon. The exploratory studies briefly discussed earlier focused on restraint use as a phenomenon and *described* patients' and nurses' perceptions of their use. However, the authors made little or no effort to generalize the findings to a population. By contrast, another type of descriptive study, termed a survey approach, is often used to gather data from a sample, with the intention of generalizing information gleaned from the sample to the population. Brett (1987) used a survey approach to examine how much nurses actually use selected research findings. An instrument consisting of brief descriptions of 14 selected research findings and Rogers' (1983) approach to measuring stages of innovation adoption was used. This tool permitted the investigator to elicit responses that indicated awareness of the findings (the knowledge or unaware/aware stage), personal evaluation of the findings (decision stage), attitudes toward implementing the findings (persuasion stage), actual personal implementation of the findings (implementation stage), and awareness of hospital policy regarding implementation of the findings (confirmation or use-always stage). According to Brett, "None of the innovations was in the unaware stage. Two were in the aware stage, seven in the persuade stage, five in the implementation stage. Only one innovation, closed sterile urinary drainage, was in the use always stage" (Brett, 1987, p. 346). This study, a simple survey design, described nonuse of established research findings, even though the nurses surveyed were aware of the findings, as a serious problem. Although the author did not suggest that her findings could be generalized to all nurses, the discussion clearly identified the nonuse of research as a continuing problem in nursing practice. The adequacy (relative size) and representativeness of the sample profoundly affect the generalizability and thus the scientific quality of survey studies.

Correlational survey designs. The objective of a correlational survey design is to describe phenomena and determine whether relationships exist among variables. A relationship refers to an association between two or more variables and is generally measured by computing special statistics called correlation coefficients. The correlation coefficient is an index that is high and positive if a strong direct relationship exists between two variables. It is zero if no relationship exists, and it is high and negative if a strong inverse relationship exists.

The details of the correlational survey design are best explained with an example. Mandel and Lohman (1987), using this design, studied the relationships of selected variables to low back pain in nurses. The survey instrument, which included a question about the occurrence of a 48-hour episode of low back pain, 6 demographic items (for example, age, sex, level of education), 6 items about medical history, 12 items about work variables, 2 questions about sports, and 6 questions about exercise, was completed and returned by 428 nurses (68% of the sample). Only 15% of the respondents reported having low back pain for the first time during the study year. Upper back and neck pain were reported by 21% and 14% of the nurses, respectively. In this study the investigators went beyond describing the phenomena of back and neck pain and attempted to identify variables associated with their occurrence. The variables most strongly related to low back pain were previous experiences of low back pain and pain in other parts of the spine or neck. Low back pain was not associated with work area. Nurses who worked in areas where more lifting of patients was involved did not report more low back pain than other nurses. Nor did age make a difference. In fact, the only variable clearly associated with low back pain, beyond pain experienced in the upper back or neck, was involvement in aerobic dance exercises. This study focused on low back pain, evaluated commonsense ideas about low back pain, and refuted the belief that repeated heavy lifting adversely affects the lower back.

Does this study indicate that upper back and neck pain caused nurses in the study to experience low back pain? Is there a cause-and-effect relationship between aerobic dance exercise and low back pain?

Ex post facto designs. Kerlinger (1973) defined an ex post facto design as follows:

> [It is a] systematic empirical inquiry in which the scientist does not have direct control of independent variables because their manifestations have already occurred or because they are inherently nonmanipulable. Inferences about relations among variables are made, without direct intervention, from concomitant variation of independent and dependent variables.*

Kerlinger defined precisely what was described earlier as "after the fact" designs. Data are gathered from subjects, and comparisons are made between groups that are constituted from the data, for example, age or sex (neither of which can be manipulated). In many ex post facto designs the same techniques of data analysis are used as for experimental designs. However, there are three important distinctions between ex post facto and experimental designs: (1) in ex post facto research there are no control/experimental group comparisons; (2) in ex post facto research the independent variable exists and cannot be manipulated by the investigator; and (3) in ex post facto research the groups are constituted on the basis of the existing independent variable, whereas in experimental research the groups are constituted by random assignment.

Fig. 4-1 illustrates the differences between simple ex post facto and experimental designs. In the ex post facto illustration the groups are based on some

---

*From Kerlinger FN (1973). Foundations of behavioral research. 2nd ed. New York: Holt, Rinehart & Winston, Inc., p. 379.

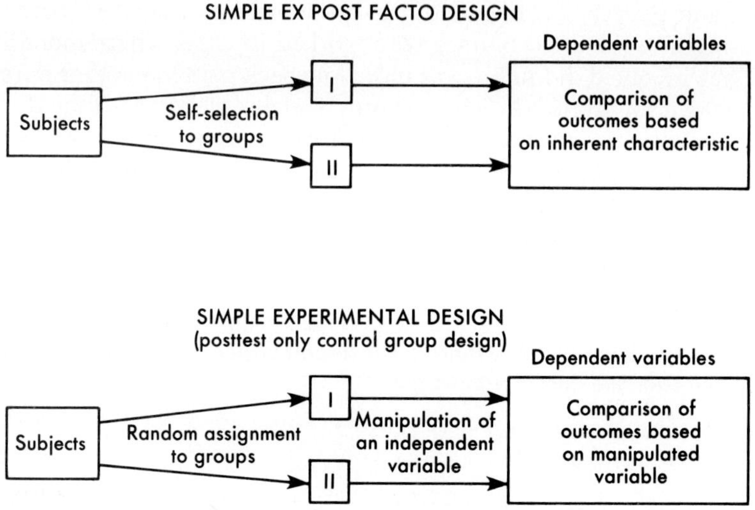

SIMPLE EX POST FACTO DESIGN

Dependent variables

SIMPLE EXPERIMENTAL DESIGN
(posttest only control group design)

Dependent variables

Fig. 4-1 Comparing simple ex post facto and experimental designs.

inherent characteristic such as age, ethnic origin, gender, or some variable that is measured in the course of collecting data. The last variable may be something like locus of control, self-care agency, extent of social supports, or diagnosis.

Megel, Langston, and Crewell (1988) used an ex post facto design to study scholarly productivity among nursing faculty researchers. Their sample (n = 96) of "leading nurse researchers" was identified by deans of nursing schools that were accredited by the National League for Nursing (NLN) and that granted master's and higher degrees. The survey instrument consisted of 13 demographic items, 32 questions about research productivity, and 49 items regarding psychological-individual factors (for example, personal preferences, age, years of experience, and rank), cumulative advantage factors (prestige of doctoral institution, mentoring, academic resources and assignments, and emphasis of department), and reinforcement factors (for example, colleagues' influence and early productivity). Descriptive information was reported on the group as a whole. Most (99%) were women, and most had spent more than 25 years in the nursing profession. The typical respondent had published slightly less than one research article per year over the preceding 3 years, had a record of increasing productivity during her career, was motivated to conduct research by peers (rather than intrinsic factors), liked conducting and writing research, had co-authored manuscripts with mentors while a graduate student, spent more time on research and publication than on teaching, and spent a substantial amount of time on administrative duties. The subjects were divided into the following four groups, based on their number of publications within the preceding 3 years:

1. No published research

2. One to four articles published
3. Five to seven articles published
4. Eight to sixteen articles published

What is the independent variable in this study?

Statistically significant differences, that is, those not due to chance, among these four groups included the following:

1. Time spent teaching in hours per week: groups 1 and 2 > 4
2. Time spent in administration activities in hours per week: group 4 > 1 and 3
3. Availability of word processing support: group 4 > 1
4. Coauthored papers: group 4 > 1
5. Number of research articles published before doctorate: group 3 > 1 and 2

It is tempting to read too much into the results of ex post facto studies. For example, from the first conclusion listed it seems logical that faculty members with heavy teaching assignments have less time to conduct research and publish their findings. However, rival hypotheses could be advanced. Perhaps those with less interest in research increase their time with students to justify their lack of research productivity. The investigators could not assert that any of the five factors listed above had a causal relationship with the level of scholarly productivity. When the subjects were placed in four groups, the real variables that caused them to fit in a group may not have been identified. Thus relationships in ex post facto research may appear to be causal when in fact this type of design cannot determine causality. In ex post facto research, investigators can strengthen their findings by investigating alternative hypotheses. In the previous example the causal nature of the findings would be bolstered if the investigators had studied other possible differences among the four groups, such as native intelligence, Graduate Record Examination (GRE) scores, writing skills, mathematical skills, and interest in research. It is important to remember, however, that identifying all possible intervening variables is virtually impossible. Kerlinger (1973) suggests that ex post facto research that does not test hypotheses or explore alternative hypotheses should be given little consideration. However, he also points out that use of statistical techniques, such as path analysis, can lend credibility to causal relationships in ex post facto research.

Suppose you wish to study as your dependent variable the health habits of two or three different groups. The groups will be constituted on some existing characteristic so that the design will be an ex post facto design. What grouping variables can you identify for such a study?

Experimental designs

True experimental designs. Three characteristics distinguish experimental research: use of a control or comparison group, manipulation of an independent variable, and random assignment of subjects to two or more groups. The experimental approach is the only one that can claim to explain causality; in experiments, "if . . . then" statements can be made. If the independent variable is implemented with one group but not with another group (commonly called the control group), *then* the dependent variable will be less (or more) in the experimental group than in the control group. For example, if relaxation training is implemented in the experimental group but not in the control group, then the observed anxiety will be less in the experimental group than in the control group. If the results of the experiment demonstrate the hypothesized relationship between relaxation training and lessened patient anxiety, the if-then relationship is supported. It is obvious that the causal variable must precede the outcome variable. However, the credibility of the experiment also depends on the control the experimenter exerts over other variables that might affect the dependent variable—in this example, patients' anxiety.

The practice of random assignment to experimental and control groups assumes that other variables will not differ in any systematic ways between the two groups. To implement random assignment, the investigator must assign subjects to groups so that each subject has an equal chance of being assigned to either group. In a study of hospital patients in a particular unit, a slip of paper with "experimental" or "control" written on it might be drawn for each patient admitted to the unit during the study period, or a coin could be flipped.

Ethical concerns dictate that potential research subjects agree voluntarily to participate in research. How should an investigator handle the procedures of random assignment if several potential subjects refuse to participate in a study?

Differences between the experimental and control group subjects tend to balance out if individuals are randomly assigned to groups. In other words, variables such as age or certain personality traits, which might affect the outcome variable, are controlled by randomization. It is important to remember that the larger the sample, the better randomization controls for extraneous variables. Theoretically, randomization completely controls for extraneous variables only when sample sizes approach the size of the population.

Common sense dictates that a few extreme cases make more of a difference in a small sample than in a large sample. Would you have more confidence in randomization in an experiment involving 20 subjects in each group or one involving 50 subjects in each group?

Thus far we have focused on the simplest sort of experimental design. Individuals are randomly assigned to experimental and control groups, an independent variable is manipulated, and the dependent variable is measured in both groups. This is called the posttest-only control group design.

Another approach to control of extraneous variables should be considered. The investigator can simply set up criteria for admission to a study that eliminate the variation of selected characteristics. For example, in a study of the effects of Lamaze childbirth preparation, an investigator might limit the sample to 20- to 25-year-old married primiparas who intend to keep their normal, healthy babies. In effect, the investigator is saying that age, parity, marital status, intact family, having the intent to keep the infant, and the infant's health status might make a difference in the outcomes and thus should be controlled. Differences in outcome variables (such as satisfaction with labor or delivery, length of different stages of labor, or decisions to breast-feed) between Lamaze-prepared primiparas and primiparas without Lamaze preparation could then be attributed more confidently to the difference in their preparation.

Would it be ethical to assign some expectant parents to Lamaze preparation and withhold this preparation from the control group? Might cooperation of subjects present a problem?

If an experiment cannot be set up, what approach might be used?

Assume for a moment that it is possible to set up an experiment to determine the effects of Lamaze preparation as just proposed. One requirement of experimental design is called separation of treatments. One group should be clearly Lamaze prepared, and the other group should be distinctly not Lamaze prepared. This is difficult to guarantee. Even if the control group mothers had no contact with Lamaze classes, expectant parents might read about preparation for childbirth or learn about coping strategies from family or friends, which would overlap with Lamaze preparation. During labor an effective nurse might coach the woman about relaxation or breathing techniques that parallel Lamaze preparation.

Separation of treatments is a real concern in setting up experimental nursing studies. For example, in a common type of study, an innovative nursing intervention might be compared with "routine nursing care" in a hospital unit. Nurses who will implement the new intervention are trained in the actions they should take, and efforts to foster uniformity are made. However, nurses commonly observe one another and discuss details of patient care. Thus contamination of treatments is possible, meaning simply that the experimental group treatment, at least in part, may also be given to the control group. That is, a nurse who should be giving routine hospital care to a control group subject might try to implement one or more features of the experimental group treatment. One way of addressing this problem is to gain the cooperation of the control group nurses so that their usual practices remain constant. Another possibility is to set up the experiment so that the two treatments are in different units or even different hospitals. But then the problem of comparability of patients, nurses, and environment must be addressed. The investigator must be prepared to demonstrate that pooling of data from several different units or agencies did not introduce error from additional extraneous variables.

Refer back to the descriptive study of use of physical restraints on medical patients (Strumpf and Evans, 1988). Suppose you decide to test the effectiveness of carefully explaining the need for the restraints to patients to gain their agreement, coupled with intensive monitoring for need to continue restraints and comfort considerations. How would you describe the experimental treatment so it would be implemented the same way with all patients in the experimental group? How would you prevent the experimental treatment from being implemented in the control group during the course of the study?

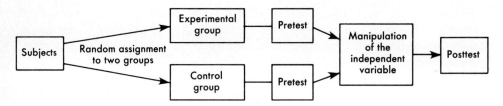

Fig. 4-2 Experimental design: pretest/posttest control group design.

Another experimental design is termed the pretest/posttest control group design. Fig. 4-2 illustrates this design, in which data are collected at two points in time rather than at the conclusion of the experimental treatment as in the posttest-only design. The subjects are randomly assigned to control and experimental groups, and the independent variable is manipulated as required, followed by posttesting. In this case, however, the investigator is dealing with a relatively small number of research subjects and does not feel confident that random assignment was effective in constituting equivalent groups. To examine the equivalence of the groups, a pretest is administered before the experimental treatment is implemented. The investigator can then use firm data to compare the two groups. If there are no significant differences in the two groups, the investigator has sound evidence that posttest differences are due to the manipulation of the independent variable. If significant differences exist in the two groups, a statistical technique called analysis of covariance can correct for pretest differences statistically. In addition, the change data for each group can be examined.

The primary problem with the pretest/posttest control group design is the effect of the pretest. It may cause subjects to change their beliefs, attitudes, or behavior so that the control group's posttest no longer reflects the outcomes of the routine care they received. The term "reactivity" describes this problem, which is discussed in some detail later in the chapter. If alternative forms of the test are available, the effects of the pretest can be ameliorated but probably not eliminated.

The problem of reactivity is addressed by adding two more groups to the experiment, resulting in the Solomon four-group design (Solomon, 1949). Fig. 4-3 illustrates this design. One control group and one experimental group receive both pretests and posttests, whereas the other pair (one experimental and one control group) receive only posttests. This approach allows the investigator to control for two additional threats to internal validity beyond reactivity—history and maturation. Internal validity refers to the action of one or more extraneous variables making a difference in the outcome or dependent variable. History refers to events other than the experimental treatment that occur between the time of pretesting and posttesting. For example, an experiment to test the effectiveness of a smoking cessation program is launched with a Solomon four-group design. Reactivity refers to the effects of data collection on the behavior

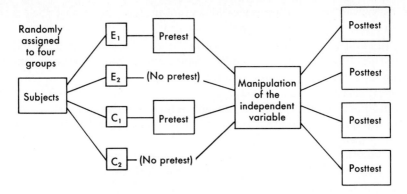

Fig. 4-3 Solomon four-group design.

of subjects. In this example the pretest might affect individuals' smoking behavior, confounding the effects of the experimental treatment. Since two groups do not experience the pretest and two groups do, the effects of the test can be examined. During the course of the program (after pretesting), a media blitz against smoking takes place in the community. The four-group design allows the investigator to assess the main effects of the media campaign on the experimental intervention by examining its effects on the control groups—one alone and one in combination with the pretest. Maturation refers to systematic effects that occur with the passage of time and may affect the outcome measures. For example, the subjects in the smoking cessation experiment may have become more concerned with health in general—or less concerned. Or, their spirit of cooperation with the experiment may have changed during its course. The four-group design allows these main effects to be analyzed.

The analyses involved in the Solomon four-group design are necessarily more complex than in designs with fewer group-treatment options. Moreover, a larger pool of subjects must be available to implement this design. If available resources permit an investigator to use the four-group design, however, the credibility of the findings is generally higher than with the other two designs above.

In some situations an extraneous variable needs to be controlled because its effects are deemed important and the samples are too small to depend on randomization for constituting equivalent groups. This variable, called the blocking variable, is used as a way of matching the patients while retaining the practice of random assignment. All potential subjects for the experiment must be measured on the blocking variable, which might be something as simple as age or as complex as severity of an illness or injury. The two subjects with the highest level of this blocking variable are identified and randomly assigned, one to the experimental group and one to the control group. The next two patients are similarly identified, and random assignment is again used. The process continues until all subjects have been randomly assigned to one group or the other. This is called a randomized block design. Analysis of these data is somewhat different than in other experimental designs that have been described, because the investigator is dealing with matched pairs.

The final type of experimental design included in this chapter is the factorial design. This design involves a multivariate approach to experimentation; that is, two or more variables are independently varied in a single study. The resulting experiment reveals more information than two separate experiments could produce. Lindquist called the factorial design, which was developed by R.A. Fisher, "among the most important contributions to experimental technique in recent decades" (Lindquist, 1956, p. 23).

Let's look at a hypothetical three-factor design. The research subjects are epilepsy patients treated at a large, tertiary medical center. The dependent variable, compliance with the medications regimen, is to be examined with respect to (1) type of teaching employed in the home visit, (2) type of medications regimen, and (3) use or nonuse of follow-up blood work. There are two experimental and one control treatment variables regarding teaching during a home visit. Three different medications regimens are being tested. The third variable is dichotomous; follow-up blood work either was or was not done. This design is illustrated in Fig. 4-4, which shows that the investigator is dealing with three levels of teaching and medications and two levels of follow-up blood work. This is a 3 × 3 × 2 design consisting of 18 cells. A fairly large sample is needed so that enough subjects are available in each of the 18 cells. The main effects of the three independent variables can be determined in one experiment rather than three separate experiments. More important, interrelationships among the independent variables in relation to the dependent variable can be studied. The techniques of data analysis become increasingly complex as the number of factors increases. If samples are adequate, factorial designs produce more information in relation to the data collected than any other type of design.

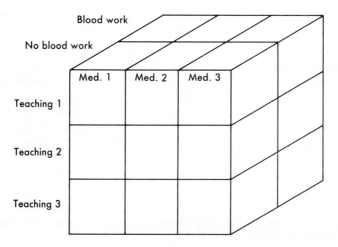

Fig. 4-4 Factorial design.

Quasiexperimental designs. A common limitation encountered by nurse scientists is their inability to select subjects randomly and assign them to control and experimental groups randomly. For example, an investigator who wants to study hospitalized medical patients might find four units in the hospital that are roughly comparable in severity and type of illnesses present. The investigator places four pieces of paper in a box, each labeled with one of the units, and draws one to be the experimental unit and another to be the control unit. A program of data collection is initiated—either pretesting and posttesting or just posttesting—and the experiment is performed, not on randomly assigned subjects, but on intact groups. Since the design does not involve randomly assigned subjects, it is quasiexperimental rather than experimental.

Could all four units be used, with two drawn as experimental groups and two as control groups? Would you impose the Solomon four-group design in this situation? Why or why not?

The first quasiexperimental design to be considered is the simplest; intact groups are used as experimental and control groups with only posttreatment data collected. Such studies are fairly common in nursing research because of the restrictions imposed by agencies where research is conducted. To use this approach, an investigator should be able to demonstrate that the two groups were reasonably equivalent on relevant variables before the experiment began. This is more difficult than it sounds because of the many factors that lead to membership in one group or the other.

The second quasiexperimental design considered here is the split group, pretest/posttest design, which involves collecting control group data from a random sample of the entire unit for a period of time. After control group data collection the experimental group treatment can be implemented with no concern about separation of treatments. For the second phase of the study, collection of experimental group data, patients must be randomly drawn from those who were not tested as part of the control group data collection process. However, the investigator must deal with at least two questions. First, are the patients, nurses, and environment equivalent during the two different periods? Second, does the experience of participating in an experiment produce responses from the nurses or the patients or both? The latter concern, referred to as the Hawthorne effect, is usually dealt with by informing both the control group and the experimental group that a study is in progress.

Additional quasiexperimental designs are possible, but the ones presented here were selected because they represent a clear difference from true experimental designs.

POPULATION AND SAMPLE

In the real world investigators are seldom able to study the entire group of subjects or objects of interest, namely the population. It would be impractical to seek information from all registered nurses, all institutionalized elderly people, or all of most other groups that interest investigators. The same is true in everyday life. We reach conclusions about people and events based on our own experience, which is necessarily a sample or a subset of the population. Thus we may conclude that today's adolescents are less studious than those a decade ago or that certain ethnic groups are clannish. Some of our beliefs are even based on others' experience, or hearsay, which is also merely a sample.

In nursing research, investigators can never know about all members of a class of patients. Therefore they gather information from a sample. A sample is a fraction of the whole group, which is the study population. The study population is the group of subjects or objects from which the sample is drawn. The larger group, which includes subjects or objects beyond the study population and which may be unknown to the investigator, is called the target population.

Another set of terms is commonly used. Sometimes the sample is drawn simply from the population (identical to the study or accessible population) and the population is part of a larger whole, called the universe (synonymous with target population). Another term for the study, or accessible, population is the sampling frame. This is merely the collection of individual units from which a sample is drawn. The terms "sample," "study population," and "target population" or "population" are used in this book. Members of the sample are termed "elements." The term "subject" commonly refers to a member of a sample involved in a study.

Identify a study population for each of the target populations listed below:

American adolescents with diagnosed diabetes

Primiparas who had Lamaze preparation

Male hip fracture patients 40 to 55 years of age

Elderly women in U.S. intermediate care facilities

Sampling can be divided into two general approaches: probability and non-probability. Probability sampling occurs when each member of a study population has an equal chance of becoming part of the study sample. Probability samples are produced by using random procedures, and nonprobability samples are constituted with nonrandom procedures.

In the discussion of study design, use of random assignment to groups was described as a necessary condition for true experiments. Distinguish between random sampling and random assignment.

Probability sampling

Simple random samples. Fig. 4-5 illustrates the relationships of three samples, A, B, and C, to a study population and to a target population. For purposes of illustration, A, B, and C are assumed to be all *random samples*. Random samples are commonly used in market surveys and political polls. In such surveys or polls the survey team is seeking information about a large group by collecting information from a random sample of that group. To employ statistics in estimating likes and dislikes or beliefs of the large group, the researchers had to draw a sample in a way that gave each member of the large group an equal chance of being selected. This is illustrated in Fig. 4-5. In the case shown in the figure the study population is the same as the target population, a rare phenomenon.

It is possible to list all collegiate and university-based nursing programs and then to list all nursing students enrolled in those programs at a given moment

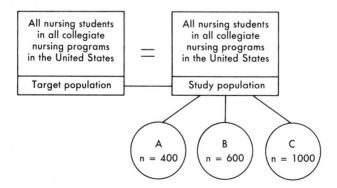

Fig. 4-5 Drawing simple random sample.

in time. From this gigantic list, or sampling frame, we can draw random samples of different sizes to learn about the nursing students in the population. If these procedures are followed, we can employ the logic of statistical inference, which is simply the ability to estimate parameters or characteristics of the study population from the characteristics of the sample. From there, we judge whether we can generalize from the study population to the target population. (In this case they are identical, but that is usually not the case.) That is, we attempt to generalize from the sample data to the target population parameters. A statistic is a characteristic of a sample, whereas a parameter is a characteristic of a population.

Let's assume that our primary interest is in the American College Testing (ACT) scores of college- and university-based nursing students in the target population, the United States. We want to know things like the highest score, the lowest score, the average score, and the median. If we have the time and funds to acquire the list described previously, each of the samples *A*, *B*, and *C* (see Fig. 4-5) is expected to be representative of the population.

Would this be practical? What alternatives can you suggest?

Logically, which sample in Fig. 4-5 would you expect to do the best job of representing the target population in relation to the parameters? Why?

The random sample drawn from this very large list is a *simple random sample.* The main features of simple random samples are that (1) they involve only one stage, (2) each object has an equal and independent chance of being drawn, and (3) the study population can be identified and listed. Since the individuals are selected at random from the total list, the investigator does not introduce any bias by choosing certain individuals or selecting individuals from one school.

Fig. 4-5 depicts a study population that is identical to the target population and three samples drawn from the study population. How likely is it that another team would draw the same individuals as are found in *A, B,* and *C?*

There are three general ways of drawing a simple random sample. One, the fishbowl technique, is to list all individuals on separate slips of paper and put them into a fishbowl.

Is the fishbowl technique practical? In terms of probability theory, how can you perform the drawing so that each object has an equal opportunity to be drawn?

Suppose that there are 9000 nursing students in the sampling frame. When the first slip is drawn, each student has 1/9000 of a chance of being drawn. For the second drawing, though, there is only a 1/8999 chance of being drawn. For the third there is only 1/8998 chance, and so on. To give each individual an equal chance, each slip that is drawn must be replaced in the fishbowl before another one is drawn.

Another approach to drawing a simple random sample is to number each individual in the master list of nursing students and go to a table of random numbers such as the one in Fig. 4-6. Without looking at the list, the researcher drops a pencil point on the table to produce a random start. The number of

5626	7018	2611	6464	7642	0207	3221	0747	1847	0583
5543	3348	4960	5694	5861	0775	0747	1090	2116	9138
1916	1697	9583	7138	0924	2503	8436	0289	4620	2996
1670	2198	3567	8587	5073	5836	8688	6444	6914	2911
6091	0902	6474	1871	1155	3387	2631	7950	3405	8059
8552	8758	0587	4347	5354	3920	5357	9977	3094	5019
9440	2797	8320	2575	7121	8524	8344	3146	4490	8939
2013	3225	0590	1919	0026	2722	2821	8134	1476	0657
7942	5234	4849	0852	2303	3266	2804	4977	8850	8485
6308	9228	6583	3685	0844	3374	1589	0799	1318	8457
4760	8252	2975	0491	7362	5151	0422	4734	4652	1739
6633	6341	2515	7964	0506	2948	3105	3790	2815	2992
2744	6578	9298	9968	2651	6407	5300	8391	9745	8423
1622	2570	5764	1518	5142	6950	2254	1367	9599	7267
6933	2126	2610	4950	0708	6446	3728	9115	4170	5455
5843	6860	9654	2039	6824	1826	9854	8722	1244	5229
7056	6496	6385	0786	8760	4372	6683	9755	2652	9435
2306	1595	5941	0660	6061	7459	5165	4493	5753	4261
0026	3479	1288	5015	1222	1473	2328	5352	7106	9152
4956	5094	7321	4452	4297	9668	8381	3246	2075	7681
2443	1551	7670	9863	2194	3724	8515	5630	9132	8084
1175	4115	9927	8922	6414	2714	3135	7990	2591	7250
3098	6376	8071	4747	7966	4291	5283	7506	2522	6893

Fig. 4-6 Table of random numbers.

digits to be read is the total number in the sampling frame. In this example it would be four digits, representing the fictional total of 9000 in the population. Any four-digit number greater than 9000 is ignored.

Reading down from the random start, which is circled, list the first 10 individuals drawn for the simple random sample.

Suppose you have a study population of only 458. What are your two options of a start from the one that is circled? To draw a sample of 100, which three-digit numbers will you ignore? Use the farthest right start and list the first 15 subjects drawn in columns of three each:

Supposing that you have access to a study population of 124, draw a random sample of 20 from Fig. 4-6. Underline the digits that represent your random start. What must you do if the three digits in your draw exceed 124? What if duplicate numbers are drawn?

The fishbowl technique and the use of a table of random numbers are tedious for drawing a sample of 400 from a population of 9000, but either approach is quite manageable for drawing a sample of 20 from a population of 124.

A third way of producing a simple random sample also requires that each individual be numbered. Instead of a table of random numbers, a computer-generated set of random numbers is used. Commonly, more numbers are generated than are expected to constitute the sample because there may be duplications that will have to be ignored.

In prospective studies (those that begin with an examination of independent variables and go forward in time to assess dependent variables), the use of random numbers, from either a table or a computer, does not necessarily involve numbering a known list of subjects. Imagine that a study focuses on hospital patients admitted for appendectomies and that you have gained the cooperation of a large, local hospital for the period January through July. You learn from prior year census data that about 95 such admissions are likely during the stated period. You assume that the patients admitted during this period are representative of the larger population who would be admitted in all such hospitals. Your task is to select a sample of 30 from among this group *at random*. The task is first to select more random numbers than you need because you anticipate that some will refuse to participate in the study, and that there may be duplicates.

Without looking, drop your pencil point on a spot in Fig. 4-6. Moving downward from your random start, select 40 two-digit numbers that are less than 85 (to use the estimate of 95 conservatively).

You need to rearrange your numbers in ascending order and eliminate any duplicates. As patients are admitted during the study period, you contact the one that corresponds to your first number and ask that person to participate in the study. The next number indicates who your second subject will be, and so on. A refusal means that you move to the next number, not the next patient.

The aim of simple random sampling is to obtain a bias-free sample of a population for the purpose of making generalizations about the population. Thus the sample should be representative of the population regarding the variables of interest. The larger the sample, all other things being equal, the better it will represent the population. In other words, the sampling error, which is the difference between the sample statistic and the population parameter, is smaller in large samples than in small samples.

Cluster random samples. Refer to Fig. 4-5. Since we have neither the time nor the money to acquire a list of all nursing students in all collegiate or university nursing programs, we decide to draw 20 schools of nursing at random from the list of all schools of nursing that are college or university based. Lists of nursing students from these 20 programs must be obtained. The second phase of the sampling process would be to draw a sample of students from the 20 lists.

Does this approach introduce bias? Does it ensure representativeness? Why or why not?

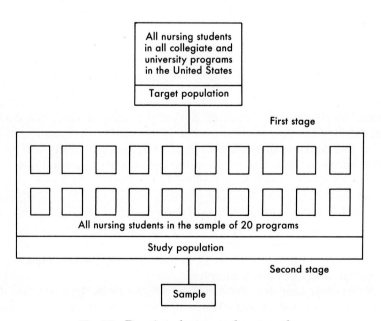

Fig. 4-7 Drawing cluster random sample.

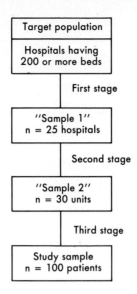

Fig. 4-8 Three-stage cluster sample.

Fig. 4-7 depicts this method of sampling, which is called cluster sampling. In our example it is a two-stage process, but additional stages can be used. For example, a target population may consist of all hospitals having 200 or more beds in a particular region. The first drawing might be from these hospitals (the study population) to produce a sample of 25. All medical-surgical units in these hospitals are then listed. The next step might involve drawing another sample, this time of 30 units from the 25 hospitals. The focus of the study may be on 100 of the female patients, aged 50 to 62 years. Or, the sampling process may involve the nurses or head nurses from these units, for example. Such a process is a three-stage cluster sampling approach and is illustrated in Fig. 4-8.

What is the list of 25 hospitals called in sampling terminology?

Is the study population the same as the target population in this example? Why or why not?

How does the work involved in this approach compare with that needed for a simple random sample?

Stratified random samples. In stratified random sampling the study population is divided into strata. Strata are simply layers or subdivisions of the
population according to some variable such as sex or educational level. For
hospitals the strata might be such characteristics as size, public or private own-
ership, or ratings of the emergency departments. Let's consider size as simply
the number of beds in the hospitals, and that we want a 50% sample of this
group of hospitals. In the population, two have more than 1000 beds (4%), six
have between 500 and 999 beds (13%), 18 have between 200 and 499 beds (39%),
and 20 have fewer than 200 beds (43%). In this simple illustration we list the
hospitals in groups according to size. Using the fishbowl technique, we draw
one of the two largest hospitals. Then, we draw three of the six with between
500 and 999 beds. Next, we draw nine from the group having 200 to 499 beds.
Finally, we draw 10 from the smallest bed-number group. The resulting sample
consists of 23 hospitals with all sizes represented in the same proportion they
were in the population. This technique, called proportionate stratified random
sampling, increases the representativeness of the sample in that each size hospital is represented proportionately.

A stratified random sample need not be proportionate. In the preceding
example one unit could have been drawn from each stratum to ensure that all
sizes would be represented. However, the resulting sample of four units would
not reflect the population proportionately.

Nonprobability sampling

Systematic samples. In some textbooks systematic sampling is described as
a technique of random (or probability) sampling. This is because it begins with
a random start. Systematic sampling is often used because it is so convenient.
We start with a list of potential subjects—the study population (or sampling
frame). If we want a 25% sample, we select every fourth member. If we want
a 20% sample, we select every fifth member, and so on. The random part of the
process is simply that we start at any accidental or arbitrary (random, not selected) point in the list.

**In systematic sampling, does every subject have an equal opportunity of being
selected?**

Is systematic sampling truly random (or probability) sampling?

Convenience samples. A convenience sample is one that is readily accessible
to the investigator. Since not all subjects have a chance of being selected, it is

not a probability (or random) sample. For example, an emergency department nurse wanted to study the compliance with discharge instructions of parents or guardians of 5- to 10-year-old children brought to the emergency department with injuries during a stated period. The parents or guardians of all children who fit the criteria of injury and age during the study period were given brief explanations of the study and asked to participate. They were informed that their participation was voluntary and that they could withdraw from the study at any time. Those who agreed to participate and actually did so constituted the sample, a convenience sample.

Surveys are often based on convenience samples. Questionnaires are mailed to potential participants, and the ones who complete the questionnaires and return them during the study period make up the convenience sample. Possibly the persons who complete and return the survey forms differ in some important way from the persons who choose not to participate in the study. The investigator should always be aware of this limitation and should report the percentage of returns obtained in a survey study.

Many published nursing studies have been based on convenience samples, and the investigators have used statistical procedures in analyzing their data. Yet randomization is a requirement for the use of statistics. In such cases the investigators have assumed that the individuals who participated in their studies were representative of all possible subjects for the studies, an assumption the reader may accept or reject.

Quota samples. Quota sampling is another type of nonprobability sampling. In this technique quotas are set for certain types of individuals, based on knowledge of pertinent characteristics in the population. Its name comes from a common practice in public opinion polls of assigning quotas to the interviewers who collect the data. The quota may be a certain number of people from a specific geographical area in a city or county. Or it may be certain numbers of men and women, interviewed in their homes, places of business, or even the streets. One well-known study was based on interviews of men and women in a certain age range who were waiting for flights in an airport terminal.

Purposive samples. The final type of nonprobability sampling this chapter addresses is called purposive sampling. Investigators purposely select individuals who are especially knowledgeable about the question at issue. For example, prominent nursing leaders may be asked to participate in a study of proposed changes in a state's nursing practice act. The study questions relate to provisions that are perceived to be most pertinent for nursing as a profession. The individuals selected are judged to be representative of some larger, unidentified population of nursing leaders, but there may be no evidence that the sample indeed represents the hypothetical population.

Purposive samples may consist of sites as well as individuals. One might look to a few elite schools of nursing to collect data for a study of conditions that foster research productivity. An in-depth study of a few carefully selected schools where excellence in research can be observed makes more sense than studying sites derived from probability sampling techniques, which might include sites of little use for the study problem.

Whom would you select to participate in a study of difficulties that must be resolved in launching doctoral programs in nursing? Why?

A summary of the probability and nonprobability techniques of sampling follows:

Probability   **Nonprobability**
Simple random   Systematic*
Cluster random   Convenience
Stratified random   Quota
                         Purposive

———

*Differences of opinion exist regarding systematic samples.

Suppose you note that many nurses pursue graduate education part-time and take as much as 10 years to obtain the master's degree. You want to determine the primary reasons for delayed master's degrees in nursing. Devise a sampling plan for this study, assuming that unlimited funding is available.

Devise a plan assuming that you have only $200 to spend.

Sample size

A general rule is to obtain as large a sample as time, availability of subjects, and funds permit. In Fig. 4-5, the largest sample, C, would provide the most precise estimate of the population parameters, and the estimate from B would be more accurate than that from A. The larger the sample, the smaller the sampling error. Sampling error is the difference between the sample statistic and the population parameter. It is inversely related to the square root of the size of the sample. Thus a sample of 900 is three times more precise than a sample of 100. Since the square roots of 900 and 100 are 30 and 10, respectively, the ratio is 3 to 1.

How much more precise (approximately) is a sample of 400 than a sample of 81? Express your answer as a ratio:

Sample size depends on a number of factors, and therefore it should be calculated for each unique research problem. Probability samples are always more representative than nonprobability samples. Thus a probability sample of 80 is no doubt superior to a nonprobability sample of 120.

As explained previously, a statistic is a sample value whereas a parameter is a population value. One purpose of statistical analysis is to estimate population parameters from sample statistics. Another is to test hypotheses. As noted earlier, a research hypothesis is simply an educated guess, generally based on a theoretical or conceptual framework derived from the literature review. Statistics can never prove a research hypothesis to be true. Instead, the hypothesis is restated as a null hypothesis, which merely asserts that there are no differences among groups or relationships among variables. Then, by rejection of this null hypothesis, support is provided for the research hypothesis.

Three null hypotheses follow. Suggest examples of research hypotheses that might have prompted them:

1. As measured by the Zilch Health Practices Inventory, there is no significant difference in the health practices of members of the university's nursing faculty and members of the university's business faculty.

2. Among adolescents, there is no relationship between impulsivity and use of mood-altering substances.

3. There is no difference between the stress burnout phenomenon in intensive care unit (ICU) nurses and non-ICU nurses.

One consideration of sample size is the control of error in accepting or rejecting a study's null hypothesis. Because of various sources of error a null hypothesis that should be accepted may be rejected. This condition of mistakenly rejecting a null hypothesis is called type I error (or alpha, α). This is a serious problem, and statisticians have found a way to control for it. Statistical tests are performed at some stated degree of precision. A research report may state that a *significance level* indicated by p, such as 0.05, was set. This means that the investigator was willing to live with a 5% possibility of a type I error. The possibility of mistakenly rejecting a null hypothesis was only 5 in 100. In other words the investigator was 95% sure that a hypothesis that was rejected should have been rejected.

Conversely, a null hypothesis that should be rejected may be accepted. This error is called a type II (or beta, β) error. Table 4-1 illustrates both problems. Investigators have sometimes accepted null hypotheses because the measurement error was too great to detect real differences when they existed. Reasons for type II errors include poor measurements (introducing error) and samples too small to demonstrate real differences or relationships when they actually exist.

The precision of the data collection instruments makes a difference in the size of the sampling error. In the calculations regarding sampling error, we were

Table 4-1 Type I and type II errors

| | Null hypothesis | |
Decision	True	False
Accept H	Correct	Type II error
Reject H	Type I error	Correct

H, Hypothesis.

really looking at sampling error as a function of measurement error. Thus a study that uses a crude measure will need to sample more subjects to obtain a reasonable estimate of a population parameter than would be needed if the data collection instrument were more precise. The less precise the tool, the larger the sample needed.

Heterogeneity of the target population in a study also affects sample size. As the number of demographic variables increases, the sample size must grow. For example, in a study of schoolchildren the independent variables sex (female and male), age (younger adolescents, defined as 12 to 14 years, and older adolescents, defined as 15 to 17 years), and socioeconomic status (low, middle, and high classes) are examined in relation to the dependent variable, health practices. Fig. 4-9 illustrates how the number of cells of subjects increases with the number of independent variables under study. There are 12 cells. If each cell has a minimum of 20 subjects, the sample will need to be at least 240 subjects. General guidelines of five to 20 subjects per cell have been recommended. Since the sample will not be equally distributed among these cells, five appears to be too small; at least 10 subjects should be included in each cell.

Another consideration concerning sample size is the type of data analysis planned. As indicated by O'Muircheartaigh and Payne (1977), if the study purpose is to develop a new attitude scale, a sample size of at least 1000 is necessary to provide a sufficient database for thorough exploration of relationships of

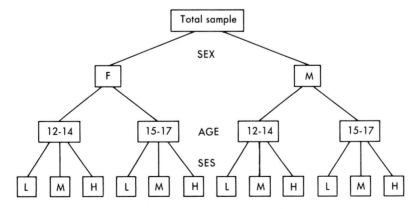

Fig. 4-9 Sample size and study heterogeneity.

attitudes, demographic factors, background, social structure, and behavior. Maranell (1974) suggests that, if the investigator wants to estimate the reproducibility of items included in a new instrument, 200 is adequate; thus the projected number of 1000 is more than sufficient.

Power analysis is a highly useful technique for determining sample size and the probability of type II error. It is also helpful in critiquing studies. If a published study reports no significant differences, the sample may have been too small in relation to the psychometric characteristics of the data collection instruments and the type of data analysis used. In such a case, power analysis can be used to determine whether studies should be replicated with larger samples.

MEASUREMENT

Measurement is the process whereby the components of phenomena under study are assigned numbers. Height and weight are expressed in terms of inches and pounds or kilograms and centimeters. The values assigned two different individuals are not arbitrary; they are based on measurement of the attributes in question, and they allow us to conclude that one individual is taller or heavier than another. Science could not exist without measurement.

Not all forms of measurement are equally precise. If biophysical instruments have been calibrated correctly and the investigator uses the instrument properly, the values obtained should be extremely accurate. This does not necessarily mean that error is avoided. The mere sight of the instruments or the investigator can influence the measurement. It has been shown that blood pressure values can be affected by the sight of the physician!

Other kinds of measures may introduce much more error. The characteristics of the data collection instrument may influence the research subject to give inaccurate information. For example, a question might be ambiguous or might put the research subject in an unfavorable light if answered truthfully. In such cases the subject may answer inaccurately because of confusion or a desire to give a more socially acceptable answer. Errors directly attributable to the instrument or measuring device are referred to as the instrument's reactivity. The topic of reactivity is considered again in this chapter. Other personal factors such as fatigue, boredom, or illness may affect the measurement process. Environmental factors may play a role: poor lighting, inadequate writing space, or excessive heat may cause scores on a paper and pencil measure to be inaccurate reflections of the true values for a given set of test subjects. Suppose that X_O represents the observed score, X_T represents the true score, and e represents the error of measurement. In this case $X_O = X_T + e$. The investigator should understand that the observed score (X_O) always differs from the true score (X_T) by some unknown quantity, the error (e). The concept of the operational definition is introduced in Chapter 3. The choice of an operational definition for each variable in a study is one of the most critical decisions in designing a study.

Validity

Three kinds of validity are relevant to the topic of measurement in nursing research. *External validity*, or generalizability, is the ability to generalize study findings to situations outside the study. The primary aim of using statistics is to allow generalization of results from a sample to a population. Sampling has a profound effect on external validity, as does scientific rigor in the design of the study.

Internal validity refers to the scientific attributes of the study—its quality. This means the extent to which the experimental treatment can be credited with causing the observed effect. Internal validity also depends on how accurately the sample represents the population. Other factors that influence internal validity are accuracy of the data collection instruments, design considerations, and statistical procedures employed. Accuracy is a synonym for internal validity.

The third kind of validity is *instrument validity*. Instrument validity is related to both external and internal validity. It refers to the precision with which the measures used in a study represent the true values of the variables, that is, how well the data collection instrument measures what it is supposed to measure. Instrument validity is closely related to but separate from internal validity, which refers to accuracy of the entire study. Instrument validity is a necessary part of internal validity, but internal validity depends on more than instrument validity. Instrument validity is also related to external validity, since it has an impact on the generalizability of the findings, but the concepts differ. Instrument validity is the focus on the following discussion.

The most obvious kind of instrument validity, hereafter called validity, is *face validity*. This is the weakest kind of validity and merely means that the instrument *appears* to measure what it is supposed to measure. Face validity is generally attained by asking a panel of experts to review the data collection instrument and judge its accuracy in measuring the targeted concepts. An investigator may construct a tool to measure the concept of burnout among intensive care unit nurses. A panel of experts determines face validity by deciding how well the items represent this concept. The items should represent the concept fully and fairly: all aspects of the concept should be included and the items should be representative. One component of the topic should not be weighted heavily by including a large number of items for it while equally important component is represented by only a few items. The items are in effect a sample of the entire population, which is the concept. In other words the items are a sample of all items that could be constructed to measure the concept or phenomenon of interest.

Content validity is similar to face validity. It is established by supporting an assertion that the components of the instrument are an accurate reflection of the essence of the concept(s). A panel of experts may give their judgments in this regard, or the investigator may base his or her claim on a literature review. Such a review reveals the essential aspects of the concept(s) that must be included in the content.

Are face and content validity objective or subjective?

Unfortunately, many nursing studies are based on data collection instruments that go no further than face or content validity. The reader must be careful not to put too much stock in such reports. Establishing face or content validity is only the first task in establishing the accuracy of a data collection tool. Another investigator may believe that such a reported measure is valid based on his or her subjective judgment. Before the instrument is used in a new study, however, more objective means of establishing its validity should be sought.

Two kinds of criterion-related validity exist. Criterion-related validity refers to a determination of accuracy based on comparing the new data collection instrument with an existing measure or criterion. One kind is called *concurrent validity*. It is based on evidence of a relationship between the new data collection instrument and an existing measure of the same concept. For example, a self-report measure of pain may be compared with physiological measures of pain such as pulse rate and blood pressure. If a measure already exists, why develop a new tool? The answer is simply that the existing tool doesn't meet the needs of the research aims and design for one reason or another. Perhaps the existing tool is long, cumbersome, or difficult to administer. In some cases an investigator may develop a questionnaire to measure concepts previously tapped only with interviews. There are many reasons for developing new data collection instruments, and their relationship to existing tools is a useful way of determining validity objectively.

Predictive validity is the other method of criterion-based validity. It is similar to concurrent validity but deals with future outcomes. Predictive validity refers to the ability to predict a future outcome from the instrument's results. For example, after a review of the literature we might expect a measure of attitudes toward health to predict future health practices among a group of high school students. If a positive, nonchance relationship exists between the results of the health attitudes scores and the later measure of health practices, we have demonstrated the predictive validity of the health attitudes tool.

Construct validity, the most powerful indicator of an instrument's accuracy, is the final type described here. Construct validity is more complex than predictive validity, and it is usually established over a period of time by several people instead of by the originator of the instrument alone. It is used to explore the relationship of the instrument's results to measures of the underlying theoretical concept(s) of the instrument.

The most common use of construct validity is in situations in which differences in two or more groups are expected to occur. For example, let's assume that we have developed an attitute measure toward computing in nursing. We have the cooperation of a class of nursing students, some of whom use computers frequently and some of whom are nonusers of computers. We hypothesize that the frequent users will score higher than the nonusers on our attitude measure. After all, they must have more positive attitudes than the other group or they would not be frequent users. The data are collected and analyzed. Using appropriate statistical procedures, we rule out chance and show that the scores of the users group were indeed higher than the scores of the nonusers group. Such a finding contributes to construct validity.

The multitrait, multimethod matrix (Campbell and Fiske, 1959) is a special application of construct validity. The scores from the instrument in question are compared with those from an instrument designed to measure the same variable by another technique; the relationships between these two sets of scores should be high and positive. Then another variable expected to measure an entirely different construct is also assessed by two methods. The results from these two measures compared with each other should be high and positive. However, when these results are compared with the scores of the first variable, the correlation should be low or even negative. To illustrate this approach, let's return to our measure of health attitudes. We choose another measure of attitudes toward health for one of the comparisons. This one is related positively to the health attitudes instrument being examined. Then we choose another construct, one that is related negatively to health attitudes. For example, we may use two different ways of measuring risk-taking behavior. The scores from these two risk-taking measures should be positively related to each other and negatively related to the two measures of health attitudes. If we obtain significant results in the predicted directions, that is, if there are positive and negative results at a nonchance level, a form of construct validity has been demonstrated. Table 4-2 reports hypothetical results for such an analysis. This approach is based on demonstrating both convergent and divergent validity. Convergent validity is demonstrated by the positive relationships among different measures of the same constructs (.854 and .765). Divergent validity is demonstrated by negative relationships among measures of vastly different constructs ($-.346$, $-.532$, $-.421$, and $-.337$).

Another question about the construct validity of a measure relates to whether it is a single, "pure" construct or measures several different constructs. For example, does our health attitudes scale measure health attitudes or health behavior? The answer to this kind of query requires a moderately large sample of test subjects to permit use of a statistical technique called factor analysis. Investigators use factor analysis to determine whether one or several factors are embedded within the measure. This statistical technique sorts items into homogeneous categories based on the research subjects' responses to the items. The categories constitute subscales of the measure. If these subscales tap different aspects of the construct, construct validity is supported. If one or more

Table 4-2 Example of a multitrait-multimethod matrix

	HeA-1	HeA-2	RTB-1	RTB-2
HeA-1	1.000	.854	$-.346$	$-.421$
HeA-2	.854	1.000	$-.532$	$-.337$
RTB-1	$-.346$	$-.532$	1.000	.765
RTB-2	$-.421$	$-.337$	.765	1.000

HeA-1, Health attitudes measured by method 1; *HeA-2,* health attitudes measured by method 2; *RTB-1,* risk-taking behavior measured by method 1; *RTB-2,* risk-taking behavior measured by method 2.

of the subscales focus on entirely different constructs, these items should be eliminated from the data collection instrument.

Validity is not a dichotomous concept—a "yes, it's there" or "no, it isn't there" phenomenon. Years may be required to show that an instrument has a high degree of construct validity. Moreover, validity is demonstrated in relation to a particular situation and specific research subjects. If the instrument is used in a different situation with different types of subjects, validity must be reestablished for the new study setting.

Reliability

An instrument's reliability is assessed in terms of stability, homogeneity, and equivalence. In relation to reliability, the first question asked is how consistently a measurement technique performs its task. We expect 10 pounds of potatoes to weigh 10 pounds on successive weighings. A person's height should be the same on successive measurements during a single day. Repeated tests on a paper-and-pencil scale regarding knowledge about aging should yield the same or nearly the same results for one person as long as nothing that alters the person's knowledge about aging takes place between tests. A measure of a stable attitude should yield comparable results, if not perfect agreement, on successive administrations to the same person. Any differences between the scores are assumed to be due to random errors. On paper-and-pencil measures the time between administrations should be long enough that the person does not remember his or her answers to the first scale, but not so long that real changes in the knowledge or attitudes being tested can take place. Periods ranging from 2 to 4 weeks are generally used with these kinds of measures. This approach to establishing the consistency of a data collection instrument is called test-retest reliability. A sample of subjects, not an individual, is used. A value for test-retest reliability can be computed when an instrument is administered to a given sample twice with an appropriate interval between the two administrations.

In a number of situations test-retest reliability is not an appropriate approach, as when real changes are expected to take place with time. Indicate which of the variables below are appropriate for use of test-retest reliability:

Variable	Appropriate?		
	Yes	No	Maybe
Trait anxiety	_____	_____	_____
State anxiety	_____	_____	_____
Attitudes toward mentally ill	_____	_____	_____
Knowledge about Alzheimer's disease	_____	_____	_____
Attitudes toward smoking	_____	_____	_____
Health beliefs	_____	_____	_____

Explain your "no's" and "maybe's":

Test-retest reliability is calculated by computing a statistic that measures relationships, called the Pearson product moment correlation coefficient (symbolized by r).

$$r = \frac{(X - \overline{X})(Y - \overline{Y})}{N \, s_x \, s_y}$$

or

$$r = \frac{N(\Sigma XY) - (\Sigma X)(\Sigma Y)}{\sqrt{[N(\Sigma X^2) - (\Sigma X^2)][N(\Sigma Y^2) - (\Sigma Y)^2]}}$$

Computation of this coefficient is straightforward but tedious: (1) scores must be tabulated, (2) a number of products and summations must be computed, (3) substitutions in the formula must be made carefully, and (4) arithmetic errors must be avoided. Statistical computer programs can compute a Pearson's r on large sets of data in fractions of a second. An example is included here based on a small dataset of 10 pairs of scores:

X	Y	XY	X²	Y²
15	13	195	225	169
18	17	306	324	289
10	12	120	100	144
17	15	255	289	225
15	15	225	225	225
14	19	266	196	361
16	20	320	256	400
16	12	192	256	144
14	15	210	196	225
20	17	340	400	289

$\Sigma XY = 2429$
$\Sigma X = 155$
$\Sigma Y = 155$
$\Sigma X^2 = 2467$
$\Sigma Y^2 = 2471$

$$r = \frac{10(2429) - (155)(155)}{\sqrt{[10(2467) - (155)(155)][10(2471) - (155)(155)]}}$$

$$r = 0.398$$

If the subjects' scores are perfectly related, the Pearson's r is 1.00. If there is no relationship between the two sets of scores, the value of r is zero. If there is a direct relationship between the two sets of values, the correlation coefficient is positive. If there is an inverse relationship between the two sets of scores, the correlation coefficient is negative. Measures with reported test-retest reliabilities above .80 are generally regarded as reliable instruments.

Two factors commonly affect test-retest reliability. One, called reactivity, occurs when the items in an instrument sensitize the test subjects to new topics to which they give further thought. This additional reflection about the topics may cause the subjects to change their responses at the second administration of the instrument.

Does reactivity cause the test-retest coefficient to be an overestimate or an underestimate of reliability?

Also, the individuals may remember the items and their answers and merely put down the same answers on the second administration of the instrument.

Would memory cause the test-retest reliability coefficient to be an overestimate or an underestimate?

Homogeneity of a data collection instrument refers to its internal consistency. To what extent do all of the items focus on appropriate concepts? In developing an instrument, an investigator usually administers a pilot version of the tool to a group of subjects and computes the correlation coefficients of each item to the total scores as a way of examining the internal consistency of the items. Items with low or negative correlations are discarded.

Split half reliability is a common approach to establishing homogeneity once the set of items has been shown to be relevant. The scores from one half of the instrument are compared with the scores from the other half—for example, the odd-numbered items versus the even-numbered items or the first half versus the second half. This approach introduces two problems. First, reliability is related to the length of a measure: the longer the measure, the more reliable. Splitting the measure into its halves necessarily produces an underestimate of reliability. Second, each way of splitting the items produces a different coefficient of reliability; an investigator may report only the highest measure ob-

tained from splitting the content in many ways. This highest value is not representative of the reliability of the instrument. It would be preferable to obtain
all possible split halves and obtain an average of these values. When the instrument has right and wrong answers, the Kuder Richardson formulas (1937)
may be used. To calculate one estimate, Kuder Richardson 20 (KR-20), the tester
must know the variance for the test, the number of items on the test, and the
number of persons getting each item correct. Then the KR-20 is calculated according to the following formula:

$$r = \frac{k}{k-1}\left[1 - \frac{\Sigma pq}{v^2}\right]$$

where k = number of items
$\quad\quad\quad v$ = variance of the test
$\quad\quad\quad p$ = proportion of persons answering the item correctly
$\quad\quad\quad q$ = $1-p$ (proportion of incorrect responses)
$\quad\Sigma pq$ = sum of p times q for each item

The variance is simply calculated as follows:

$$v^2 = \frac{(X - \overline{X})^2}{n}$$

The KR-20 is appropriate for any test that has right and wrong answers; the
item difficulties are taken into account and may differ substantially. If the items
can be assumed to be fairly uniform in difficulty, a simplified formula, Kuder
Richardson 21 (KR-21), can be used. KR-21 is calculated according to the following formula:

$$r = \frac{k}{k-1}\left[1 - \frac{\overline{X}\left(1 - \frac{\overline{X}}{k}\right)}{v^2}\right]$$

Table 4-3 illustrates the computations for both Kuder Richardson formulas
from a single set of data. Since the items are not very uniform in difficulty, the
values of KR-20 and KR-21 differ substantially. Under these conditions the test
will not show a very high coefficient of reliability, nor are the conditions right
to substitute KR-21 for KR-20.

These reliability values are so unacceptable that revision of the existing test
would not be productive. However, if the reliability of a measure is promising
(say, above .70 or .72), it can be improved by any of the following means (Ebel,
1965):

1. Adding more items
2. Improving the homogeneity of the items
3. Administering the test to more heterogeneous groups
4. Administering the test as a timed test so that not all examinees finish in
   the allotted time

Table 4-3 Computation of the Kuder Richardson formulas

					Scale items						
	1	2	3	4	5	6	7	8	9	10	T
Subject											
01	1	1	0	1	1	1	1	1	1	1	9
02	1	1	0	1	1	0	0	1	0	0	5
03	1	1	0	1	1	0	0	1	1	1	7
04	1	1	1	1	1	0	0	1	0	0	6
05	1	1	0	1	1	0	1	1	1	1	8
06	0	0	1	0	1	0	0	1	0	0	3
07	1	1	0	1	0	0	1	1	0	0	5
08	1	1	0	1	1	1	1	1	1	1	9
09	1	1	0	1	1	0	1	1	1	1	8
10	0	1	1	0	1	0	1	0	1	1	6
Total correct	8	9	3	8	9	2	6	9	6	6	66
p	.80	.90	.30	.80	.90	.20	.60	.90	.60	.60	
q	.20	.10	.70	.20	.10	.80	.40	.10	.40	.40	
pq	.16	.09	.21	.16	.09	.16	.24	.09	.24	.24	1.68

Mean = 6.6; variance = 3.44.

$$\text{KR-20: } r = \frac{10}{9}\left(1 - \frac{1.68}{3.44}\right) = 0.57$$

$$\text{KR-21: } r = \frac{10}{9}\left[1 - \frac{6.6\left(1 - \frac{6.6}{10}\right)}{3.44}\right] = 0.39$$

5. Revising items so that items with a midrange difficulty index replace very easy or very difficult items
6. Revising items to improve the discrimination indexes

The first four methods of improving reliability are self-explanatory. The last two—the difficulty index and discrimination index—should be examined further. Both of these indexes are commonly computed as part of an item analysis obtained from a computer program. The difficulty index of an item is the proportion of examinees who get the item correct; the difficulty indexes in Table 4-3 are simply the p values, showing that items 1, 2, 4, 5, and 8 are very easy and items 3 and 6 are very hard. Items almost no one gets correct or those almost no one misses are not effective in spreading out a group's scores to indicate varying levels of ability or comprehension.

The discrimination index is a measure of the relationship of an item to the total score when there are correct and incorrect answers. It varies depending on how well subjects who score well on a test and those who score poorly on a test perform on each item.

Cronbach's alpha (1984) is a more general approach to determining internal consistency. Unlike the Kuder Richardson formulas, Cronbach's alpha can be computed for measures that have no right or wrong answers, such as attitude scales. When computer programs are used for item analyses, the Cronbach's alpha is usually computed, and it is interpreted the same way as other measures of internal consistency. Values of .80 and up are considered acceptable. Alpha is tedious to calculate from raw data because the variances of all items and of the total measure must be calculated as shown in the following formula (Cronbach, 1984):

$$\alpha = \left(\frac{k}{k-1}\right)\left[1 - \left(\frac{\Sigma v_i}{\Sigma v_T}\right)\right]$$

where k = number of items on the scale
Σv_i = sum of item variances
Σv_T = variance of the total scores on the scale

The final form of reliability to be considered is equivalence. Equivalence is the extent to which two measures or two (or more) raters agree. As an example of the former situation, two nursing interventions—an experimental treatment and a control treatment—are implemented in an experimental study. The differential effects are to be determined by the results of pretests and posttests of the dependent variable. If two versions of equivalent tests are administered instead of the same measure being administered twice, the investigators can be more confident that the posttest scores have not been influenced by prior exposure to the measure. But the two measures must truly be equivalent. Such forms are called parallel forms, and their equivalence is determined by administering both measures to a large group of subjects and comparing the scores on each version by means of a correlation coefficient. The correlation coefficient should be very high—.90 or more. In instrument credentialing the developer may use item analysis data (such as discrimination and difficulty indexes) to select items for each of the parallel forms to make them equivalent.

The second situation in which equivalence is important occurs when two or more investigators collect data by means of observation. When any two observers' data are compared, interrater reliability is being determined. If the instructions for making observations are clear and the raters are attentive to their task, the relationship should be quite high—perhaps more than .80. A simple correlation coefficient can be calculated. Another, less accurate approach is to calculate the percentage of agreement as a proportion of the number of possible decisions. This approach is less accurate because it results in a proportion of about .50 simply by chance if a dichotomy (only two options) is involved. Thus an overestimate of interrater agreement is likely.

Sensitivity

The sensitivity of a data collection instrument reflects how well the measure detects differences among research subjects when real differences exist. The discrimination index described previously is an indicator of an instrument's sensitivity. The average discrimination index (which is calculated for each item) provides the investigator with an objective measure of an instrument's sensitivity. In general, measures of biophysical variables are more sensitive than measures of behavioral variables. Differences in subjects' weights can be detected with greater accuracy than can differences in their attitudes toward aging, their health practices, or their social support systems.

Sensitivity is discussed earlier in the text in relation to type I and type II errors. A type I error (alpha or α) occurs when a null hypothesis is mistakenly rejected. The investigator concludes that a significant difference or relationship was found in a study when in fact there were no real differences. A type II error (beta or β) occurs when a null hypothesis is mistakenly accepted. The investigator declares that no significant differences or relationships were found when in fact real differences existed.

Which type of error occurs when the data collection instruments are not as sensitive as they should be? Why?

As measurement error decreases, what happens to sensitivity?

Reactivity

Reactivity refers to changes in the values of a variable that take place as a consequence of the way it is measured. Reactivity occurs when an individual's blood pressure rises at the sight of the nurse or physician who is about to measure it. Patients or nurses who know they are being observed as part of a study may behave in abnormal ways. Research subjects who are being interviewed may be affected by the interviewer's personality or manner, a situation that changes their behavior and perhaps their responses. Certain questionnaire items may focus on information the subject finds embarrassing to disclose; the subject's responses are affected by the presence of those items. Careful attention in the design of a study should be given to possible reactivity. Reactivity may be cited as a limitation in a study, but the magnitude of the error introduced by reactivity cannot be estimated.

Range

Range refers to the scope of a data collection instrument. A desirable range is one that measures from the individual scoring the least possible up to and including the individual who scores the most possible. On an instrument with desirable range, no individual should score zero or obtain a perfect score. If either occurs, the instrument is not functioning as it should to discriminate among subjects or to measure their highest attainment regarding the variable of interest.

Objectivity

The results from a data collection instrument or procedure should not depend in any way on extraneous variables. Investigators strive to eliminate subjectivity in a study. Let's look at the possibility of cultural bias. There has been considerable concern about the use of the Scholastic Aptitude Test and intelligence tests in decisions about higher education for subjects of various backgrounds. Since the tests were designed primarily for white, middle-class students, they may not provide accurate measures for subjects from different cultures; that is, they may be culturally biased and therefore not objective. The nurse should be aware of this source of error in data collection. As in the case of the Scholastic Aptitude Test, it may be a function of the content of the instrument. However, it may occur in studies that use interviews or observation because of the investigator's "set." In our perceptions of reality, all of us are influenced, sometimes unconsciously, by our beliefs and experience. When using a data collection instrument, the investigator must always be aware of this problem and make an effort to be objective. Objective data collection tools are those that can glean the same data for a given group from two or more independent administrations of the instrument. An objective observation checklist is one that will be filled out the same way by two or more observers watching a given subject for a stated period of time.

Practicality

For an instrument to be a valid reflection of an attribute, its content should be understood by the investigator and by all research subjects. Observers and interviewers should recognize and guard against sources of error that may be inherent in their data collection techniques. Research subjects should understand the questions or tasks posed for them. Any ambiguity should be eliminated from measures. A question should be so clear that it is like a stimulus to which an individual can give only one response. The data collection instrument should be appropriate for the research subjects in terms of their ability and readiness to furnish the required data. Age, reading level, health status, and emotional status of subjects are pertinent considerations.

Another facet of practicality is the demands made on the research subjects. Nonintrusive procedures are preferable to intrusive ones. Short questionnaires are preferable to long ones. Bland questions are preferable to sensitive or intimidating queries. Data collection techniques must be assessed carefully in terms of their potential risk—either physiological or psychosocial—to the potential subjects. Ethical considerations, discussed briefly in Chapter 3, dictate that risk not be imposed capriciously or without the subjects' informed consent. The purpose of institutional review boards is to ensure that research on human subjects is carried out under conditions of minimal risk, benefit to society and the research subjects involved, and informed consent. Informed consent means that the subject has full knowledge of any potential risks of participation in a study and understands that he or she can terminate participation at any point in the study. Practicality cannot be attained unless ethical considerations have received adequate attention. Appropriate debriefing procedures should be included in designs that affect the psychological status of research subjects.

Efficiency is the third aspect of practicality in measurement. Both the investigator's and research subjects' time should be considered valuable. The cost of various approaches should be weighed. Only information that is necessary for the research should be elicited. It is surprisingly easy for an investigator to get sidetracked and ask for information that is nice to know rather than essential to know. In the literature review the investigator will probably have found several approaches to data collection about relevant variables. In selecting tools for a study, a primary consideration is adequacy. Does the instrument measure the variable in a complete, consistent, and balanced way? Validity, reliability, sensitivity, and objectivity are essential features of adequacy. Another consideration should be its practicality, including its efficiency.

METHODS OF DATA COLLECTION

Nursing research may be regarded as a series of decisions (see Fig. 2-3). What topic should be studied? How should the study topic be delineated and delimited? What dependent and independent variables will be studied? What approach should be used: exploratory, descriptive, ex post facto, quasiexperimental, or experimental? What is the optimal population that can be sampled for the study? Most of these decisions are based on information gleaned in the literature review; some reflect the investigator's personal interest and resources.

After the literature review the investigator should state the research problem fully and precisely, identifying the concepts that will be studied. An essential component of the problem statement is the set of conceptual and operational definitions of the variables to be studied. Generally the literature provides the investigator with some choices. Several sources are used to develop a theoretical framework or a conceptual framework for the study. It is up to the investigator to determine which materials should be included and which should receive primary emphasis.

The literature review also provides information about methods of data collection used by other investigators. There may be several possibilities for each study variable. For example, the researcher might find that pain has been measured in a number of ways. Reading (1980) described a comparison of four pain measures. One was a Present Pain Intensity (PPI) verbal report consisting of the adjectives "mild, discomforting, distressing, horrible, excruciating" (p. 120); another was a visual analogue scale consisting of a 10 centimeter line with the extremes labeled "no pain at all" and "worst pain imaginable" (p. 120); the third was a 10-point horizontal scale with anchor points consisting of the adjectives "none . . . mild . . . moderately distressing . . . very distressing . . . unbearable" (p. 120); the fourth simply asked the research subjects to rate on seven-point scales some specific pain adjectives (such as throbbing, pulling, stinging, aching, tiring, and annoying) from the McGill Pain Questionnaire (Melzack, 1975). Other researchers have used totally different approaches such as physiological measures, observation checklists, and analgesics requested. The resources required for each of these measures vary widely. Can the investigator observe each patient or obtain reliable physiological measures at appropriate times? If the subjects are young children, will they be able to give reliable self-reports of pain they experience? Perhaps a nonverbal tool such as the "Oucher" (Beyer and Aradine, 1986), in which photographs of children experiencing increasing levels of pain are used, would be the best choice.

The next decision concerns the research question and the pertinent variables it identifies. Following in importance are the population and sample, the design selected for the study, and the investigator's resources. The total time subjects are expected to commit to a research project must also be considered. If a large number of variables are to be studied, finding efficient ways of eliciting data is important. In this section we look at the main methods nursing investigators use to collect data.

Existing records

A cardinal rule of data collection is to use existing records whenever possible. In studies of hospitalized patients, for example, admission data, charts, incident reports, and nursing notes contain potentially useful data. Long-term care facilities and visiting nurse associations maintain extensive records. Industries keep records on employees' health and absenteeism. If schoolchildren are the study subjects, the school records should be reviewed before data collection begins to see what information is readily available about such factors as growth, family status, immunizations, and absences because of illness. The investigator should never waste subjects' time and efforts by asking for data obtainable from available sources. If existing records furnish part of the data in a study that might, for example, also employ interviews with the patients, of course the agency's, patients', and physicians' permission must be received before data gathering.

In retrospective studies, records are the sole sources of data. The data may cover extensive periods. In this type of research it is usual to adopt careful procedures for recording data anonymously, and the researcher needs to obtain permission only from the agency involved. An excellent example of this kind of research is the study of hospitalized patients' falls by Janken, Reynolds, and Swiech (1986). The purpose of the study was to determine characteristics that could be used at admission to identify patients at risk for falling. The authors gathered data from incident reports to identify patients 60 years of age and over who had fallen during hospitalization. They used patients' charts and admission data to identify another sample who were similar to the fall sample but had not fallen during hospitalization. The entire study was retrospective and used existing records. The authors found that the fall group was distinguished by general weakness, decreased mobility of the lower extremities, sleeplessness, incontinence, confusion, depression, and substance abuse. Certain other variables such as impaired vision, which conventional wisdom would suggest to be predictive of falls, did not emerge as relevant to an assessment of patients at risk for falls.

The limitations these investigators described are common to retrospective studies and point to difficulties commonly experienced in using existing records for research. Since the study was retrospective, it relied on chart documentation;

therefore some variables such as alcohol abuse, fall history, and depression were probably underreported. In the course of their study of nonfall patients, the authors learned that one had fallen but no incident report had been filed— another source of error. They also noted that some relevant variables may not have been recorded at all.

Existing records are particularly useful for longitudinal studies in which data about research subjects can be gathered for several years. The investigator should always remember, however, that the data were not recorded for research purposes and therefore omissions or mistakes—serious sources of error—cannot be checked. Moreover, retrospective studies often involve data recorded by different personnel with different habits and styles of reporting information. Such factors as location of certain information within the total record or the use of abbreviations may cause special problems.

Biophysiological measures
At one time biophysiological instruments were used only by nurses who were also physiologists, and primarily in animal studies. This area of investigation still produces valuable knowledge for nursing practice. However, since the 1960s, when the American Nurses' Association urged nurses to concentrate on clinical research because clinical settings are typically equipped with a wide variety of instruments designed to measure physiological functions, it was inevitable that increasing numbers of nursing studies would use biophysiological measures. Although some investigations have used biophysiological instruments (such as biofeedback instruments) as independent variables, the focus of this discussion is on their use as dependent variables. Such instruments furnish valuable research data for many nursing studies. Gift and Soeken (1988) reported that 13% of the studies published in *Nursing Research, Research in Nursing and Health,* and *The Western Journal of Nursing Research* in 1986 involved the use of physiological measures, and 60% of the studies published in *Heart and Lung* in 1986 involved the use of physiological measures. However, they noted a dearth of reports about the accuracy, precision, and sensitivity of instruments used, and they urged that investigators stop assuming that these characteristics are present when physiological measures are used. They also noted the need to establish selectivity, stating that "the selectivity of electrocardiographic signals permits detection of electrical signals generated by the myocardium from those generated by skeletal muscles . . . but . . . are changes in the intracranial pressure the result of position changes or the result of the touch involved in turning the person?" (Gift and Soekin, 1988, p. 130). Table 4-4 lists the sources of errors in physiological measures identified by Gift and Soeken (1988) and examples of each.

When behavioral measures are reported in study findings, investigators usually report the evidence of validity and reliability, and perhaps additional criteria for judging the precision and relevance of the instruments used. Similarly, when biophysiological measures are used, investigators should report the accuracy, precision, and sensitivity of their equipment in relation to the sources of error listed previously. Information about the procedures and techniques employed

Table 4-4 Sources of error with physiological instruments

Source	Example
Environment	Temperature of the room on spirometer readings (Perks, Sopwith, Brown, Jones, and Green, 1983)
User	Random encouragement of subjects during pulmonary function tests (Gift and Soeken, 1988)
Subject	Lack of full subject effort in spirometric determination of pulmonary function (Sobol and Emergil, 1964)
Administration	Changing supplies, for example, from prefilled syringes to a closed injectate system, to inject the solution for determining thermodilution cardiac output (Barcelona, Patague, Bunoy, Gloriani, Justice, and Robinson, 1985)
Machine	Improper calibration procedures or failure to calibrate the instrument (Gift and Soeken, 1988)
Interpretation	Improper heating of the element (Gift and Soeken, 1988)

should also be given. An exemplary journal article, in which the investigators meticulously identify types of equipment, standards for its use, and actions taken to ensure its calibration, is that by Hayman, Meininger, Stashinko, and Gallagher titled, "Type A Behavior and Physiological Cardiovascular Risk Factors in School-Age Twin Children," published in the May-June 1988 issue of *Nursing Research.*

Many nursing studies use objective, biophysiological measures to seek answers to nursing research problems. For example, Beard (1982) studied a sample of 105 college students to answer four questions:

1. What are the relationships between interpersonal trust, life events and coronary heart disease risk factors?
2. Is there a difference in the level of interpersonal trust, life events, and coronary heart disease risk factors of young (age 20-35) and older (age 50-65) adults?
3. Are there interactions between interpersonal trust, life events and age?
4. What are the major contributing factors of risk?*

Life events and interpersonal trust were operationalized as pencil-and-paper measures. Additional data collected were subjects' blood pressure, height, weight, pulse, pulse pressure, mean arterial pressure, and the biochemical indexes of creatine phosphokinase level, glutamic-oxaloacetic transaminase level, and electrolyte balance.

Beard found statistically significant relationships between interpersonal trust and life events, blood pressure, obesity, and exercise. Differences in the magnitude and direction of relationships among variables were found between the younger and older age groups. The major risk factors identified included blood

---

*From Beard M (1982). Trust, life events and risk factors among adults. *Advances in Nursing Science* 4:33.

pressure (both diastolic and systolic), mean arterial pressure, body mass index, age, pulse, pulse pressure, cholesterol and triglyceride levels, and family history.

Observational measures

The use of observation as a data-gathering technique is described extensively in Chapter 5, which is devoted to qualitative research. In such studies the investigator may introduce varying amounts of structure from none at all, with the observer recording field notes on whatever he or she sees, to highly structured observations, which may use time- or event-sampling techniques. Before the observation begins, the investigator must define precisely what will be observed and how it will be recorded. In time sampling the observer records communications (verbal and nonverbal) and actions at specified intervals and for a specified time. For example, an observer may collect data about the interactions between a new mother and her baby every 3 minutes with observation periods limited to 30 seconds each. The remaining 2½ minutes of each 3-minute period is used to record the observations.

What advantages and disadvantages do you see in the time-sampling approach?

By contrast, an event-sampling approach might involve recording behavior every time the new mother makes a verbal comment or response to her baby. The observation periods continue as long as the verbal behavior or event occurs, hence the term "event sampling." Recording must be completed between events.

What advantages and disadvantages do you see in the event-sampling approach?

Additional structure may be introduced into an observational approach. Instead of simply recording that a behavior occurred or did not occur, the investigator may use a checklist or rating scale that provides a score. For example, Fegley (1988) studied two methods of preparing 61 children for radiological procedures—either intravenous pyelograms (IVPs) or cystourethrograms (VCUGs)—to find out their distress, cooperation, and information-seeking behavior. One method of preparation was termed contingent and consisted of answering the children's questions and encouraging additional questions until the children's curiosity was satisfied. In the other method, termed noncontingent, the children were given predetermined information about the radiological procedures. Four dependent variables were studied: searching for information, an upset score (1 to 5), a cooperation score (1 to 5), and a distress score. The first three variables were measured by a nurse's observations during the procedure. Two upset and cooperation scores were obtained for each subject—one while the child was being put on the table and one during the intrusive procedure. The distress score was obtained by questioning each child after the procedure had been completed. The contingency group spent significantly less time searching for information than the noncontingency group. There were no differences in the upset, cooperation, or distress scores between the two groups. However, the older children in both groups were more cooperative and less upset and reported less distress than the younger children. Thus observation was used effectively in testing hypotheses about preparation of children for radiological procedures.

No validity or reliability information was reported in relation to the measures used. How could these attributes be established? What is your opinion of using only one nurse observer?

Interviews and questionnaires

Both interviews and questionnaires are used to elicit information from research subjects; the data consist of self-reports. Varying amounts of structure may be used in both approaches. Interviewers commonly elicit demographic data and then ask questions pertinent to the research topic. The questions may be designed specifically for the investigation, or they may consist of one or more scales, either alone or embedded within other items. Closed or open-ended questions may be asked. A closed question is one in which the respondent is forced to choose from options, whereas an open-ended question allows the respondent to answer the question in any way she or he sees fit. Examples of each approach to obtaining information about basic nursing education follow:

Closed question:
　1. Please check (√) the answer that describes your basic nursing education:
　　　a. _____ Associate degree
　　　b. _____ Diploma
　　　c. _____ Baccalaureate degree
　　　d. _____ Master's degree
Open-ended question:
　1. What was your basic nursing education?

　　Before an interview study begins, all interview protocols should be standardized as much as possible. The interviewer's approach should be defined carefully so that the same tones and statements are used with all research subjects. It is neither practical nor desirable to require that exactly the same wording be used throughout an interview. One advantage of the interview process is that the interviewer can follow up on specific information given by different subjects in different ways. Still, the probes that will be used and the depth of the interview should be established in advance. It would not be desirable to have different interviewers asking questions about respondents' answers (using probes) while other interviewers take the first answer given and leave it at that.

Sequence is important in devising a formal interview guide, usually called an interview schedule. First the interviewer should explain the project and ask whether the subject has any questions about it. The interviewer should try to establish rapport with the subject. Since nurses use interviewing techniques frequently in practice—for example, in taking a history or making an assessment—the interview approach in research is relatively easy for them to implement. Bland information should always be sought before sensitive questions are posed. No more detail should be elicited than will be used. For example, an interviewer who wants to divide subjects into young adults, middle-aged adults, and older adults should ask if the person is between 21 and 40 instead of requesting an exact age. The same approach should be used when seeking income data.

Many studies have used interviews as the primary data collection method. One study of burn patients used interviews to examine gender differences regarding functional disability, disfigurement, social resources, coping responses, and psychosocial adjustment (Brown, Roberts, Browne, Byrne, Love, and Streiner, 1988). These authors also determined the relationships between psychosocial adjustment and gender, burn severity, time since the burn, functional disability, disfigurement, social resources, and coping responses. Chart reviews were used to gather data about the burn event, and the subjects were interviewed to obtain information on sociodemographic variables, social resources, coping, and psychosocial adjustment to the burn. Interviewers used observation to rate the extent of functional disability and disfigurement. In addition to the demographic data (such as age, marital status, and employment status) gathered in the interviews, four scales were administered: a Social Participation Scale and a Social Support Scale, both developed by Davidson and colleagues (Davidson, Bowden, and Feller, 1981), an Indices of Coping Responses Scale (Moos, Cronkite, Billings, and Finney, 1984), and Derogatis and Lopez's Psychosocial Adjustment to Illness Scale (PAIS) (1983). The authors found that persons of both sexes had adjusted to their burn injury. For men, functional disability was the most important variable related to adjustment. For women it was greater use of problem-solving coping responses. The interview approach was particularly appropriate for this study because of the nature of the sample—individuals with burn injuries. Responding to interview questions was easier for them than completing a questionnaire.

Questionnaires are most commonly mailed, although they can be administered to groups such as students or participants in a workshop or conference. This has the advantage that total group participation is much more likely than with mailed questionnaires. However, the investigator should make it clear that participation is voluntary and should answer any questions. Individual distribution of a questionnaire in a hospital or other health care agency is also fairly

efficient and gives the research subjects additional incentives to participate because of the personal contact and opportunities for questions. Before administering a questionnaire by any approach, the investigator should conduct a pilot
test of the instrument to be sure that questions are clear and answerable.

What is wrong with the following questionnaire item?

Please circle the response that best describes your use of microcomputers:
a. No use
b. Little use at home or school
c. Moderate use at home or school
d. Heavy use at home or school

**Reconstruct possible answers that will correct these problems. Use as many
responses as you wish.**

Please circle the response that best describes your use of microcomputers:

**Would the question above or the question "How much do you use
microcomputers?" be easier to analyze? Why?**

Because of the prevalence of the use of mailed questionnaires, we should
take note of some of the difficulties and potential solutions in this approach.
First, the cover letter must be carefully designed. It should be respectful, concise,
and clear. The letter should attempt to motivate the respondents to participate

in the study. Sometimes the importance of the health problems being addressed or the population at risk is sufficient incentive to participate. An honest estimate of the time required for participation should be provided. In some cases investigators may wish to offer participants a report of the study. Provisions for confidentiality or anonymity should be spelled out. Preaddressed, stamped envelopes should be enclosed for responses. If the research is funded or sponsored by a prestigious organization, this fact may encourage participation.

The design of a questionnaire affects its appeal. It should be free of errors, and the printing should be clear and attractive. Colored stock might be used for different parts of a survey instrument. The questionnaire should appear as brief as possible. If funds permit, printing a questionnaire in a booklet form makes it look more professional and shorter than a typewritten, photocopied instrument. The instrument can be divided into several sections if appropriate, and a new set of numbers can be used for each section. Thus, in scanning the questionnaire, the potential participant never gets to items with high numbers like 80! If code numbers are affixed to the questionnaire with a master list retained by the investigator, the questionnaire should explain that these numbers are merely for follow-up to send the participant a reminder in case of a nonresponse or a report of findings if offered. Follow-up reminders do increase the return rate, especially if the reminder letter is accompanied by a second copy of the questionnaire and a second preaddressed, stamped envelope. Follow-ups are generally mailed to nonrespondents about 2 weeks after the initial mailing. If no code numbers are used, the reminder must go to the entire mailing list; in this case it should contain an appeal for nonrespondents and an expression of appreciation to respondents. More than one reminder can be used. The first reminder may be just a postcard sent only a week after the initial mailing, in hope that the potential participants still have the original mailing. Then 2 weeks later an additional letter, questionnaire, and preaddressed, stamped envelope may be mailed.

The nursing literature contains many examples of questionnaire studies. Savage, Cullen, Kirchoff, Pugh, and Foreman (1987) examined nurses' responses to do-not-resuscitate (DNR) orders in 10 of the perinatal centers of a single state's hospitals. The so-called Baby Doe regulations, mandating treatment of all infants regardless of condition and implemented in 1983, have three exceptions: if a patient is chronically and irreversibly comatose, if treatment would only prolong dying, and if treatment would be virtually futile in terms of survival and therefore inhumane (Rhodes, 1985). The purpose of the study by Savage and co-workers was to determine how many of the centers had DNR policies for patients in neonatal intensive care units and what factors influenced nurses' decisions to comply with a DNR order.

A three-part questionnaire was used, with fixed-response items (closed questions) designed to determine the nurses' awareness of a DNR policy and their attitudes toward it. The second part consisted of four hypothetical situations involving babies with different expected outcomes. Attitudes toward resuscitation of each infant were measured by means of semantic differentials. A semantic differential is simply a set of bipolar adjectives with a scale line drawn between them. Examples of items used in the DNR study are as follows:

good ____|____|____|____|____|____|____ bad

harmful ____|____|____|____|____|____|____ beneficial

The respondent checks a space indicating how close to either extreme he or she wishes to place an attitude. Scaling varies, but in this example $+1$, $+2$, and $+3$ were used for the three favorable responses and -1, -2, and -3 were used for unfavorable responses. Checkmarks in the center were assigned a value of zero.

How would you score the checkmarks below?

harmful ____| X |____|____|____|____|____ beneficial

powerful ____|____|____|____|____|____| X powerless

happy ____|____| X |____|____|____|____ unhappy

Nurses were also asked to rate, on a seven-point scale from extremely improbable to extremely probable, how their peers would respond to each situation. After a review of ethical considerations and a pilot study, questionnaires were distributed to 30 nurses. Responses were obtained from 90% after a second follow-up reminder. Eighteen reported having DNR policies in their hospitals. Factors related to compliance with the DNR orders were agreement that the infant should not be resuscitated ($n = 24$) or respect for the parents' wishes ($n = 19$). The ratings of peer responses were more often related to nurses' decisions not to resuscitate than were the attitudes as measured by the semantic differential items.

Vignettes

The nurses in the DNR study were given hypothetical descriptions of four infants and asked to make decisions about these cases. These were very short vignettes, or short descriptive sketches. Several nurse scientists have used vignettes to study stereotyping behavior. One of the more recent studies was that reported by Ganong, Coleman, and Riley (1988). They named a hypothetical pregnant woman "Sara Holmes" and presented information about her to two groups of nursing students in two sessions each, one a verbal description and the other a videotape of a nurse interviewing Sara. The information was identical except that Sara was married in the group 1 version and unmarried in the group 2 version. After hearing the verbal report about Sara, each group of nursing students completed two scales: a 40-item First Impressions Questionnaire (FIP) and an 118-item Family Role Stereotype Instrument (FRSI). After seeing the video-tapes, they completed another instrument, a nine-item Predicted Behavior of a Hospitalized Adult (PBHA).

The results were interesting. The FIP consists of six subscales: evaluation, potency, activity, satisfaction/security, personal characteristics, and stability. The married Sara was rated more favorably than the unmarried Sara on all subscales except activity. The students characterized the married Sara as an advocate for children, supportive, and reliable, whereas they characterized the unmarried Sara as promiscuous, liberal, unhappy, and undereducated. Similar differences prevailed after the students viewed the videotape. Students predicted that the unmarried Sara would have a more difficult time if hospitalized than the married Sara.

Use of vignettes allowed the investigators to discern nurses' different atti-tudes about married and unmarried pregnant women indirectly. Such an ap-proach is more likely to reveal true attitudes than a direct question, which often receives an answer the respondent thinks is socially desirable (that is, non-prejudiced).

What research problem areas can you identify that would be amenable to a vignette approach?

Diaries and critical incidents

Other approaches to obtaining self-report data are diaries and critical incidents. Diaries are an appropriate source of research data when the subjects can be motivated to describe their behavior or thoughts on an ongoing basis. For ex-ample, Perry (1981) studied the effectiveness of a specific rehabilitation program designed for patients with chronic bronchitis and emphysema. Patients kept daily records of symptoms experienced and treatments employed for 4 weeks before their participation in exercise and self-care rehabilitation programs. After the rehabilitation program they resumed keeping diaries for 8 weeks. These posttreatment diaries were compared with the pretreatment diaries. Symptoms such as difficulty raising phlegm, tight chest, increased shortness of breath, fatigue, sleep difficulties, and wheezing decreased significantly after treatment. The number of "good days" increased significantly. Subjects' reports of treatments showed significant increases in their use of breathing, relaxation, and general exercises, postural drainage, purposeful positioning, increased fluid intake, intake of hot fluids, and rest. A sample of 20 patients (of 31) completed the 11-month study. One reason the study avoided the heavy attrition frequently associated with this type of data collection was that the investigator structured the diaries to make them easy to write. (The structured approach also made analysis easier.) Moreover, the rehabilitation program was highly successful in ameliorating the research subjects' symptoms—an important incentive for them to continue with the study.

The Perry study illustrates two advantages of diaries as a mode of data collection. First, longitudinal data can be gathered without the continual involvement of the investigator, and second, participants' reports are more spontaneous and thus more likely to reveal differences over time.

Identify a situation and research subjects that would be appropriate for use of diaries as a data collection technique.

The critical incident technique was originated by Flanagan (1956), who used it in educational research. In his "Performance Record for the Personal and Social Development Program," children's behavior was recorded on a form that illustrated such concepts as personal adjustment, responsibility and effort, and creativity and initiative. This technique has been used in a variety of ways in nursing research. For example, part of Thomas' study (1984) of primiparas involved an interview 4 weeks after the infant was born. New mothers were asked to identify the most stressful event or situation that occurred during labor and delivery and also the most stressful event or situation that occurred during the first month post partum. The descriptions were critical incidents—they represented the extremes in the mothers' experiences. Results consisted of identification and descriptions of the most stressful events or situations during the two time periods. Concerns about the safety and well-being of the baby dominated the labor-delivery stresses, and feelings of fatigue and overwhelming responsibilities were most prevalent in the postpartum collection of stressors (Thomas, 1984).

Use of the critical incident approach requires that the investigator ask for information in a timely manner. Most authorities agree that asking for recollections of events before the previous 6 months is unrealistic, although psychologically salient events may be recalled for a very long time.

To whom would you direct requests for critical incidents to determine nursing actions most valued by surgical patients?

Q sorts

The Q sort, a scaling technique developed by Stephenson (1975), can be used in a number of ways. Respondents are asked to sort a set of cards into clusters according to criteria explained by the investigator. The scaling may reflect dimensions such as agreement and disagreement, most important and least important, or most like me and least like me. The investigator may instruct subjects to sort cards into a specific number of clusters and may even restrict subjects' decisions about how many cards can be placed in each cluster. Normally, anywhere from 50 to 150 cards are involved in a Q sort. Subjects usually find Q sorts more interesting to do than questionnaires or other printed data collection instruments. Another advantage of Q sorts is their versatility. The primary disadvantage of the Q sort is that it is time consuming because it is generally administered on a one-to-one basis.

Larson (1986) used the Q sort approach in studying cancer nurses' perceptions of caring. She developed an instrument called the CARE-Q, which consisted of six subscales: is accessible (6 items), explains and facilitates (6 items), comforts (9 items), develops a trusting relationship (16 items), anticipates patients' needs (5 items), and monitors and follows through (8 items). The sample of cancer nurses was asked to sort these 50 cards into seven clusters. The most important items were placed in cluster seven and the least important in cluster one. Means and standard deviations were computed for each item. The most important items included the following: listens to patient, touches when comforting is needed, allows expression of feelings, and gets to know the patient as an individual. The least important items were these: is professional in appearance, suggests questions for the patient to ask the doctor, is cheerful, and offers reasonable alternatives.

Projective techniques

Projective techniques provide stimuli to research subjects in such a way that a variety of responses are elicited. Generally the investigator provides a task, such as drawing or interpreting a picture, that requires the subject to respond in a uniquely personal manner. The manner of response reflects the person's needs, personality characteristics, attitudes, or values. Although the interpretation of data derived from projective techniques usually requires training in clinical psychology, it is an approach nurses can learn to use.

Sentence completion is a projective technique that has been used by health professionals to measure subjects' attitudes toward the elderly. Examples of sentence beginnings are "When I think of spending an afternoon with an 83-year-old man, I . . . " and "The most distinctive trait of elderly men is. . . ."

In an interesting study in which a projective technique was used to learn about children with cancer, a nurse scientist spent a summer working with a psychologist to learn to interpret the drawings she obtained from children (Scungio, 1984). The purpose of the study was to determine the relationship between self-concept and social activities of children with leukemia and healthy children. Self-concept was measured by the Piers Harris Test (1967), Human Figure and Self Figure drawings, the Wish Expressions Test, and a semistructured interview. Social activities were measured by the Children's Social Activity Scale. On the Piers Harris measure, children with leukemia demonstrated a significantly lower self-concept than did healthy children. On the drawing measure that was interpreted by projective techniques, children with leukemia put in two more emotional indicators than healthy children did, and they also drew more close relatives whereas the healthy children drew more friends. On their wish test children with leukemia reported health-related wishes significantly more often than healthy children did (Scungio, 1984).

REFERENCES

Barcelona M, Patague L, Bunoy M, Gloriani M, Justice B, and Robinson L (1985). Cardiac output determination by the thermodilution method: comparison of ice temperature injectate versus room temperature injectate contained in prefilled syringes or a closed injectate delivery system. *Heart and Lung* 14:232-235.

Beard M (1982). Trust, life events and risk factors among adults. *Advances in Nursing Science* 4: 26-43.

Beyer J and Aradine C (1986). Content validity of an instrument to measure young children's perceptions of the intensity of their pain. *Journal of Pediatric Nursing* 1:386-395.

Brett J (1987). Use of nursing practice research findings. *Nursing Research* 36:344-349.

Brown B, Roberts J, Browne G, Byrne C, Love B, and Streiner D (1988). Gender differences in variables associated with psychosocial adjustment to a burn injury. *Research in Nursing and Health* 11:23-30.

Campbell DT and Fiske DW (1959). Convergent and discriminant validation by the multitrait-multimethod matrix. *Psychological Bulletin* 56:81-105.

Cronbach LJ (1984). *Essentials of psychological testing*. 4th ed. New York: Harper & Row, Publishers Inc.

Davidson T, Bowden M, and Feller I (1981). Social support and post burn adjustment. *Archives of Physical Medicine and Rehabilitation* 62:274-278.

Derogatis L and Lopez M (1983). *PAIS and PAIS-SR administration, scoring and procedures manual*. Baltimore: Johns Hopkins School of Medicine, Clinical Psychometric Research.

Dube A and Mitchell E (1986). Accidental strangulation from vest restraints. *Journal of the American Medical Association* 256:2725-2726.

Ebel RL (1965). *Measuring educational achievement*. Englewood Cliffs, NJ: Prentice Hall.

Fegley B (1988). Preparing children for radiologic procedures: contingent versus noncontingent instruction. *Research in Nursing and Health* 11: 3-9.

Flanagan J (1956). *Teachers' guide for the personal and social development program*. Chicago: Science Research Associates.

Ganong L, Coleman M, and Riley C (1988). Nursing students' stereotypes of married and unmarried pregnant clients. *Research in Nursing and Health* 11:333-342.

Gift AG and Soeken KL (1988). Assessment of physiologic instruments. *Heart and Lung* 17:128-133.

Janken J, Reynolds B, and Swiech K (1986). Patient falls in the acute care setting: identifying risk factors. *Nursing Research* 35:215-219.

Kerlinger FN (1973). *Foundations of behavioral research*. 2nd ed. New York: Holt, Rinehart & Winston, Inc.

Kuder GF and Richardson MW (1937). The theory of the estimation of test reliability. *Psychometrika* II:151-160.

Larson P (1986). Cancer nurses' perceptions of caring. *Cancer Nursing* 9:86-91.

Lindquist EF (1956). *Design and analysis of experiments in psychology and education.* Boston: Houghton Mifflin Co.

Mandel J and Lohman W (1987). Low back pain in nurses: the relative importance of medical history, work factors, exercise, and demographics. *Research in Nursing and Health* 10:165-170.

Maranell G (1974). *Scaling: a source book for behavioral scientists.* New York: Aldine Publishing Co.

Megel M, Langston N, and Crewell J (1988). Scholarly productivity: a survey of nurse faculty researchers. *Journal of Professional Nursing* 4:45-54.

Melzack R (1975). The McGill pain questionnaire: major properties and scoring methods. *Pain* 1:277-299.

Moos R, Cronkite R, Billings A, and Finney J (1984). *Health and daily living form manual.* Palo Alto, Calif: Social Ecology Laboratory, Veterans Administration.

O'Muircheartaigh C and Payne C (1977). *Exploring data structure: the analysis of survey data.* New York: John Wiley & Sons Inc.

Perks W, Sopwith T, Brown D, Jones C, and Green M (1983). Effects of temperature on Vitalograph spirometer readings. *Thorax* 38:592-594.

Perry J (1981). Effectiveness of teaching in the rehabilitation of patients with chronic bronchitis and emphysema. *Nursing Research* 30:219-222.

Reading AE (1980). A comparison of pain rating scales. *Journal of Psychosomatic Research* 34:119-124.

Rhodes A (1985). "Baby Doe" rules: implications for nurses. *Maternal Child Nursing Journal* 10:405.

Rogers E (1983). *Diffusion of innovations.* 3rd ed. New York: Free Press.

Savage T, Cullen D, Kirchoff K, Pugh E, and Foreman M (1987). Nurses' responses to do-not-resuscitate orders in the neonatal intensive care unit. *Nursing Research* 36:370-373.

Scungio J (1984). The relationship of self concept and social activities of leukemic and healthy children. In King I, ed. *The world of work: research in nursing practice.* Indianapolis: Sigma Theta Tau.

Sobol B and Emirgil C (1964). Subject effort and the expiratory flow rate. *American Review of Respiratory Disease* 189:402-408.

Solomon R (1949). An extension of control group design. *Psychological Bulletin* 46:137-150.

Strumpf N and Evans L (1988). Physical restraint of the hospitalized elderly: perceptions of patients and nurses. *Nursing Research* 37:132-137.

Thomas B (1984). Stress and coping with childbirth among primiparas. In King I, ed. *The world of work: research in nursing practice.* Indianapolis: Sigma Theta Tau.

Yarmesch M and Sheafor M (1984). The decision to restrain. *Geriatric Nursing* 5:242-244.

REFERENCES FOR FURTHER STUDY

Anderson G, McBride M, Dahm J, Ellis M, and Vidyasager D (1982). Development of sucking in term infants from birth to four hours postbirth. *Research in Nursing and Health* 5:21-27.

Campbell D and Stanley J (1963). *Experimental and quasi-experimental designs for research.* Chicago: Rand McNally College Publishing Co.

Clayton G (1987). Evaluating measuring instruments. *Nurse Educator* 12:9.

Cook T and Campbell D (1979). *Quasi-experimentation: design and analysis issues for field settings.* Chicago: Rand McNally & Co.

Cronenwett L (1987). Increasing the cost-effectiveness of research in clinical settings. *Journal of Nursing Administration* 17:4-5.

Diers D (1979). *Research in nursing practice.* Philadelphia: JB Lippincott Co.

Diers D (1987). On research in nursing practice. *Image* 19:106.

Doolittle N (1988). Stroke recovery: review of the literature and suggestions for future research. *Journal of Neuroscience Nursing* 20:169-173.

Downs F (1987). The time of our lives. *Nursing Research* 6:331.

Frank B (1986). Choosing a methodology—investigating the process of nursing education. *Nurse Educator* 11:6-7.

Haller K (1987). What's the best sample size? *Maternal Child Nursing* 12:448.

Hinshaw A (1988). Practice and research are natural partners. *American Nurse* 20:4.

Hinshaw A (1988). Using research to shape health policy. *Nursing Outlook* 36:21-24.

Lawson L (1988). Building research credibility. *Journal of Nursing Administration* 18:7, 24.

Lewis M (1988). Attribution and illness. *Journal of Psychosocial and Mental Health Services* 26:14-17, 21, 35.

Martin K (1988). Research in home care. *Nursing Clinics of North America* 23:373-385.

McBride A (1987). Developing a woman's mental health research agenda. *Image* 19:4-8.

McCranie E, Lambert V, and Lambert C (1987). Work stress, hardiness, and burnout among hospital staff nurses. *Nursing Research* 6:374-380.

Munro B (1988). Research priorities. *Clinical Nurse Specialist* 2:44.

Norbeck J (1988). International nursing research in social support: theoretical and methodological issues. *Journal of Advanced Nursing* 13:173-178.

Richardson S (1988). Health promotion practices. *Journal of Pediatric Health Care* 2:73-78.

Smeltzer S (1988). Research in trauma nursing: state of the art and future directions. *Journal of Emergency Nursing* 14:145-153.

Smith D (1988). Collaboration in nursing research—a multidisciplinary approach. *International Journal of Nursing Studies* 25:73-78.

Washington CC and Moss M (1988). Pragmatic aspects of establishing interrater reliability. *Nursing Research* 37:190-191.

Williams M (1988). Fear of research. *Research in Nursing and Health* 11:69-70.

CHAPTER 5

Analyzing qualitative data

Objectives

After completing this unit of study, students will be able to:

1. Define qualitative data
2. Define and describe content analysis
3. List at least three uses of content analysis in nursing research
4. Identify at least four data collection techniques that might produce qualitative data
5. Identify and describe five units of content analysis
6. List desirable attributes of qualitative data analysis
7. Devise categories for content analysis in several ways and at several levels
8. Use single- and multiple-digit codes in analyzing qualitative data
9. Distinguish between two levels of content analysis and perform each
10. Use the correct conventions in reporting results from analysis of qualitative data

Qualitative data consist of information derived from communication or observation of behavior. Since nurses are expert at interviewing and observing others' behavior, it is not surprising that qualitative studies are gaining popularity in nursing research. Because qualitative research focuses on human perceptions, beliefs, attitudes, and experiences, the investigator must confront the subjects on a personal level. The information may take the form of a transcribed interview, a diary, an organization's minutes, nurses' notes, responses to open-ended questions in a questionnaire, or field notes recorded by an observer. Such data cannot be readily summarized or directly subjected to any quantitative analysis techniques. Sometimes these data provide descriptive or even theoretical materials that remain in narrative form. Qualitative data in ethnographic or phenomenological studies provide interesting and meaningful information without being quantified. For many purposes, however, the narrative materials must be reduced to create categories or classes that can be tabulated, summarized, and interpreted.

The quantification of qualitative data is called content analysis or data reduction. The five possible units of analysis are words, themes, characters, items, and space or time (Berelson, 1971). Word counts simply indicate the presence of particular words. For example, the number of times the word "budget" is used in a politician's speech can be counted as an indicator of his concern about fiscal policy. Themes are entire ideas or thoughts. "Allows expression of feelings" is an example of a theme concerning nurses' behavior. Characters refer to people; this unit is used most often in analysis of literary or journalistic material. Items are entire messages from the research subjects or a complete record of their behavior. Items are often used when the research purpose dictates that equal weight be given to each subject's data. Space and time refer to the amount of space given a topic in written materials and to the amount of time given to a topic in a speech, debate, or oral interaction. Because they have proved most useful for human research purposes, themes and items are the most commonly used units of analysis in nursing research.

The aim of content analysis is to organize a mass of information into meaningful classes, generally with some degree of quantification. Qualitative analysis is the most subjective, and in some ways the most demanding, of all approaches to data analysis. Analyzing qualitative data is like grading an essay question, whereas analyzing quantitative data is more like scoring answers to completion, multiple-choice, or true-false questions. Essay questions are easier to formulate than objective test items, but the answers to essay questions are harder to analyze and interpret.

The nursing literature contains an extensive dialogue about the relative merits of using qualitative data and quantitative data for specific research designs (Duffy, 1987; Knafl, Pettengill, Bevis, and Kirchoff, 1988; Smith, 1983; Swanson and Chenitz, 1982). The commentaries cited and others ultimately suggest that neither approach is superior. Rather, each technique is uniquely suited to particular research aims and problems, and they should be viewed as opposite ends of a continuum, as shown in Fig. 5-1. Qualitative and quantitative data often are gathered together as complementary parts of a study.

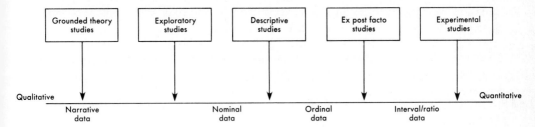

Fig. 5-1 Qualitative and quantitative data as a continuum.

PURPOSES OF QUALITATIVE DATA ANALYSIS

Qualitative data analysis has five broad purposes: instrument development, identification of relevant variables or hypotheses in a little-known field, description, hypothesis testing, and theory development. These categories are not always distinct in nursing research. A study that is primarily exploratory in design may also generate descriptive information. Another study might be designed to test hypotheses generated from a theoretical framework; such a study also serves theory development. On the other hand, the hypotheses to be tested may have been derived from a conceptual framework, and the purpose of the study may be to challenge or verify prior findings rather than to test a theory.

Instrument development

Data may be gathered to construct a single-item or a lengthy, multiple-item data collection instrument. To develop a data collection instrument from qualitative data, the investigator attempts to obtain information that will represent the concepts or constructs adequately and representatively. The qualitative data should represent the population of information in the same way that a sample represents a population of research subjects.

Identification of relevant variables and hypotheses

Sometimes an investigator wants to study a topic but can find little guidance from the literature to formulate research questions or hypotheses. In this situation the level of inquiry should probably be an exploratory study. The investigator identifies a population that can logically provide the information and asks the subjects open-ended questions about the phenomenon of interest. The identification of relevant variables by content analysis of the qualitative data can produce information about pertinent variables and possible relationships among them. These results can be used to move to a descriptive level of study or even to the formulation of hypotheses for testing.

The Delphi method is another form of data collection that produces qualitative data. The Delphi technique is a method for the systematic collection and analysis of judgments, beliefs, or ideas on a topic through a series of questionnaires interspersed with feedback of summarized group data (Delbecq, Van de Ven, and Gustafson, 1975). It was developed in management science to improve decision making by pooling information from individuals in widely separated locations. A purposive sample is selected, usually not more than 25 individuals, and these potential subjects are sent an explanation of the study and an invitation to participate. Two or three rounds of questions are submitted to participants with each round except the first based on information gleaned from prior responses.

Description

Descriptive studies may be based on quantitative data, qualitative data, or a combination of the two. A survey study may consist mainly of a questionnaire that yields readily coded answers such as never, sometimes, frequently, and always. The bulk of the data produced is ordinal (see p. 153) and can be analyzed with quantitative techniques. These quantitative data may be the only data in the study. However, the investigator may ask research subjects to answer an open-ended question or describe a critical incident to elaborate and illustrate the topic under study. In such a study the descriptive nature of the questionnaire items is complemented by examples from the respondents' experience in reply to the open-ended question or critical incident items. In other cases the entire dataset of a descriptive study is derived from open-ended questions either on a questionnaire or in an interview and qualitative data analysis is the sole technique used.

Hypothesis testing

Contrary to common notions, qualitative data analysis can be used to test hypotheses. Although the hypothesis testing may focus on explanations or predictions that evolve from theories, qualitative data analysis can be used to confirm or refute relationships among concepts or differences among groups. If some form of data reduction can be implemented to allow the investigator to compute relationships or compare groups, qualitative data can be analyzed to test hypotheses.

Theory development

Theory development from analysis of qualitative data may take two forms: testing existing theories and discovering theories from grounded theory analysis. The former consists of studying nursing phenomena in the context of a theory. The theory may be taken from another discipline such as psychology or sociology, or it may be from nursing. The discovery of theories from grounded theory analysis was developed by Glaser and Strauss (1967) and aims to discover theory by means of constant comparative analysis. The study starts with a question about the factors in a situation and the relationships among them. Only as data analysis proceeds are concepts formed and relationships identified. The ideas is to produce theory "grounded" by the data.

PROCEDURES AND PROBLEMS
Instrument development

The procedures for conducting qualitative data analysis to develop a data collection instrument are straightforward. The information may be used to construct statements about attitudes or beliefs, with the possible answers placed on a scale from strongly disagree to strongly agree. In construction of a multiple-choice item, the open-ended question is formulated carefully and the resulting data are reduced to a stem and foils, which are really just the categories derived from the data reduction. (A stem is a part of a sentence or a question. Foils are phrases that complete a sentence or answer a question.) For example, a nurse educator designed a follow-up study of graduates of the master's program and wished to include a question about reasons for choosing the graduate program. To furnish information for constructing a closed question, a sample of 12 current graduate students answered the question posed in Problem 5-1.

Problem 5-1

Developing an item from qualitative data

"Why did you choose to enroll in this graduate program?"

01 My husband is doing his residency here.
02 Because I heard such good things about the program from a friend who got her master's here 4 years ago.
03 Well, costs are reasonable, and I wanted to stay close to my parents who aren't well.
04 My fiance is a graduate student in Business. He has 2 more years and I think I can finish before we leave.
05 I'm interested in administration and can get the program I want.
06 I have friends already in the program—that's the main reason.
07 Two nurses that I graduated with convinced me that I should come here rather than stay in Chicago.
08 I want to teach, and the program description indicated that I would get good preparation for a faculty role here.
09 The ease of getting part-time employment influenced me.
10 My husband works here; we've lived here for 6 years. I couldn't consider any other programs really.
11 After graduating from the baccalaureate program here, I took a job in Texas, but came back here to work 2 years ago. I'm continuing to work while I take classes. I wish I had started the program earlier.
12 My mother, who is very ill, lives nearby; I see my parents often and help Dad a lot.

The 12 statements above constitute the dataset for developing the desired question. In deciding how to code these data, consider all five possible units of analysis: words, themes, characters, items, and space or time. The purpose of the analysis dictates that you look at ideas, since they require a phrase or sentence for expression. Words, characters, and space or time are logically inappropriate for this task. If you try to use items (that is, the entire response from each individual) as the unit of analysis, you cannot deal with subject 03's

Problem 5-1, cont'd

Developing an item from qualitative data

response accurately because this answer contains two different ideas. Coding one omits the other. Therefore themes are probably the most useful unit of analysis for this problem because all of the responses contain one or more themes.

Read the entire set of responses to get a feel for the data. Identify and separate the narrative materials into themes. Draw a bracket around each single idea in the responses and draw a line through irrelevant material. Number the themes. Reread the themes and try to develop categories. In this problem six categories have been identified for you. Place the number of each theme opposite the category in which it belongs:

Residence of spouse/fiance
Reasonable costs
Friends' influence
Family's influence
Desired field of study
Employment

How many responses contain more than one theme?

How many responses contain irrelevant material?

Did you have any trouble placing each theme in a category?

Is there more than one category that would fit any of the themes?

If you had trouble finding a place for any themes or deciding which spot was right in Problem 5-1, you need to revise the categories. There should be only one category for each theme. In research terms, the categories must be exhaustive and mutually exclusive, a cardinal rule of content analysis. In this example there is one problem area. "Residence of spouse/fiance" is somewhat redundant to "Friends' influence" and "Family's influence." To be mutually exclusive in its most precise sense, the *influence* categories need to exclude *residence* specifically, or the *residence* category should be eliminated and the themes in the *residence* class moved to the appropriate *influence* themes. However, collection of additional data might produce a response that refers to the residence of the subject rather than that of a spouse or significant other. With this in mind we should probably define *influence* as excluding *residence* and retain the *residence* category. Problems such as this point to the need to define and delimit categories. Each category must be defined precisely as to what it contains; it also must be delimited as to what it does *not* contain. If classification of qualitative data is to be as scientific and objective as possible, the criteria for including and excluding themes for the different categories must be clear. The aim is to define categories so carefully that another coder will reach the same conclusions as the original coder. Defining the categories carefully and completely contributes to the reliability and replicability of the data analysis.

In constructing a closed item, the nurse educator merely listed the categories in some logical order and added the final foil "Other (please specify) _____" in case not all possible responses were listed. The larger the sample, the more likely that all possible answers are identified.

The construction of an entire data collection instrument instead of just one item can also be an outcome of qualitative data analysis. In some cases, ideas or themes on a subject are derived from the literature, and a table of specifications may be constructed before information is obtained from a sample of appropriate subjects. In other cases the literature search may stand alone as the source of items. In developing an instrument to measure nurses' attitudes toward computing, Thomas (1988) constructed a table of specifications from a logical analysis of computer applications in nursing, validated by a literature search. The table of specifications reproduced in the table on p. 134 provided the framework for generating items that were then judged for validity by a panel of experts. Actual statements made by nurses and nursing students constituted the bulk of the items, although a number of items were constructed by the author and panel members, based on their own observations. Such a table of specifications may be used to obtain balance in the data collection tool; items should be constructed to reflect each cell in the table. For example, items that fall in cells A.2 and C.3 are as follows:

A.2 _____ Acronyms for computer terms like JCL and SPSS-X make computing very hard to understand.

C.3 _____ The most sensible use of computers in hospitals is for billing and staffing rather than more complex administrative tasks.

Write the letter and number from the cells in the table on p. 134 that are appropriate for each of the following statements.

_____ **Statistical programs can perform analyses that would require too much effort without computers.**

_____ **Most computer-assisted instruction programs are so difficult to use that they result in frustration rather than learning.**

_____ **I would like to use computers more to save time in my work.**

_____ **I'm afraid to depend on computer output where patient care is concerned.**

_____ **The use of computers dehumanizes nursing care.**

Attitudes toward computing in nursing: a table of specifications

		Applications			
Factors	A General	B Research	C Administration	D Practice	E Education
1 Effective/ineffective					
2 Comprehensible/incomprehensible					
3 Flexible/inflexible					
4 Dependable/undependable					
5 Affect/disaffect					
6 Appropriate/inappropriate					

Identification of relevant variables or hypotheses

The use of qualitative analysis in exploratory studies has been relatively common. In such studies too little is known about the field of inquiry to formulate precise research questions or hypotheses. Exploratory studies are needed to clarify issues, identify relevant variables, and formulate research questions or hypotheses. The research purpose for such a study is usually stated as a declarative sentence: "The purpose of this study is to identify . . . " or " . . . to explore . . . ."

In a retrospective, hospital-based study, Janken, Reynolds, and Swiech (1986) used existing records to identify variables associated with patient falls in an acute care setting. They noted the general belief that nurses could assess patients on admission to a hospital to identify how likely they were to fall but determined that age was the only characteristic that had been associated convincingly with patient falls. Overrepresentation of elderly people in the fall category had been documented (Swartzbeck and Milligan, 1982; Walshe and Rosen, 1979), but other factors such as confusion, sensory deficits, and selected medications had been identified as risk factors without being studied adequately (Janken, Reynolds, and Swiech, 1986). These investigators studied the charts of 331 patients 60 years of age and older who fell and of 300 who did not fall, tabulating characteristics recorded at admission for all patients in the study. For the patients who fell they also recorded factors noted in the charts during the 24 hours preceding the fall. For the nonfall group's second chart audit they recorded information for a random 24-hour period during each subject's hospital stay. The analyses of these data by cross-tabulation and computation of chi squares revealed 10 admission day variables and 11 fall/random day variables that distinguished the fall group from the nonfall group. Seven of the variables—general weakness, decreased mobility of the lower extremities, sleeplessness, incontinence, confusion, depression, and substance abuse—appeared on both lists (Janken, Reynolds, and Swiech, 1986). Although the investigators noted the limitation that considerable variance remained unexplained, this study is a good example of an exploratory study that identifies variables and produces useful information for nursing practice.

Problems 5-1 and 5-2 illustrate the type of data to which content analysis can be applied at the manifest level or the latent level. The manifest level of analysis focuses on the actual meaning of the narrative materials. In it, there is no attempt to judge attitudes, motives, or any underlying meanings and currents the data may contain; the analysis goes no further than the surface meaning of the statements. By contrast the latent level of content analysis looks for selected underlying meaning. In such a study the researcher attempts to make inferences from the data about the attitudes, feelings, or motives of the participants. Analysis at the latent level involves much more subjectivity on the part of the investigator and is generally less reliable than analysis at the manifest level (Fox, 1982).

Identification of variables and description

Problem 5-2 presents a dataset that was generated in answer to the request, "Please describe problems experienced with the monthly, mandatory drug re-

view in your long-term care facility." The brief dataset that follows was extracted
from a large number of responses to a questionnaire study about the mandatory
monthly drug review in Iowa's long-term care facilities (Thomas and Price, 1987).

Problem 5-2

Identifying variables from qualitative data

"Please describe problems experienced with the monthly mandatory drug
review in your long-term care facility."
01 Dr. negative about being told what he can or can't do. For example,
   maximum dose of Xanax is 2 mg/24 hours . . . his resident gets 3 mg and is
   doing fine.
02 Time and follow-up.
03 Time consuming . . . isn't always an effective review.
04 Nurses were not signing properly, and this was corrected.
05 I think the drug review has been very beneficial in reducing the number of
   medications being given to residents.
06 Physicians don't respond to the recommendations and get angry if we
   phone them after sending the report.
07 Time.
08 Traffic jam at charts when review is under way.
09 Physicians do not keep up with medications and side effects when ordering
   meds. There is not always a diagnosis for the medication ordered.
10 The regulations state that the review will be done by an RN in an ICF. I
   strongly disagree . . . our pharmacist does them and is trained in this area.
11 The form is cumbersome . . . could be more compact and flexible.
12 Sometimes it's difficult to present a problem to a physician without getting
   his ego involved. It's difficult also to know if we're doing an adequate job
   because it's never assessed by an outsider.
13 None.
14 Nurses monitoring their own work . . . following up on
   antibiotics . . . giving required doses . . . accurate time and stop
   dates . . . gaps in vitals charting.
15 Doctors like to keep orders PRN and not be told to make it a different
   order.
16 We now have three pharmacies supplying drugs. This makes it more
   difficult for the pharmacist consultant.
17 Cost of hiring the pharmacist to do the review—our pharmacist was overly
   rigorous in doing the review and subsequent pharmacist too casual in his
   approach. Lack of time for Director of Nursing to do comprehensive review
   prompted us to seek pharmacist to do review.
18 Only one of our doctors pays any attention to the recommendations. The
   others make monthly visits to their patients and feel that this is all that's
   needed. Also feel that they do not have any patients on large enough
   dosages to warrant blood work.
19 It is very time consuming, and I feel that every 3 months would be
   adequate.

Identifying variables from qualitative data

20 Very time consuming, and it creates a terrific jam at the nurses' station.
21 Physicians in this area like PRNs. Difficult removing the prescription when the acute condition subsides.
22 Some difficulty with the pharmacy to keep the med sheets updated.
23 Really we don't have many problems except for some physicians who order 20 to 30 drugs for one patient and will not discontinue any.
24 Not sure what is required.
25 Whether to consider more than six meds an irregularity when doctor considers all drugs necessary.

Read through the dataset and bracket the themes, deleting extraneous material as before. Instead of numbering the themes, use the double-digit codes for the categories listed in the table on p. 139, assigning a two-digit code to each theme. Let's use the first statement as an example:

11

[Dr. negative about being told what he can or can't do.] [For example, maxi-

13

mum dose of Xanax is 2 mg/24 hours . . . his resident gets 3 mg and is doing fine.]

In a large dataset, notes summarizing the data are made in the margins of the transcriptions as the analysis proceeds. In this problem you merely need to count the themes in each category and fill in the n column in the table on p. 139. You recall that n is simply the frequency associated with each response. Next, compute a percentage of the total for each n; that is, divide each n by the total and multiply the quotient by 100. Which main category contains the highest percentage of themes?

Is your analysis at the manifest or latent level?

Problem 5-2, cont'd

CONTENT ANALYSIS REPORT

Write a report of the information you have derived from the content analysis. Each "level one" theme can constitute a paragraph starting with the one containing the most responses.

A frequency distribution of themes in two levels

Level One	Level Two	n	%
1. Physician	1. Resents the drug review regulations		
	2. Disagrees with regulations		
	3. Ignores recommendations		
	4. Reminders or prodding causes anger		
	5. Lacks up-to-date information on drugs and side effects		
	6. Orders drugs without recording a diagnosis/orders excessive drugs		
	7. Defensive (ego-involved) about recommendations		
	8. Likes PRNs		
	9. Fails to order needed laboratory work		
2. Nurse	1. Failure to sign reports properly		
	2. Problems monitoring own work		
	3. Gaps in charting vital data		
3. Pharmacist	1. Too rigorous		
	2. Too casual		
	3. Failure to keep med sheets up to date		
4. Time/cost	1. Review: time consuming		
	2. Follow-up: time consuming		
	3. Lack of time limits effectiveness		
	4. No time for DON to do it		
	5. Cost of hiring pharmacist to do it		
5. Medications	1. Antibiotics problematic . . . not always given at right dosage, time or duration		
	2. Rx not removed when condition subsides		
6. Procedures	1. Traffic jam at charts/nurses' station		
	2. Adequacy never assessed by an outsider		
	3. Obtaining drugs from three pharmacies increases difficulties		
7. Regulations	1. Review by nurse when pharmacist is more qualified		
	2. Cumbersome form		
	3. Every month too frequent . . . three months often enough		
	4. Requirements not clear		

Problem 5-2, cont'd

Identifying variables from qualitative data

Another investigator might disagree with the categorization scheme displayed in the table. For example, the theme "Medications" might be eliminated because theme 5.1 might be assigned to the nurses' category and 5.2 to the physicians' category. Before qualitative data are analyzed, the categories should be defined and delimited so that two coders would reach the same decision about placement of themes. For purposes of this problem, use the themes as they are listed.

You could also analyze these data to examine the attitudes of the directors of nursing about physicians' responsiveness (or nonresponsiveness) to the mandated drug review. In such an analysis, you would be studying underlying meanings from the nurses' statements.

Is this an example of content analysis at the manifest or latent level?

A third coding level could be added to the table to allow for this analysis. Such a coding scheme will produce a three-digit code for each theme. A third code can be added to each coded theme. However, it is apparent that only nine categories refer to physicians. In such a situation the investigator has two options: to use themes as before and include a special code for "not applicable" as well as "neutral" or to use items for this analysis instead of themes. Try using the entire response of each participant (items as the unit of analysis) to rate them according to the following scale:

1 = Very unfavorable
2 = Somewhat unfavorable
3 = Neutral, ambiguous, or not applicable
4 = Somewhat favorable
5 = Very favorable

Your set of 25 numerical ratings should be placed in the left margin of the problems list on p. 136. These ratings can be described and summarized in several ways. For example, a mode can be reported, or a frequency distribution by ratings can be constructed, including both numbers and percentages. Compute some quantitative results and write a paragraph or two to describe the participation of physicians in the mandated monthly drug review, incorporating the quantitative results along with the qualitative findings.

Hypothesis testing

Use of the Delphi technique is usually a kind of exploratory study, although descriptive information is always produced and hypotheses are sometimes

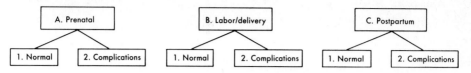

Fig. 5-2 Coding scheme for Delphi study.

tested. Several nursing investigators have used this method to identify research priorities. Lindeman (1975) used a huge sample (by Delphi standards—investigators usually deal with no more than 25 subjects in Delphi studies) of 433 participants to identify the most acute clinical research needs as perceived by nurses in Veterans Administration hospitals. The research needs were compared among groups of panelists and by focus. Four rounds of questionnaires were used.

Thomas (1984) used the Delphi technique to identify and examine ideas for research on childbirth formulated by two samples, one a group of Lamaze instructors and the other a group of maternity nurses. Fig. 5-2 depicts the categories that emerged. The second and third rounds of this study asked participants to set priorities among the research ideas and to rank their importance.

An uncertainty coefficient (a statistic for comparing ratings produced by two groups of research subjects) was computed to test the hypothesis (which was supported) that the priorities of childbirth educators would differ significantly from those identified by maternity nurses.

Problem 5-3

Identifying research ideas from Delphi data

A small portion of Thomas's data (1984) is reproduced below. Using the categories depicted in Fig. 5-2, bracket themes and place them in appropriate categories by writing the proper code above each item. For example:

A.1

01   [What techniques in childbirth education are perceived to be most effective by the mothers? Least effective by the mothers?]

In this example, since most effective and least effective are extremes of one concept, the entire response is categorized as a single theme.

01   What techniques in childbirth education are perceived to be most effective by the mothers? Least effective by mothers?

02   How extensive are elective inductions? What are the reasons for them?

03   What are the advantages and disadvantages of ambulation during labor?

04   What factors affect mothers' and fathers' responses to emergency cesarean births?

Problem 5-3, cont'd

Identifying research ideas from Delphi data

05   What stresses do new parents experience as a consequence of lack of extended families?

06   Is a realistic picture of childbirth given in childbirth education classes?

07   What is the impact of observers (for example, students) in the delivery room? Is it best for the family?

08   What are the effects of the setting on bonding, for example, hospital delivery room? Birthing room? Home delivery? On the parents' feelings about the childbirth experience?

09   What are the advantages and disadvantages of fetal monitoring?

10   How are plans to breast-feed affected by an emergency cesarean birth? To what extent is the mother given support to do so?

11   Is there a relationship between incidence of vaginal and uterine prolapse in later years and whether episiotomies were performed at delivery?

12   What factors does a mother consider when deciding between general and spinal anesthesia for a cesarean birth?

13   Does childbirth education affect the incidence of postpartum depression among new mothers?

14   How can collaboration between physicians and other professionals be improved for the benefit of families?

15   Are there differences in childbirth preparation related to whether the childbirth educator is a nurse?

16   How do fathers feel about attending a cesarean birth when it is scheduled? When it is not scheduled?

17   How helpful or effective would it be for the labor nurse to help new mothers reconstruct their labor and delivery experiences?

18   What effects does childbirth education have on parenting?

How many themes are there?
Which themes caused you the most problems? Why?

Summarize these data.
Are all of these questions stated in researchable terms? If not, which ones
aren't?

A useful basic reference on the Delphi technique is the book by Delbeqc,
Van de Ven, and Gustafson (1975). It contains a complete description of the
process and provides instructions and special tips for making a Delphi study a
success. The following steps in the process were adapted from the book:

1. Formulate the questions and plans for two or three follow-up sets of
   feedback and further questions.
2. Conduct a pilot test of the questions using participants who are like the
   planned Delphi group.
3. Decide who the respondent group will be, how large it will be, and
   whether participants will be anonymous.
4. Perform the sampling or selection process to identify Delphi participants.
5. Obtain commitments to participate from the respondent group.
6. Formulate decision rules for handling the data at each stage of the Delphi
   study.
7. Before proceeding, decide whether the three critical conditions for a successful Delphi study are present:
   a. Adequate time
   b. Participant skill in written communication
   c. High participant motivation

The five purposes of qualitative data analysis overlap. For example, identification of variables necessarily describes phenomena and identifies relevant
factors in the situation, as discussed previously. Moreover, there are qualitative
studies or portions of studies whose main purpose is description, that is, pro-
vision of illustrative information about findings that are primarily quantitative.

In the report about the mandated drug review in long-term care facilities,
Thomas and Price (1987) used critical incidents to elicit information that illustrates
both positive and negative outcomes of the drug review. The main focus of the
study was on problems in completing the drug reviews, but the investigators
also wanted information about both positive and negative outcomes of the drug
review. These data added a balance and richness to the problems identified by
respondents and to the quantitative results of the study and made the findings
more useful and interesting to readers, as the following excerpts show:

1. A patient on diuretics was being given salt tablets.
2. A patient was on six regular medications and five PRNs.

3. A patient's digoxin level was way over the toxic level, but the order remained unchanged.
4. A patient on naproxen died of a hemorrhage after the physician refused to discontinue the drug in spite of bleeding problems.*

Some authors think only of quantitative data analysis when testing hypotheses. Many investigators use qualitative data analysis for hypothesis testing and achieve interesting results. Problem 5-3 illustrates the use of qualitative data analysis for hypothesis testing.

Theory development

Existing theory. Browner (1987) used qualitative data analysis to test stress-coping theories. The hypothesis was that staff members who reported having more supportive, work-based social networks would also report better health than those with less supportive social networks. The hypothesis was developed from a conceptual framework consisting of a body of work revealing social support as a mediator between work stress and its deleterious effects on health. Participant observation and semistructured interviews produced the qualitative data gathered from 21 mental health staff members. The observational data were used to characterize behavior in the work setting such as activities associated with patients' waking up, grooming, and eating, verbal interactions, help-seeking behavior, and the nature of conflicts and their modes of resolution. Through interviews, information was gathered about sources of perceived stress and satisfaction at work and about five types of social support (information, material, appraisal, emotional, and normative). These data were coded and analyzed to rank the social support and cohesiveness of the four units of staff members. The coding gave each unit a numerical value representing its relative degree of social support and cohesiveness. The quantification of these data allowed the investigator to compute correlation coefficients. The variable "health" was measured by staff's responses to the Cornell Medical Index Subscale scores. The investigator's hypothesis that staff with stronger social networks would report better health than staff with weaker social networks was supported. In addition, the study produced useful descriptive data about work-related stresses and sources of satisfaction that were reported by the research subjects.

The Browner study (1987) of stress, social networks, and health is an example of testing a hypothesis to support both a conceptual framework and an existing theory. Fig. 5-3 illustrates the theoretical relationships of stressors, mediating variables, and health that have emerged from the vast body of work stimulated by Selye's initial description of the fight or flight syndrome (Selye, 1948).

Lazarus's theory of cognitive appraisal focuses on the type of stressor encountered, its perceived threat, and secondary appraisal of the threat as determining the individual's coping responses (Lazarus, 1966). Many studies have supported this theory. In extending the theory, Antonovsky (1979) studied sur-

---

*From Thomas B and Price M (1987). The effectiveness of monthly drug reviews in Iowa's long-term care facilities. *Journal of Gerontological Nursing* 13:17-21.

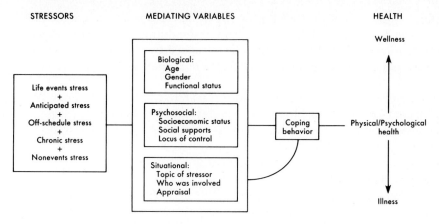

STRESSORS   MEDIATING VARIABLES   HEALTH

Wellness

Life events stress
+
Anticipated stress
+
Off-schedule stress
+
Chronic stress
+
Nonevents stress

Biological:
Age
Gender
Functional status

Psychosocial:
Socioeconomic status
Social supports
Locus of control

Situational:
Topic of stressor
Who was involved
Appraisal

Coping
behavior

Physical/Psychological
health

Illness

Fig. 5-3 Stressors, mediating variables, and health.

vivors of the Nazi holocaust in World War II and identified a human characteristic he called "hardiness." He asserted that hardiness enabled some people to withstand stress without harsh effects on their health, whereas others, without this characteristic, became ill or disabled.

Nurses have also conducted research to test these theoretical relationships. Hardiness and other phenomena were studied in samples of nurses who worked in intensive care units and those who worked in other units (Keane, Ducette, and Adler, 1985). Burnout, hardiness, control, and challenge were measured with quantitative instruments to test the theory represented in Fig. 5-3. In this same study qualitative data were gathered to test Wiener's theory of attribution (Wiener, 1979, 1983). Wiener asserted that a person's perception of being in control or lacking control determines how that person copes with stressors. Open-ended questions were used to assess how the nurses felt about their work. Answers were subjected to content analysis to determine the degree of controllability indicated by the response.

Is this the manifest or latent level of analysis? Why?

The responses were scored as entire items, with a 3 assigned to controllable factors, a 2 assigned to intermediate factors, and a 1 assigned to uncontrollable factors. The nurses attributed both success (72%) and failure (64%) to controllable factors. There was no relationship between the success scores and burnout, but there was a significant relationship for failure: "nurses who were experiencing more burnout believed that failures were caused by events they could not control" (Keane, Ducette, and Adler, 1985, p. 235), which lends support to Wiener's attribution theory.

Grounded theory. Grounded theory research, the process of analyzing qualitative data for theory development, was developed by Glaser and Strauss (1967). This technique uses terminology new to most students of nursing research, as well as most investigators trained in quantitative research methods. Having a mentor or adviser who is experienced in grounded theory is important when learning this process.

Before beginning data collection, the investigator makes a conscious effort to eliminate his or her preconceived beliefs about the phenomena under study. This is called bracketing. The aim is to let the data dictate identification of concepts, linkages, and ultimately grounded theory.

The methodology of analyzing narrative data is called constant comparative analysis, meaning that each piece of data is constantly compared with every other piece of relevant data. Data produced by interviewing or observation may be summarized by the investigator from notes or from verbatim transcriptions. The investigator attempts to identify the most pertinent concepts and assigns codes to each one. The codes assigned to these qualitative data are generally gerunds—action words ending with "ing" such as evading, supporting, obstructing, or assisting. As data are coded, the investigator's ideas about the importance of certain variables or about possible relationships among them are recorded in a process called memoing. The basis for the coding scheme is constantly reviewed. Other ways of coding may emerge as more useful than the original scheme.

Once concepts have been identified and related, the investigator searches the literature for information about the phenomena under study. This sequence is in contrast to most other approaches to research, in which the literature review precedes formulation of the research problem. As the process continues, certain concepts take on more importance. These concepts are called core variables.

As the core variables appear, higher-order codes may be assigned and the discovery of relationships may produce either confusion or, if logical, preliminary hypotheses or a preliminary theory. The process is one of inductive reasoning. If the reasons for a relationship are not apparent, additional data or further study of the literature may clarify the situation. In some cases a third variable, not originally identified, is involved and must be discovered to clarify the linkage.

The theory must be tested by attempting to explain or predict relevant relationships based on still more data. Sometimes additional data dictate that a theory be modified or even discarded. The aim is to integrate the study findings with information in the literature so that a theoretical framework emerges. Another strategy in addition to memoing is diagramming. Diagramming is visually representing discovered relationships. The diagram portrays core variables and the relationships among them as shown in Fig. 5-3. Such a diagram is included in the description of Chenitz's work (1983) that follows.

The theoretical framework is self-correcting; that is, the framework is generated from and grounded in the data gathered up to any point in the study process. Adjustments are made to accommodate new information from additional data and from comparisons made with the literature. Theoretical codes are identified and used to define concepts precisely so that theory grounded in the data can be developed.

Chenitz (1978) studied the experience of nursing home admission from the perspectives of both the staff and the patients. Synopses of this study were published in 1983 and 1986. She gathered data by interviewing and observing 30 mentally alert older adults. She also interviewed staff members and consulted physicians and the patients' medical records.

The field notes produced theoretical memos, which Chenitz placed in categories. Eventually the memos were linked to produce grounded theory regarding the individuals' moves into nursing homes: the nature of their responses to admission, conditions predictive of negative responses, consequences of negative responses, and nursing interventions (both successful and unsuccessful) for dealing with negative responses. Elderly persons' responses to admission were viewed on a continuum from acceptance to resistance; this construct is portrayed as the dependent variable in Fig. 5-4.

Importance was defined as the centrality of the admission in the elders' struggles for autonomy, that is, how much the admission would limit their choices. Legitimation was defined as understanding an acceptable reason for the admission and came from physicians, nurses or social workers, family, friends, or the older adults themselves. Desirability refers to elderly persons' perceptions of nursing homes as desirable or undesirable. Voluntary nature is

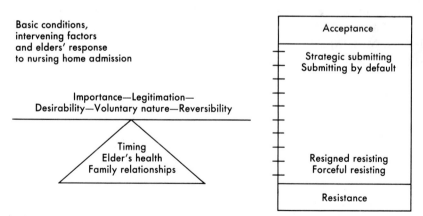

To varying degrees, elders accept nursing home admission if they believe it is necessary, legitimate, desirable, the result of their own decision, and for a short time. Elders who see admission as undesirable, involuntary, and permanent usually resist.

Fig. 5-4 Chenitz's theoretical diagram.

From Chenitz W (1983). Entry into a nursing home as status passage: a theory to guide nursing practice. *Geriatric Nursing* 4:95. Copyright 1983, American Journal of Nursing Company. Reprinted with permission from *Geriatric Nursing.*

self-explanatory. Reversibility refers to whether the elders saw themselves as in a nursing home until death or only for a short stay. Time, the elder's health, and family relationships are shown in Fig. 5-4 as intervening variables. All of these variables have potential effects on the basic conditions listed above.

One possible outcome, strategic submitting, represented acceptance from two stances: either the older adult regarded the stay as temporary and tolerated conditions at the nursing home, or the stay was necessitated by recognizably deteriorating health status and the elder's attempts to maintain aspects of former life-style were at least somewhat successful. Another outcome, submitting by default, was primarily associated with preoccupation: the elder had suffered a loss, usually of a spouse, that precluded consideration of the move to the nursing home, or the person was otherwise preoccupied with pain or worry.

The data showed that acceptance was associated with satisfaction of more than one of the basic conditions and that the most important of these conditions were reversibility and voluntary nature.

Two forms of resistance emerged from the data, as shown in Fig. 5-4. Resigned resisting emerged from states such as expressions of distress and sadness to states reflecting utter hopelessness and waiting to die. Forceful resisting was even more serious; the elders so categorized were refusing to carry on activities such as bathing or eating and were indulging in antisocial behaviors such as hitting, throwing food, or verbal abuse. Chenitz described the consequences of resistance on staff, family, and the older adult and devised a practice theory to guide nurses and family members. The resister was viewed as being in crisis, and nursing interventions designed to resolve the crisis were described. As Chenitz wrote, "The test of the theory is whether it will assist nurses to frame their practice with elders entering nursing homes and assist educators who teach nurses about long-term care" (1986, p. 225). As with any theory, its usefulness rests on its ability to guide, explain, and predict.

This brief description of Chenitz's work attempts to portray the interesting processes employed in grounded theory research. Such studies require imagination, careful work, and strong analytical skills. The dataset may consist of 500 or more pages of narrative. Yet theory development studies often focus on datasets of that size. Some are much larger. The student might ask, how much data are enough? The usual response is that data collection continues until the data are saturated. This means that data collection starts to produce redundant data; nothing new is being generated. These factors preclude the inclusion in this book of an illustrative problem for grounded theory analysis.

USING COMPUTERS

Using computers is a basic component of quantitative research but is somewhat less common in qualitative research. Yet computers can save considerable time and effort. This section briefly describes how one software package for microcomputers can take the tedium out of qualitative research.

ZyIndex, a powerful database system developed by the ZyLab Corporation, is designed to process narrative materials, such as correspondence, bibliographies, or datasets, for qualitative data analysis. Let's assume that we have an extensive collection of transcribed interview data. We have read the entire dataset and have developed a preliminary set of theoretical codes. As we begin work on the data, we simply create text files using any word-processing program that can produce American Standard Code for Information Interchange (ASCII) files. These are files ZyIndex can read. From the ASCII file, ZyIndex's Index Program creates an Index List that stores information about the file in which each word appears, as well as each word's location relative to all other words in the file. The file corresponds to a category of the theoretical codes. Files can be indexed as the investigator chooses, at a single level or at several levels.

The other component of ZyIndex, the Search Program, gives the investigator the ability to search the files for all instances of a single theoretical code or for any word, combination of words, or characters. Combinations of letters and numbers can be used to devise multilevel codes, and the files can be searched rapidly for the narrative materials entered with the specified codes. For example, stressors experienced by a particular population are being studied by interviews of a random sample of the population. Each stressor identified by research subjects is coded in three ways: (1) what is it about? (for example, crisis, chronic stress, everyday hassle), (2) who is involved? (family, friends, business colleagues, acquaintances, strangers), and (3) how much control does the subject feel over the stressor? (great, some, little, none). Each category of each level is

Table 5-1 Summary of operators for ZyIndex search requests

Operator	General use	Example
?	Single-character wild card*	wom?n retrieves woman, women
*	Multicharacter wild card[a]	auto* retrieves automobile, automatic, autos, etc.
OR	Enlarges search	Geriatric OR gerontology retrieves files containing either word
AND	Narrows search	Radiation AND cancer retrieves only files containing both words
AND NOT	Narrows search	Cardiac AND NOT monitor retrieves files that contain cardiac but do not mention monitor
( )	Combines operators	(baby OR infant) AND nutrition retrieves any file that contains baby or infant and also contains nutrition
W/n	Helps define abstract concepts	(client OR patient) W/10 (compliance OR concordance) retrieves files that contain one of the first words within 10 spaces of one of the second words
OR NOT	Enlarges search	Adult *or not* (infant *or* baby) retrieves any file containing adult and also files that do not contain infant or baby

[a] A question mark represents any letter.

assigned a number or letter. One category might be everyday hassles with business colleagues in which the subject perceives little or no control over the stressor. If this category were labeled E32, a search request specifying this code would be entered. A few seconds later all files with this code would be displayed on the computer screen. The investigator can print out the files or any part of them in any order. If more useful codes develop as the investigation proceeds, the files can be modified. All files containing a word or phrase can be brought to the screen. Again, all or parts of the files can be marked and printed out, facilitating the construction of new theoretical codes. Changes can be made in a part of the collection of files or in the entire dataset.

ZyIndex search requests can be expanded or narrowed by means of the operators displayed in Table 5-1.

The package can handle large datasets and allows investigators to find specific files or information quickly. All database software packages have potential for managing a collection of qualitative data, but the capabilities of each must be assessed, since their power and size vary substantially. Any word-processing software that has a "find" command can be used for storage and retrieval of qualitative data. Using a microcomputer package such as ZyIndex takes much of the drudgery out of qualitative data analysis.

REFERENCES

Antonovsky A (1979). *Health, stress and coping.* San Francisco: Jossey-Bass Inc, Publishers.

Berelson B (1971). *Content analysis in communication research.* New York: Free Press.

Browner CH (1987). Job stress and health: the role of social support at work. *Research in Nursing and Health* 10:93-100.

Chenitz W (1978). *Acceptance of the standards of geriatric nursing practice and perceptions of satisfaction and stress in practice by geriatric nurses.* Unpublished doctoral dissertation. New York: Teachers College, Columbia University.

Chenitz W (1983). Entry into a nursing home as status passage: a theory to guide nursing practice. *Geriatric Nursing* 4:92-97.

Chenitz W (1986). Entry into a nursing home as status passage: a theory to guide nursing practice. In Chenitz W and Swanson J (eds). *From practice to grounded theory.* Menlo Park, Calif: Addison-Wesley Publishing Co, Inc.

Delbeqc A, Van de Ven A, and Gustafson D (1975). *Group techniques for program planning.* Middleton, Wis: Green Briar Press.

Duffy M (1987). Quantitative and qualitative research: antagonistic or complementary? *Nursing and Health Care* 8:356-357.

Fox D (1982). *Fundamentals of research in nursing.* 4th ed. Norwalk, Conn: Appleton & Lange, pp 391-412.

Glaser BG and Strauss AL (1967). *The discovery of grounded theories: strategies for qualitative research.* Chicago: Aldine Publishing Co.

Janken J, Reynolds B, and Swiech K (1986). Patient falls in the acute care setting: identifying risk factors. *Nursing Research* 35:215-219.

Keane A, Ducette J, and Adler D (1985). Stress in ICU and non-ICU nurses. *Nursing Research* 34:231-236.

Knafl K, Pettengill M, Bevis M, and Kirchoff K (1988). Blending qualitative and quantitative approaches to instrument development and data collection. *Journal of Professional Nursing* 4:30-37.

Lazarus R (1966). *Psychological stress and the coping process.* New York: McGraw-Hill Inc.

Lindeman CA (1975). Delphi survey of priorities in clinical nursing research. *Nursing Research* 24:434-441.

Selye H (1948). *The stress of life.* New York: McGraw-Hill Inc.

Smith JK (1983). Quantitative versus qualitative research: an attempt to clarify the issue. *Educational Researcher* 12:6-13.

Swanson J and Chenitz W (1982). Why qualitative research in nursing? *Nursing Outlook* 30:241-245.

Swartzbeck EM and Milligan WL (1982). A comparative study of hospital incidents. *Nursing Management* 13:39-43.

Thomas B (1984). Identifying priorities: research on childbirth. *Journal of Obstetric, Gynecological and Neonatal Nursing* 13:400-408.

Thomas B (1988). Development of an instrument to assess attitudes toward computing in nursing. *Computers in Nursing* 6:122-127.

Thomas B and Price M (1987). The effectiveness of monthly drug reviews in Iowa's long-term care facilities. *Journal of Gerontological Nursing* 13:17-21.

Walshe A and Rosen H (1979). A study of patient falls from bed. *Journal of Nursing Administration* 18:31-35.

Wiener B (1979). A theory for motivation for some classroom experiences. *Journal of Educational Psychology* 71:3-25.

Wiener B (1983). Some methodological pitfalls in attribution research. *Journal of Educational Psychology* 75:530-543.

REFERENCES FOR FURTHER STUDY

Chenitz WC and Swanson J, eds (1985). *Qualitative research in nursing: from practice to grounded theory.* Menlo Park, Calif: Addison-Wesley Publishing Co Inc.

Fagerhaugh S (1973). Getting around with emphysema. *American Journal of Nursing* 73:94-99.

Glaser BG and Strauss AL (1966). The purpose and credibility of qualitative research. *Nursing Research* 15:56-61.

Glaser BG and Strauss AL (1968). *Time for dying.* Chicago: Aldine Publishing Co.

Goodwin LD and Goodwin WL (1984). Qualitative vs. quantitative or qualitative and quantitative research? *Nursing Research* 33:378-380.

Leininger M, ed (1985). *Qualitative research methods in nursing.* Orlando, Fla: Grune & Stratton Inc.

McCall G and Simmons JL, eds (1969). *Issues in participant observation: a text and a reader,* Reading, Mass: Addison-Wesley Publishing Co Inc.

Miles M and Huberman A (1984). *Qualitative data analysis: a sourcebook of new methods.* Beverly Hills, Calif: Sage Publications.

Oiler C (1982). The phenomenological approach in nursing research. *Nursing Research* 31:178-181.

Parse R, Coyne B, and Smith M (1985). *Nursing research: qualitative methods.* Bowie, Md: Brady Communications Co.

Quint JC (1966). Awareness of death and the nurse's composure. *Nursing Research* 15:49-55.

Sims LN (1981). The grounded theory approach in nursing research. *Nursing Research* 30:357-359.

Stern P (1980). Grounded theory methodology: its uses and processes. *Image* 12:20-23.

Wilson HS (1977). Limiting intrusion—social control of outsiders in a healing community: an illustration of qualitative comparative analysis. *Nursing Research* 26:103-111.

ZyIndex (1983). Chicago: ZyLab Corp.

CHAPTER 6

Analyzing quantitative data to describe phenomena

Objectives

After completing this unit of study, students will be able to:

1. Identify the aims of descriptive statistical analyses

2. Identify and describe commonly used descriptive statistics such as the frequency distribution, mean, standard deviation, mode, range, and median

3. Describe the concepts skewness, kurtosis, and normal curve

4. Compute commonly used descriptive statistics, given a dataset

5. Describe the preliminary and primary roles of computers in data analysis

6. Complete problems in descriptive data analysis such as describing samples and reporting questionnaire findings

7. Use computers efficiently in calculating descriptive statistics

8. Interpret computer output regarding descriptive statistics

9. Construct tables and graphs to report findings of descriptive data analysis

10. Discuss the results of data analysis in terms of specific research purposes

ESSENTIAL STATISTICAL CONCEPTS
Aims of statistical analysis

Statistics is the science of compiling facts or data of potentially numerical nature to reveal important information about phenomena. It is a science that allows us to reduce large masses of data into more manageable and interpretable forms. Statistics is the source of much that we know about health, illness, caregivers, and patients. It is a tool used by investigators to make sense out of the phenomena they study.

The choice of test statistic depends in part on the level of data involved. Interval and ratio data are the highest levels of measurement; they represent scores or values that have equal intervals between the score or value points. Ordinal data are variables that can be ranked from lower to higher, but the intervals between values are not equal. Nominal data consist of different categories (such as religions) that cannot be ranked in any way.

Statistics is used for many purposes. This chapter focuses on the use of statistics to describe phenomena. Statistical description is employed (1) to generalize from sample statistics to population parameters (this can properly be termed inferential statistics as well as descriptive statistics), (2) to clarify comparisons in a set of data, and (3) to summarize data from surveys and case studies. Additional uses of statistics in examining relationships and comparing groups are addressed in Chapters 7 and 8.

Statistics can be used to describe survey data from a sample that will be generalized to a study population. For example, a team of investigators might collect data in a large community by means of a telephone survey. A survey is a study of a relatively large number of subjects about specific variables, events, or situations. Careful sampling techniques are employed so that survey results can be generalized to the study population, the community. This is one aim of statistical analysis: making inferences about a study population based on data gathered from a sample. Descriptive information about the sample is assumed to apply to the study population. For example, a survey might deal with parents' perceptions of priorities in the role of the school nurse in the community's elementary schools. If less than 30% of the survey respondents perceives the primary role of the school nurse to include health promotion activities, the investigator could state that these results reflect community perceptions. The accuracy of this inference depends on the sample size and representativeness, the error involved in data gathering, and possible biases introduced by the interviewers. This survey could be extended to compare the attitudes of parents of elementary school children with those of school nurses. The investigators could gather parallel information from the nurses and compare the data with information gleaned from the parents' interviews. In our hypothetical survey the results might be startling—it would not be surprising if more than 90% of the school nurses perceived their primary roles to include health promotion.

Descriptive statistics can also be used to summarize data from case studies. Nursing literature still contains many examples of case studies that were conducted for descriptive purposes, although they are less common than they once were. These are intensive studies of a relatively small number of subjects about specific variables or situations. In many instances the results of case studies are reported in narrative terms with no attempt to quantify findings. In other cases behavior over time is sampled in quantitative terms and the reports of such studies display data in tables similar to those used in surveys.

Frequency distributions

A frequency distribution is a way of summarizing data to make it more meaningful. The researcher summarizes data by arranging values in order of increasing or decreasing size and tabulating the frequencies and perhaps additional information such as percentages to display data in an organized fashion. How detailed the summaries are depends on the research purposes of the survey.

A community survey might focus on the prevalence of selected illnesses. The team of investigators interviews a random sample of adults. At the conclusion of the study each member of the team produces many pages of notes representing the information gathered in the interviews. As raw data the survey results are too voluminous and disorganized to be meaningful. No one can read the pages of research notes and reach valid conclusions about the prevalence of various kinds of illnesses or the incidence of certain illnesses among special groups such as adolescents or the elderly. Statistics permits the team to summarize the data, making the information easier to understand.

If a summary of only the overall incidence of illness in the community is desired, the investigators merely need to construct a list of illnesses and tabulate the occurrence of each from the data. For example, they could devise a mutually exclusive and comprehensive list of illness categories and use hash marks to represent each time an illness, such as respiratory disease or cardiovascular disease, was reported. Mutually exclusive categories require that each category be unique, not overlapping any other category in any way. Comprehensive means that the list of categories is adequate for all possible cases; it is exhaustive. Tabulation by categories describes and summarizes the data by means of the statistical tool called frequency distribution. The ratio, proportion, or percentage of each frequency value to the whole is also important information. An incidence of 12 in a total of 350 (3%) is quite a different result from an incidence of 12 in 94 (13%).

Tabulating the occurrence of different categories is just the first step in con-

Table 6-1 Community survey results: morbidity

Illness	Frequency	Cumulative frequency	Percent	Cumulative percent
Cardiovascular	32	32	32	32
Reproductive	14	46	14	46
Gastrointestinal	17	63	17	63
Respiratory	19	82	19	82
Neurological	18	100	18	100
TOTAL	100		100	

structing frequency distributions. Table 6-1 illustrates a frequency distribution, showing that the cumulative frequency, the percentage, and the cumulative percentage are also calculated and tabulated. For purposes of illustration, the list of illnesses in Table 6-1 should be considered both mutually exclusive and comprehensive.

In Table 6-1 a total of 100 patients was selected to simplify the calculations. The leading type of illness is clearly cardiovascular disease, whereas reproductive illness is reported least.

What frequency of respondents reported respiratory diseases?

What percentage?

More detailed information could be tabulated to compare certain subgroups within the sample. The categories of illnesses could be analyzed on the basis of different age groups. Each age group would have to be defined in years so that the responses would be placed in one and only one category.

What is wrong with the scheme that follows?

Group 1	Infants	0-2 years
Group 2	Young children	2-11 years
Group 3	Adolescents	12-18 years
Group 4	Young adults	19-35 years
Group 5	Middle-aged adults	36-55 years
Group 6	Elderly adults	56-99 years

Using a corrected list of categories, the researchers could prepare frequency distributions for each class based on the illnesses reported to the interviewers. In addition to describing the results in more detail than the overall summary described above, the researchers can make comparisons. Table 6-2 shows the data from Table 6-1 in terms of age groups. The cumulative frequencies and cumulative percentages were omitted from this table. For comparative purposes

Table 6-2 Community morbidity data by age group (frequencies and
              percentages*)

Illness	Group 1 n	Group 1 %	Group 2 n	Group 2 %	Group 3 n	Group 3 %	Group 4 n	Group 4 %	Group 5 n	Group 5 %	Group 6 n	Group 6 %
Cardiovascular	0	0	0	0	1	3	2	6	14	44	15	47
Reproductive	0	0	1	7	2	14	3	21	3	21	5	36
Gastrointestinal	1	6	2	12	1	6	1	6	4	24	8	48
Respiratory	2	11	2	11	3	16	3	16	4	21	5	26
Neurological	1	6	0	0	1	6	3	17	5	28	8	44

n, Number.
*Percentages were calculated based on the total for each group by illness category. Percentages
based on the entire group are the same as the frequencies.

only the frequencies and percentages are needed to convey the relevant information about subgroups of the sample.

The numerical results that report incidence of respiratory diseases among
adolescents can be compared with similar data from any other subgroup, such
as the elderly.

Is the incidence of respiratory diseases greater in infants or in adolescents?

Which group reported the highest percentage of cardiovascular illness?

Which group had the lowest percentage of gastrointestinal illness?

Problem 6-1

Frequency distribution

Listed on p. 157 are the ages of a sample (n = 80) of patients with rheumatoid
arthritis. Construct a frequency distribution from these data in the table that
follows.

Problem 6-1, cont'd

The data

62	54	48	60	58	59	57	56
50	61	49	53	57	48	59	63
60	50	53	59	65	49	54	53
58	54	62	58	64	63	59	60
51	48	56	49	50	64	56	57
55	58	60	54	55	61	49	64
62	50	56	57	48	60	65	48
50	51	54	53	51	63	53	48
60	54	55	52	48	62	61	64
56	51	49	64	62	55	64	61

What is the smallest value in the list? The largest?

The difference between the smallest and largest values is called the range and defines the boundaries of the frequency distribution. The term "range" is used for both the difference and the spread between the maximum and minimum values. It is a measure of variability or dispersion, not central tendency.

Frequency distribution

Age	Frequency	Cumulative frequency	Percent	Cumulative percent
48				
49				
50				
51				
52				
53				
54				
55				
56				
57				
58				
59				
60				
61				
62				
63				
64				
65				

Sometimes the range of values to be tabulated is too large to be manageable. For example, we may wish to tabulate age data with a minimum value of 20 and a maximum value of 74. The range is the spread or the difference between these two values: $74 - 20 = 54$. Tabulating each age value separately requires a list of 55 age values. In such cases a frequency distribution of *grouped* data should be constructed.

First the interval size must be determined. In this example a total of about 15 intervals is deemed appropriate. In general, there should be at least six and no more than 20 classes. The range (54) is divided by the number of intervals (15) to obtain a quotient of 3.60. In such a case either 3 or 4 can be used as the interval size. Odd-numbered interval sizes are more convenient than even-numbered ones because the midpoints of the odd-numbered intervals are always whole numbers. The lowest interval should start with a value that is at least as low as the lowest value in the table and is also a multiple of the interval size— in this case 3. For the example of ages ranging from 20 to 74, the lowest interval should be 18-20. The last interval should contain the highest value listed in the array of ages—in this case 74.

Problem 6-2

Intervals

List the entire set of intervals that will include all possible data for this example in three or four columns:
18-20

Graphic presentation of frequency data

The four common ways to present summarized data graphically are bar graphs, frequency polygons, histograms, and pie graphs. These graphics are used frequently in nursing research to describe samples or present findings simply, accurately, and forcefully.

Bar graphs can be used when the data are nominal or ordinal, as well as interval. Nominal data consist of discrete categories such as different religions,

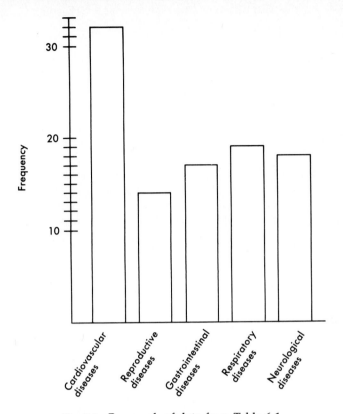

Fig. 6-1　Bar graph of data from Table 6-1.

and ordinal data consist of values that can be ranked, such as the clinical performance of a small group of nursing students. A bar graph can be constructed from the nominal data in Table 6-1. Fig. 6-1 illustrates the bar graph from the frequencies of these data.

　　Table 6-1 and Fig. 6-1 convey the same information to the reader. In this case the frequencies and percentages are the same because the total number of cases tabulated was 100. In most cases, however, the frequencies and percentages are different and the investigator must choose which one to use in constructing a bar graph. Thus in most cases tables contain more information than bar graphs display. It is common practice to use frequencies when the group's size is less than 100 and percentages when it is more than 100.

　　If data are interval level, such as the ages tabulated in Problem 6-1, a frequency polygon such as Fig. 6-2 can be constructed with these steps:

1. Draw a horizontal axis, x (the abscissa), and a vertical axis, y (the ordinate). The point at which they meet is the zero point for the scales running along either axis.
2. Label each axis. Use the y axis for the frequencies of measures and the x axis for the values of the measurement scales.
3. Place a break in the axis if the scale does not progress steadily from zero

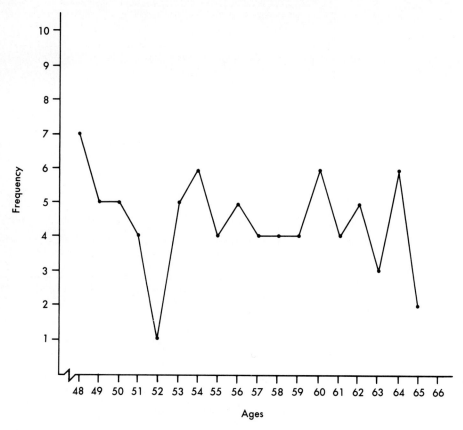

Fig. 6-2 Frequency polygon of ages from Problem 6-1.

to succeeding values. For example, in Fig. 6-2 a large amount of space would be wasted if the horizontal scale included all numbers from zero to the first actual value reported, which was 48. The break in the abscissa indicates that there were no values between 0 and 48.

4. Plot each value and connect the dots with straight lines.

Frequency polygons can also be constructed from grouped data. For any one of the intervals, an assumption is made that, if all the values in that interval were averaged, the average would be equal to the midpoint of the interval. The midpoints are marked off on the x axis, and the points are plotted in the same way for the intervals as for individual values.

Frequency polygons can be used for comparative purposes. For example, an investigator might collect scores of middle-aged and elderly women on a measure of depression. Both sets of scores can be graphed on a frequency polygon to judge the similarity of the scores of the two groups. Fig. 6-3 illustrates this type of graph with fictitious data.

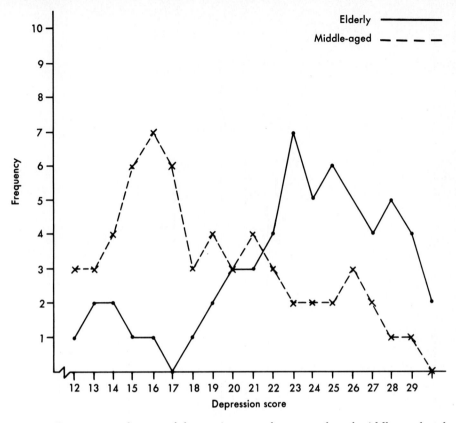

Fig. 6-3 Frequency polygons of depression seen from samples of middle-aged and elderly women.

Which group has more people at the higher score values?

Which group includes the highest recorded score?

Which group has the lowest?

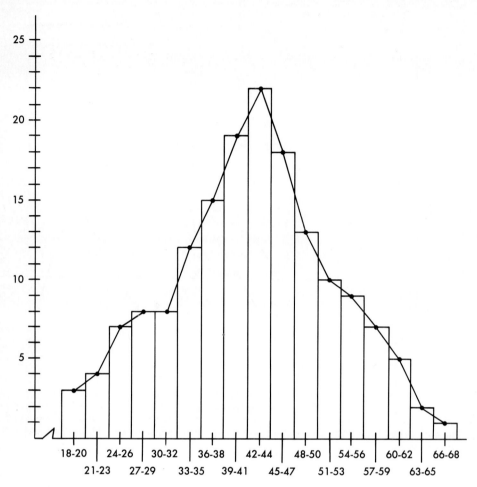

Fig. 6-4 Frequency polygon and histogram from grouped data.

Note that the graph for the middle-aged sample peaks to the left of center while the graph for the elderly peaks to the right. Neither is symmetrical. "Symmetrical" refers to a balanced curve whose midpoint is at the center of the curve. By contrast, a skewed distribution is unbalanced, and the midpoint is not centered. Since the shape of a distribution is important in the applied science of statistics, attention is given to this topic later in the chapter.

Another type of graph, the histogram, is similar to the frequency polygon. The x and y axes are used in the same ways as for a frequency polygon. The difference lies in how the frequency values are plotted. Fig. 6-4 shows a frequency polygon and a histogram that were plotted from the following grouped data:

Interval	Frequency	Interval	Frequency
18-20	3	45-47	17
21-23	4	48-50	13
24-26	7	51-53	10
27-29	8	54-56	9
30-32	8	57-59	7
33-35	12	60-62	5
36-38	15	63-65	2
39-41	19	66-68	1
42-44	22		

Either graph could be constructed from the information given in the other one.

Which interval contains the highest frequency of values? Its midpoint?

The lowest? Its midpoint?

The final type of graph to be illustrated is the pie graph. This is simply a circle in which the 360 degrees are used to represent the entire sample, that is, 100% of the values. The data from Table 6-1 are displayed in the pie graph shown in Fig. 6-5. Each percentage is expressed as a decimal number (by moving the

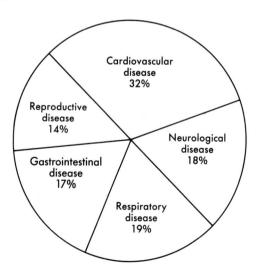

Fig. 6-5   Pie graph of Table 6-1 data.

decimal point two places to the left) and multiplied by 360 to convert the value to degrees. A protractor is used to allocate the portion of the circle to each category.

Measures of central tendency

A measure of central tendency is a statistic that makes it possible to represent some of the information in a set of data as a single value. Often it is desirable to produce a statistic that provides information about the most frequent values in the distribution or about some middle or typical values. Three measures of central tendency—the mode, the median, and the mean—are described in this section.

The mode is the simplest measure of central tendency in a distribution. The mode is simply the value of the score that occurs most frequently in the distribution. It is not the frequency that is largest, but the value associated with that largest frequency. Fig. 6-6 illustrates the concept of mode (or modal value).

What is the mode? The minimum?
   Mode:
   Minimum:
What is the mode for the data displayed in Fig. 6-1?

A given distribution can have two or more modes. The general term for a distribution with two modes is bimodal; the general term for a distribution with more than one mode is multimodal. The mode is particularly useful in describing

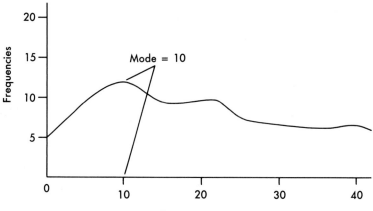

Fig. 6-6 Illustration of mode.

Table 6-3   Years of experience of registered nurses in hospital X (n = 43)

Years' experience	Frequency
1-3	12
4-6	9
7-9	10
10-12	5
13-15	2
16-18	3
19-21	2

phenomena that are at the nominal level of measurement because neither the mean nor the median can be used with such data.

The median is the value in an ordered distribution above which and below which half the values fall. It is the middle score in a set of scores that has been sorted by size. In the set of values 23 28 33 36 42, the median is 33. Many other distributions with a median value of 33 could be developed, for example, 15 26 33 45 62 or 29 31 33 56 79. The median is insensitive to the extreme scores in the distribution; it is the middle score and does not take into account the magnitude of other scores. In an even-numbered group of values the median is the average of the two middle scores. Thus, in the series 26 29 32 34 37 40, the median is (32 + 34)/2 = 33. The median does not actually exist in this set of scores.

In some sets of grouped data the interval containing the middle value is unique and the median is easy to locate. In other sets of grouped data the frequency is more than one for the middle category and calculation of the median becomes a bit more complex. Table 6-3 reports such a distribution and can be used to illustrate the procedure.

In the array of data in Table 6-3, since there are 43 nurses in all, the midpoint of the data is at the point of the twenty-second nurse, which means that it falls in the interval 7-9. Here we must turn to the concept of true limits. By definition the true limits of the interval containing the median are 6.5 and 9.5. Since there are 21 cases in the first two intervals, the twenty-second individual is the first one in the specified interval: 6.5-9.5. Thus we must multiply the lower true limit by $\frac{1}{10}$ to obtain 0.65. The median is then 6.5 + 0.65 = 7.15.

Why can't there be a median for nominal data? Give illustrations from the data in Table 6-1.

The third measure of central tendency, the arithmetic mean, is both the most complex and the most familiar of these measures. Sometimes people use the terms "mean" and "average" interchangeably, but this is misleading because average is such an imprecise term. Average is often used to represent typical as in "average person." Clearly, "average person" is not the same as "mean person." Average is also used to denote normal as distinct from abnormal in relation to some characteristic such as appearance.

The mean can be calculated only for data that are at the interval or ratio level of measurement. Its computation requires that values be added, and addition is meaningful only for numbers with equal intervals between each value. It is simply the sum of a set of values divided by the number of values (n) in the set. The mean is represented by X bar: $\overline{X}$. The Greek letter sigma (Σ) stands for "sum of," X stands for each person's score or value, and the formula for calculating the mean is as follows:

$$\overline{X} = \frac{\Sigma X}{n}$$

To find the mean of a group of scores, we merely add the scores and divide the sum by the number of scores in the set of data. Thus the mean for these scores (45 36 76 54 60 34 28 48 39 47) is 46.7 because this is the quotient from the sum (467) divided by n (10).

Table 6-4 illustrates the calculation of the mean from an ungrouped frequency distribution where X represents the values or scores, f represents frequency, and fX represents the product of the value and the frequency.

The mean, unlike the median, is affected by extreme scores. In fact, the mean is affected by every score in the distribution. Thus it is commonly used when interval or ratio level data are involved.

Measures of dispersion

The measure of dispersion that is easiest to understand is one we defined in relation to constructing frequency distributions, the range. It is the difference between the smallest and largest values in a distribution. A teacher might be

Table 6-4 Calculating a mean from an ungrouped frequency distribution

X	f	fX	Calculations
26	1	26	
28	3	84	$\overline{X} = \frac{\Sigma fX}{n}$
30	2	60	
32	4	128	
36	3	108	$\overline{X} = \frac{536}{16}$
42	2	84	
46	1	46	
	n = 16	$\Sigma fX = 536$	$\overline{X} = 33.50$

interested in the range or spread of scores on a given test. A nurse might be interested in the spread of a patient's vital signs during hospitalization.

The range of a grouped set of data is the difference between the midpoint of the highest interval and the midpoint of the lowest interval. In the following set of data, the two midpoints are 22 and 34; therefore the range is 12:

21-23
24-26
27-29
30-32
33-35

Since a single extreme score can change the range dramatically, the range is considered an unstable measure of dispersion. For example, in the two lists of scores below, an extremely low value was placed in the first set and an extremely high value was placed in the second set.

Set 1: 22   54   65   68   70   75   83   85   87   90
Set 2: 55   57   64   66   68   74   78   84   96   115

Except for the low value of 22 in the first set of scores and the high value of 115 in the second set, the two distributions are similar. Extreme values can occur in successive samples, causing large sampling fluctuations. The larger the sample, the more likely that it contains extreme values. Because of the range's limitations, other measures of dispersion are used more frequently.

The most widely used measure of dispersion is the standard deviation, commonly abbreviated as SD. The standard deviation is a kind of mean of the deviations of all values from the mean of those values. Its calculation takes into account all values in a set of data. Table 6-5 illustrates the calculation of the standard deviation for a set of 10 values. The first step is to tabulate all of the values and compute the mean. Next, the difference score, or deviation score,

Table 6-5   Calculation of standard deviation

Value X	Deviation from mean $x = X - \bar{X}$	Squared deviation $x^2 = (X - \bar{X})^2$
12	0	0
11	−1	1
14	2	4
16	4	16
13	1	1
15	3	9
10	−2	4
8	−4	16
12	0	0
9	−3	9
$\Sigma X = 120$	$\Sigma x = 0$	$\Sigma x^2 = 60$

$\bar{X} = \Sigma X/n = 12$

$SD = \sqrt{\Sigma x^2/n} = \sqrt{60/10} = \sqrt{6.00} = 2.45$

that is, the value minus the mean, is computed for each value. They always sum to zero. The next step is to square each of the deviation scores; the negative sign is lost in this step. Next, these squared deviation values are summed. The sum of squared deviation scores is divided by the number of scores, and the square root of this quotient is taken. This is the standard deviation. In research involving interval-level data, the standard deviation is often reported along with the mean to describe the variable in terms of both central tendency and dispersion.

The quotient of the sum of squared deviation scores divided by the number of scores is called the variance. Obviously it is the square of the standard deviation. The variance is used in calculating some inferential statistics, but it is not reported routinely in describing data. We will consider the standard deviation and measures of central tendency further as we look at shapes of distribution.

Shapes of distributions

As explained previously, a frequency polygon is a line graph derived from plotting frequencies of grouped or ungrouped data. If the sample is progressively increased so that the length of the lines between points is progressively decreased, finally the number of points approaches infinity, the lines become shorter and shorter, and the frequency polygon approximates a smooth curve. If the left half of the curve is a mirror image of the right half, the curve is said to be symmetrical. A special kind of symmetrical curve is called the normal distribution. The concept of the normal distribution was formulated by Gauss to represent the regularity that many physical characteristics exhibit. For example, the heights of most adults fall in a given range, say, from 62 inches to 74 inches; the bulk of values from a set of height data falls between these two limits. There are some individuals who are shorter or taller than the stated boundaries. Thus the normal curve that represents the physical property, height, peaks at its center and decreases toward either side. Fig. 6-7 illustrates the normal curve, showing that the mode, median, and mean coincide. Note also that the standard deviation divides the curve into six segments. These segments account for 99.72% of the area under the curve instead of 100%. The normal curve is a

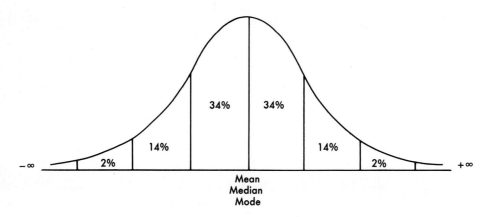

Fig. 6-7 Normal curve.

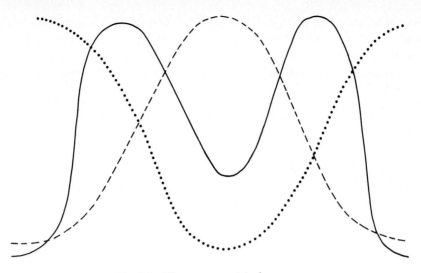

Fig. 6-8 Three symmetrical curves.

theoretical distribution, and as such it extends to infinity in both directions; the curve never intersects the baseline. About 68% of the area under the curve falls within one standard deviation of the mean, about 95% of the data fall within two standard deviations of the mean, and over 99% of the data fall within three standard deviations of the mean.

Other symmetrical curves are illustrated in Fig. 6-8. In each case the mean is the axis of symmetry, and it is always equal to the median. However, the curve may be bimodal, as the solid line in the example shows.

A distribution that is not symmetrical is called skewed. It is positively skewed if the bulk of the area under the curve lies to the left of the center; that is, most of the data falls at the low end of the curve. It is negatively skewed if the bulk of the data falls at the high end of the curve. Fig. 6-9 illustrates skewed distributions.

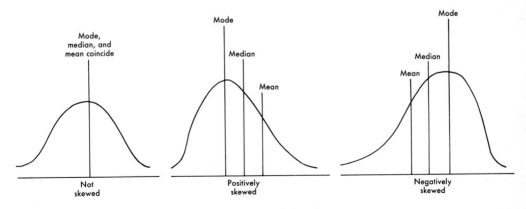

Fig. 6-9 Skewness of distributions.

Distributions also vary in relation to peakedness. This attribute is called kurtosis. Fig. 6-10 illustrates the three kinds of distributions, leptokurtic (peaked), mesokurtic (moderate), and platykurtic (flat). Leptokurtic curves indicate a high concentration of scores at or near the mean value. Mesokurtic distributions are those having a spread of values throughout the range of the distribution. Platykurtic distributions indicate a fairly equal concentration of values across the entire range of possible values.

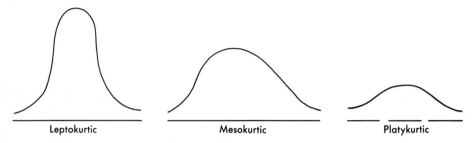

Leptokurtic   Mesokurtic   Platykurtic

Fig. 6-10   Three kinds of distributions.

USING COMPUTERS TO ANALYZE DESCRIPTIVE DATA
Computer capabilities

Computers have taken the drudgery out of data analysis. There are three main sizes of computers: micro, mini, and maxi. Microcomputers are the best known although they were the most recently developed. Microcomputers are stand-alone machines containing microprocessors that can perform a variety of tasks, depending on what the computer program, or software, directs. Some word-processing, database, or spreadsheet programs can be used to prepare manuscripts and collections of information such as a set of addresses or income and expenditures. There is also software designed to help the user learn about a topic—computer-assisted instruction (CAI).

Our interest is in still another kind of software, that which can perform statistical analyses. Some statistical programs require the use of a microcomputer with a hard disk because they need considerable memory for successful operation. Others require only ordinary amounts of memory, and floppy diskettes are adequate for both the programs and the data the investigator enters for each study.

Larger computers include intermediate and large time-sharing computers: minicomputers and maxicomputers (or mainframe computers). A time-sharing computer is one large enough to handle the work of many users at the same time. Time-sharing computers have a very large main memory and extensive disk capacities.

Investigators must code their data for computer analyses. Data must be numerical. Data for different variables such as age and years of experience must be entered in different columns so the computer can treat each separately. In general, computer-based statistical analyses require that the investigator inform the computer about three things: the statistical program to be used, the number and labels (if used) of variables to be analyzed, and the locations of variables to be analyzed. When using time-sharing computers, the investigator must also be identified as a legitimate user of the system, usually by means of identification numbers, project numbers, and passwords. This information allows the computing center to bill costs to the investigator and to keep users' work separate. The problems in this book are designed for use with computer-based statistical programs such as MYSTAT, MINITAB, SAS, Statistical Package for Social Sciences (SPSSX), and BMDP Statistical Software or for the microcomputer versions of MINITAB, SAS, SPSSX, or BMDP.

Coding data

Data must be coded for computer analysis, since the computer can handle only numbers. Sometimes the numbers are meaningful, such as age in years, height in inches, or weight in grams. In other cases numbers are assigned arbitrarily to discrete categories. For example, the investigator might assign females the value of 1 and males the value of 2. Computer analysis of these data allow the researcher to report the numbers and percentages of females and males in the sample.

The investigator usually specifies data according to columns so that the computer can be directed to analyze certain variables in specified ways. The columns assigned to the variables are often incorporated into the questionnaire, interview guide, or observation checklist so that data entry can proceed directly from the data collection instrument. This practice not only saves time but also lessens the chances for errors that are possible when data must be recopied from one form to another for data entry. Fig. 6-11 displays the coding for three items.

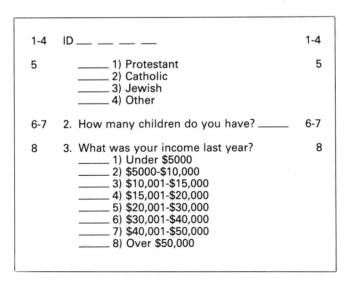

Fig. 6-11 Coding scheme.

The columns for the identification number and the variables are placed in both margins in Fig. 6-11; most investigators use one of these schemes but not both. The number of columns for an identification number or variable must be adequate for the largest possible value that can be obtained. Thus columns 1 to 4 allow us to collect data from subjects 0001 through 9999. The numbers are placed as far right in the field as possible; this is called right justifying the data. This practice prevents the computer from reading 0010 as 0001, 0100, or 1000.

In some cases, such as in an anonymous survey, it may seem unnecessary for the investigator to code identification numbers. However, omitting them is poor practice. If unusual values appear in the analysis, the investigator can use the identification number to check the coded data with the raw data on the data collection instrument.

In item 1 of Fig. 6-11, numbers were assigned to discrete categories. These are arbitrary; the religions could be listed in any order. A space for "other"— for persons whose religions are not listed— is included. An "other," "no opinion," or "don't know" might be necessary for many items. It assists the researcher in identifying *each* subject in terms of the variables in question.

If the categories in a question can be rank ordered, they should be placed in either ascending or descending order. For example:

Item 4: Please rate your health

_____ 1. Poor

_____ 2. Fair

_____ 3. Good

_____ 4. Excellent

In queries such as this the investigator should make a conscious decision about whether the respondent should be forced to choose a stated response. If the answer to this question is no, an alternative of

_____ 5. Don't know

should be added to the item.

How would an answer of "Catholic" to item 1 in Fig. 6-11 be coded?

For item 2 most of the respondents will report fewer than 10 children, but it only takes one respondent reporting 10 or more to require two digits for the coding plan. For answers of one to nine, the data must be right justified by placement of a zero in front of the digit. If a coder indicates that a three belongs in column six instead of column seven, the computer will read it as 30 children instead of three children.

How would an answer of three to item 2 be coded?

In item 3 the investigator is asking for information many people consider too personal to divulge. In such a case, asking for a category rather than an exact income value increases the likelihood of receiving a usable answer.

What response will be given by an individual having an income of $18,000?

With reference to Fig. 6-11, what numbers would you place in columns 1 to 8 for the third subject in a survey who reported that he is Catholic, has four children, and falls in income category 5?

Columns	(1)	(2)	(3)	(4)	(5)	(6)	(7)	(8)

Data entry

Data entry should not begin until the investigator has reviewed the data collection forms or coding forms for errors and omissions. Items that appear perfectly clear to the investigator may be ambiguous to research participants. A pretest may eliminate some of these problems by suggesting revisions needed in the data collection instrument. However, some problems of accuracy or interpretation may remain. Data must be examined carefully for these kinds of problems. The investigator must decide when data are not accurate or complete enough to include in the results. In some cases omissions are given special codes so that a "no response" category can be tracked. In other cases vital data may be missing and the investigator may have no choice but to omit a subject's entire set of responses.

Use of a *fixed format* is recommended for laying out the data for all timesharing statistical packages except MINITAB. Fig. 6-11 illustrates an approach to a fixed format. This simply means that the data for specific variables are put in the same columns for all subjects. In Fig. 6-11 the number of children that survey participants have will always be found in columns six and seven. A new line is used for each subject. The alternative is called freefield format or simply free format. With freefield format, data are entered in the same sequence for all subjects with blanks or commas placed between the variables. Freefield formatting does not require the use of right justification. However, it has important disadvantages. It is easy for the person entering the data to lose track of where he or she is. Moreover, it is virtually impossible to scan data on the computer screen for errors.

Statistical packages for time-sharing computers generally require users to enter their data with a program called a text editor. This is a computer program that allows persons to enter data, called files. Once the files have been entered, they should be saved. At that point or some later date the files may be edited or modified. On IBM computers with operating systems in the OS family, the most common text editor in current use is WYLBUR. WYLBUR has two modes: a command mode that allows the user to take actions such as renumbering, saving, or editing files or moving lines about, and a collect mode that allows the user to create or add to files. On VAX computers with VMS operating systems, the text editor is usually called EDT.

Statistical packages for microcomputers have built-in data entry systems. These frequently require freefield data entry; that is, the investigator is directed to enter the data in a given sequence with a blank or comma entered between each pair of variables. One time-sharing statistical package, MINITAB, uses this approach exclusively.

Regardless of the type of computer or statistical package used, the investigator should take great care in entering data. The computer treats all values entered as accurate representations of variables. Computers do what they are instructed to do, and they churn out erroneous analyses with no error messages if mistakes have been made in data entry.

Generally investigators learn to use only one statistical package along with its appropriate text editor because most of the programs will do all that most people need. Any of the three main programs, SAS, SPSSX, and BMDP, can produce all the statistical analyses a nurse scientist might want. Moreover, it is confusing to use more than one package. However, if change of location means changes in computing resources, investigators often must learn a new system. The various statistical packages are similar enough that knowledge of one will help in learning another.

Preliminary data analysis

Once data have been entered, two types of preliminary analyses should be completed before use of statistical programs geared to answer research questions. First, any errors in the data must be corrected. Second, the distributions of data should be viewed with respect to the assumption of normality that many parametric statistical analyses require. Investigators often run a statistical program that produces frequency distributions, plots, or histograms to meet both of these needs. The only types of errors detected by these programs are outliers — impossible values that lie outside the ranges of possible values for the variables. For example, if 56 is mistakenly entered instead of 65 for an age, the error will not be detected unless 56 is outside the possible range of values for the variable. In a sample of elderly subjects whose ages should be 62 and over, the error of 56 will be noted. From the printout of the file as well as the frequency distribution printout, the investigator can return to the raw data, find the identification number of the subject, and make a correction to the affected columns' numbers. Eliminating errors prevents mistakes in research results and wasted time in analyzing uncorrected data.

In relation to the shape of the distribution, some statistical tests require normality whereas others (nonparametric statistics) are distribution free. That is, nonparametric statistics can be used when distributions are skewed in either direction. For a number of years, parametric statistics were used only with data that were known to be at least interval level and nonparametric statistics were used with ordinal and nominal variables. However, many studies have shown that the use of parametric statistics with ordinal data yields virtually the same results as those obtained from the use of nonparametric statistics. Some authorities assert that the real issue is the shape of the distribution, not the level of measurement. Thus there are advocates for using parametric statistics for ratio, interval, and ordinal data if the sample size is 30 or more and reserving nonparametric statistics for nominal data or small samples of ordinal data (Armstrong, 1981; Nunnally, 1978; Popham and Sirotnick, 1973; Munro, Visitainer, and Page, 1986). The more conservative approach, however, reserves parametric statistics for ratio and interval level data.

Problem 6-3

Describing a sample

The purpose of the study is to determine how frequently nurses employed in a state's visiting nurse associations (VNAs) engage in continuing nursing education, both formal and informal. A random sample of the nurses employed in VNAs at the time of the study was drawn and totals 20. The investigator wants to describe the sample in terms of the variables listed below. Indicate each variable's level of measurement as N (nominal), O (ordinal), or I (interval).

Variables:
    I. Age _____
   II. Ethnicity _____ (1 = Caucasian, 2 = Black, 3 = Hispanic, 4 = Other)
  III. Religion _____ (1 = Catholic, 2 = Jewish, 3 = Protestant, 4 = Other)
  IV. Years since obtaining RN license _____
   V. Years since last formal nursing education _____
  VI. Highest nursing education _____ (1 = AD, 2 = Diploma, 3 = BSN)
 VII. Years employed as a visiting nurse _____
VIII. Marital status _____ (1 = Unmarried, 2 = Married)
  IX. Number of children _____

Complete two tables, one for nominal data (including type of basic nursing education, which might be treated as an ordinal variable) and another for interval data. Write a brief paragraph for each table describing the samples in terms of the variables tabulated in each.

Describing a sample

The data

I	II	III	IV	V	VI	VII	VIII	IX
33	1	1	12	12	3	8	2	2
24	1	2	4	4	1	2	1	0
26	3	1	6	5	2	3	2	0
29	2	3	8	8	3	7	1	0
37	1	3	17	12	2	9	2	3
45	1	1	23	23	3	14	1	0
32	1	3	12	12	1	1	2	2
41	2	3	20	20	2	8	2	1
28	1	3	6	6	3	4	2	1
33	2	3	12	12	3	6	2	2
42	1	1	22	10	3	9	2	4
30	3	1	11	11	1	2	1	0
27	1	3	6	6	1	2	1	0
38	2	3	18	18	1	6	1	0
22	1	2	1	1	3	1	1	0
26	1	3	3	3	3	2	1	0
35	1	3	13	13	3	11	2	2
31	2	3	9	9	3	7	2	1
34	1	2	12	9	3	5	2	0
47	1	1	27	24	3	12	2	0

Use a computer-based statistical package program to complete the tables that follow.

Distribution of nominal level data

Variable	n	%

Problem 6-3, cont'd

Distribution of interval level data

Variable	Range	Mode	Mean	Standard deviation

Write a brief paragraph to describe the sample:

Describing observed phenomena

Observing maternal-infant attachment interactions

Ainsworth (1973) and Holaday (1981) studied maternal interactions with well
and chronically ill infants by means of nonparticipant observation. The
following simulated study was suggested by Holaday's report in the
November-December 1981 issue of *Nursing Research* (vol. 30, pp. 343-348). The
theoretical framework for this study was Bowlby's assertion (1960) that infants'
crying behavior is genetically programmed to elicit closeness and protective
responses from the mother. Crying and other infant behavior that brings the
mother to the infant represents attachment behavior.

The research problem for this simulated study is to describe maternal-infant
interactions when premature infants cry. Because the purpose of this problem
is simply to illustrate a descriptive study based on observation data, the data
collection and analyses are less complex than those Holaday used. Holaday
made four 4-hour visits to each of six mother-infant pairs in which the infants
were chronically ill. Observation record forms were completed for each of the
visits. Holaday compared her results with those of a published study about 26
mother-infant pairs whose babies were healthy (Bell and Ainsworth, 1972). The
interactions of interest were the mothers' responses to infants' crying episodes.
Your task is to analyze the simulated data that follow and answer some specific
questions about the results. Data consist of coded data from 4 hours of
observation for each of four premature infant-mother pairs.

Data were coded in six columns according to the following coding guide. A
dashed line in the data table simply means that crying did not take place
during that hour.

   I. Pair (1 to 4)/hour (1 to 4)
   II. Episode (numbered in sequence) and duration of cry (in seconds)
   III. Delay: Mothers' response times in seconds/episode
   IV. Proximity to mother: 1 = within 5 feet of mother in same room
                              2 = over 5 feet from mother in same room
                              3 = another room
   V. Event preceding cry: 1 = noxious stimulus
                            2 = mother puts infant down
                            3 = bathing
                            4 = feeding
                            5 = dressing
                            6 = sleep
                            7 = mother moves out of sight
                            8 = nothing observed
   VI. Interventions: 1 = approach, no verbal, no touch
                        2 = approach, verbal, no touch
                        3 = approach, no verbal, touch

4 = approach, verbal and touch
5 = pick up and hold
6 = pick up and pat
7 = verbal, no approach
8 = offer pacifier or toy
9 = feed
10 = remove noxious stimulus
11 = change diaper
12 = bathe
13 = put down for nap
14 = ignore
15 = other

Result of intervention: Crying continued = CC
Crying stopped = CS

The data

I	II	III	IV	V	VI
1-1	1-248	1-18	2	2	5-CS
	2-54	2-54	3	2	14-CS
1-2	1-38	1-16	3	6	5-CS
	2-64	2-24	2	8	4-CC
	3-220	3-15	1	1	10-CC
1-3	1-114	1-78	2	8	5-CS
	2-86	2-3	1	4	9-CS
	3-33	3-17	2	8	5-CS
	4-52	4-12	2	7	4-CC
1-4	1-182	1-44	3	8	7-CC
	2-43	2-43	3	7	1-CC
	3-89	3-14	2	8	2-CC
	4-112	4-20	1	8	9-CS
2-1	1-242	1-92	3	2	5-CS
	2-97	2-16	2	3	12-CS
	3-22	3-14	1	5	5-CS
	4-66	4-23	3	7	11-CS
2-2	----	----	---	---	-----
2-3	1-312	1-68	3	8	4-CC
2-4	----	----	---	---	-----

Observing maternal-infant attachment interactions

The data

I	II	III	IV	V	VI
3-1	1-58	1-12	1	1	8-CS
	2-18	2-18	2	8	2-CS
	3-68	3-18	1	2	4-CS
3-2	----	----	---	---	-----
3-3	1-75	1-24	3	8	4-CC
3-4	1-110	1-39	3	6	5-CS
	2-22	2-4	1	4	6-CS
	3-314	3-102	3	8	5-CC
	4-82	4-30	3	7	2-CC
	5-418	4-36	3	1	10-CC
4-1	----	----	---	---	-----
4-2	1-116	1-18	1	1	10-CS
	2-38	2-30	2	8	6-CS
	3-114	2-28	2	8	9-CS
4-3	1-69	1-28	2	8	6-CS
	2-19	2-10	1	8	11-CS
4-4	1-112	1-14	2	8	7-CC
	2-168	2-28	3	2	4-CC
	3-34	3-20	1	8	6-CS
	4-142	4-28	2	8	5-CC
	5-126	5-42	3	2	14-CC

Seven variables will be entered to compute descriptive statistics about these data. The first variable will be the pair number/hour number (PNHN); the second will be crying time in seconds (CRY); the third will be the mothers' delays in seconds (DEL); the fourth will be the proximity code (PROX); the fifth will be the event code (EVE); the sixth will be the intervention code (INT); and the seventh will be the outcome code (OUT: CS = 1, CC = 2). Use a computer-based statistical program to answer the following questions.

What was the longest crying spell?

How many times were mothers in a different room from their infants when the crying began?

What was the shortest delay? The longest?

What was the least used intervention(s)?

Complete analyses in order to fill in the table that follows.

Mothers' delays and duration of infants' cries

Variable	n	Minimum	Maximum	Mean	Standard deviation
Delay (seconds)					
Cries (seconds)					

Cross-classify the data to answer the following questions.
What interventions were used most when crying stopped?

When it continued?

Describing survey results

A survey of continuing nursing education

In Problem 6-3, 20 subjects were analyzed to describe the sample of VNA nurses. Suppose now that these 20 subjects completed brief questionnaires about their participation in continuing nursing education activities, both formal and informal. Possible answers for six questions were N = never, S = sometimes, and A = always. These responses are to be coded 1, 2, and 3, respectively. The total score reflects participation in continued learning. The six items are displayed in the table that follows. You are to analyze the data and complete the table. Answer the questions about the total score that follow the table. The total score was included in the coded data in this problem, but the computer could have created this variable—as you will see in the next problem. Write a brief paragraph reporting your findings. The coded data are as follows.

The data

Subject	Items						
	1	2	3	4	5	6	T
01	3	3	2	2	3	1	14
02	2	2	2	2	2	2	12
03	3	3	2	1	1	1	11
04	2	2	1	1	1	1	8
05	3	1	1	1	1	1	8
06	3	3	3	2	3	1	15
07	2	2	2	2	1	1	10
08	3	3	3	3	3	1	16
09	2	2	1	1	1	1	8
10	3	3	3	3	3	2	17
11	3	2	2	2	2	1	12
12	3	2	1	1	1	1	9
13	3	3	1	2	2	1	12
14	3	2	1	1	2	1	10
15	2	1	1	1	1	1	7
16	2	2	2	1	1	1	9
17	2	3	3	3	3	1	15
18	1	2	2	2	1	1	9
19	3	3	3	3	3	2	17
20	3	2	2	2	1	1	11

Use a frequency distribution program from a statistical package to complete the table that follows.

Continued learning activities of community nurses (n = 20)

Item	N		S		A	
	n	%	n	%	n	%
I attend state nurses' association meetings.						
I attend regional community nurses conferences.						
I attend at least three continuing nursing education programs a year.						
I attend at least three in-service nursing education programs a year.						
I read at least one nursing journal each month.						
I complete a credit course in nursing each year.						

Describe the attendance of this sample at professional meetings:

Has a nursing background given these nurses a habit of reading professional journals regularly?

Use appropriate statistical programs to answer the following questions.

1. What is the range of scores for these 20 subjects?

2. What is the mode of total scores?

3. What is the mean of the total scores?

4. What is the standard deviation of the total scores?

Comparing subgroup responses to a survey

Differences in health habits by gender

A school nurse wanted to plan health education based on existing needs and
surveyed health habits of upper elementary school students by means of a brief
questionnaire. Each of the statements in the table of health practices required a
response of disagree (D:1 point), neither disagree nor agree (N:2 points), or
agree (A:3 points). These 10 statements were followed with a single question
about gender (G), which was coded "1" for female and "2" for male.

The data

ID	Number of question										G
	1	2	3	4	5	6	7	8	9	10	
01	3	2	1	3	3	3	2	2	2	1	2
02	2	1	1	1	2	3	3	1	1	1	2
03	1	3	3	3	1	3	3	3	1	1	1
04	3	3	3	3	3	3	3	3	3	2	1
05	1	1	3	2	3	3	3	2	1	3	1
06	3	2	3	3	3	2	1	2	3	2	2
07	3	3	3	3	1	1	3	3	3	3	1
08	1	3	3	3	2	2	1	1	3	3	1
09	3	3	1	1	1	2	1	3	1	1	2
10	1	1	1	2	3	2	1	1	2	1	2
11	3	2	2	2	2	3	1	3	3	3	1
12	2	1	1	3	3	2	1	3	3	3	1
13	3	3	3	2	2	3	2	3	2	2	1
14	2	2	3	1	2	3	2	3	3	2	2
15	3	3	2	2	3	3	3	3	3	2	1
16	1	1	1	1	2	3	3	2	2	1	2
17	3	3	3	2	2	2	1	3	1	3	2
18	3	3	2	2	1	1	1	1	3	3	1
19	3	3	3	1	1	3	3	1	3	1	1
20	1	1	2	3	3	3	1	2	3	3	2
21	3	2	3	3	2	1	2	2	2	2	2
22	3	3	2	3	1	3	1	3	1	3	1
23	2	2	3	1	1	2	3	3	3	3	1
24	3	1	1	3	3	3	1	3	3	3	1
25	3	3	2	1	1	3	3	3	1	3	2
26	2	2	3	3	1	1	1	3	3	1	1
27	2	3	1	1	3	2	1	2	1	1	2
28	2	3	3	3	3	3	2	3	3	1	1
29	3	1	1	3	2	3	1	2	3	3	2
30	1	3	3	3	2	1	1	1	3	2	2

Planning is always the first step in data analysis. You probably noticed that a total health practices score was not included in the data. Computer-based statistical programs will do this for you. Such a maneuver is called creating a new variable by transformation. Follow the directions of your statistical package to create this new variable.

Use appropriate commands to complete the following table.

Health practices of elementary school children

Item	DA		N		A	
	n	%	n	%	n	%
I am careful to get enough sleep.						
I take a bath or shower daily.						
I enjoy games and other exercise.						
My weight is about right.						
I get yearly dental checkups.						
I try to include the basic four food groups in my diet every day.						
I avoid sweet snacks.						
I brush and floss my teeth after meals.						
I avoid smoking and other drugs.						
I have good posture.						

On which areas of health teaching should the school nurse concentrate?

What is the mean of the total health practices scores?

The standard deviation?

The highest score?

Problem 6-6, cont'd

Differences in health habits by gender

The lowest score?

Cross-classify these data by gender, using a computer-based statistical program. Make a table to display the frequencies of the boys' and girls' responses. Do any of the results for boys and girls differ markedly? If so, write a paragraph to report the distributions of responses for the items that differed.

In this chapter various ways of summarizing data and extracting information from the data are presented. The use of computer-based statistical programs takes the drudgery out of data analysis, making it fun and rewarding. The techniques used in this chapter are limited to descriptive statistics—techniques for producing information from the data. These techniques are useful in describing samples or measures in any kind of study or in describing phenomena as the main purpose of a study.

REFERENCES

Ainsworth M (1973). The development of infant-mother attachment. In Caldwell B and Ricciuiti H, eds. *Review of child development research*. Chicago: University of Chicago Press.

Armstrong G (1981). Parametric statistics and ordinal data: a pervasive misconception. *Nursing Research* 30:60-62.

Bowlby J (1969). *Attachment*. New York: Basic Books Inc, Publishers.

Holaday B (1981). Maternal response to their chronically ill infants' attachment behavior of crying. *Nursing Research* 30:343-348.

Munro BH, Visitainer MA, and Page EB (1986). *Statistical methods for health care research*. Philadelphia: JB Lippincott Co.

Nunnally JC (1978). *Psychometric theory*. New York: McGraw-Hill Inc.

Popham WJ and Sironik KA (1973). *Educational*

statistics: use and interpretation. New York: Harper & Row, Publishers Inc.

REFERENCES FOR FURTHER STUDY

Conover W (1971). *Practical nonparametric statistics*. New York: John Wiley & Sons Inc.

Jacobsen B (1981). Know the data. *Nursing Research* 30:254-255.

Knapp R (1985). *Basic statistics for nurses*. 2nd ed. New York: John Wiley & Sons Inc.

Kviz F and Knafl K (1980). *Statistics for nurses: an introductory text*. Boston: Little, Brown & Co Inc.

Shelley S (1984). *Research methods in nursing and health*. Boston: Little, Brown & Co Inc.

Siegel S (1956). *Nonparametric statistics for the behavioral sciences*. New York: McGraw-Hill Inc.

Suter W (1987). Approaches to avoiding errors in data sets. *Nursing Research* 36:262-263.

CHAPTER 7

Analyzing data to examine relationships

Objectives

After completing this unit of study, students will be able to:

1. Define inferential statistics
2. Identify the purposes of inferential statistics
3. Identify common measures of association, such as Pearson's r, Spearman's rho, Kendall's tau, and measures related to chi square, and explain why they are useful
4. Explain the limitations of chi square as a measure of association
5. Interpret tables, reporting correlations correctly
6. Choose appropriate measures of association for a variety of problems and conditions
7. Calculate a variety of correlation coefficients for small-sample problems
8. Use statistical computer packages to compute a variety of correlation coefficients for problems with samples of any size
9. Interpret the output of statistical computer programs used for correlation analyses
10. Present results from correlation analyses effectively

INFERENTIAL STATISTICS

In the previous chapter the use of descriptive statistics and computer programs to analyze them is discussed. In some situations, however, descriptions are not enough. Instead of answering questions about descriptive statistics from samples to generalize to study populations, we wish to use samples to tell us about relationships of variables in study populations. In this chapter the focus is on *inferential statistics* designed to show associations between two or more variables. Inferential statistics are those that allow investigators to reach conclusions about relationships among variables or differences between groups in populations from samples. Some of the most frequently asked questions in nursing research are related to relationships among variables. Is there a relationship between age and satisfaction with nursing care? Is there a relationship between self-concept and health practices? Is there a relationship between type of surgical procedure and effectiveness of preoperative teaching? These and many similar questions can be answered through the use of inferential statistics designed to examine relationships.

MEASURES OF ASSOCIATION

Analysis of data to examine the possibility of relationships between two or more variables is called correlational analysis. Statistics that serve this purpose are called correlation coefficients. Many correlation coefficients have been developed; the discussion in this chapter is limited to those summarized in Table 7-1. As the table shows, each measure has conditions that must be met for its proper use. The first step in analyzing data for the purpose of examining relationships is to select the appropriate correlation coefficient for the conditions that prevail in the study. Selection of an improper test is a waste of time and effort and leads to erroneous conclusions.

In correlation studies, appropriate inferential statistics are usually employed to determine whether the relationship between two or more variables is closer than would occur by chance. A condition of no relationship whatsoever will produce a correlation coefficient of zero in the absence of error. However, errors introduced by such factors as sampling and measurement may produce a correlation coefficient different from zero—either positive or negative—even when no real relationship exists. The investigator wants to determine whether the nature and extent of the relationship between the two variables are due to chance or a real association between the two variables. Is the relationship greater than would occur by chance? To control for a possible error in concluding that results are statistically significant, investigators set a level of significance. This is called an alpha level, and it controls type I error. Setting the alpha level at .05 or .01 is a way of determining whether the correlation coefficient is large enough to rule out chance with a 95% or 99% confidence, respectively.

If an association is truly present, what is the direction of the relationship—direct or inverse? A direct (positive) relationship occurs when an increase or decrease in one variable results in a corresponding increase or decrease in the other variable. An inverse (negative) relationship occurs when an increase in one variable results in a decrease in the other variable and vice versa. Thus the

Table 7-1 Summary of correlation coefficients

Statistic	Abbreviation	Parametric or nonparametric?	Required conditions
Pearson's product moment correlation	r	P	Normal distributions; ratio/interval data; random sampling; linearity
Spearman's rank order correlation coefficient	rho	N	Distribution-free; ordinal data; random sampling
Kendall's rank correlation	tau	N	Distribution-free; ordinal data; random sampling
Contingency coefficient	C	N	Distribution-free; ordinal/nominal data; random sampling; no zero cells
Phi	phi	N	Distribution-free; ordinal/nominal data; 2 × 2 contingency table; no zero cells
Cramer's V	V	N	Distribution-free; ordinal/nominal data; no zero cells

sign of a correlation coefficient indicates the direction (direct or inverse) of a relationship.

Would you expect the relationships between the following pairs to be direct (D), inverse (I), or absent (A)?	**Height and weight**	_____
	Pulse rate and excitement	_____
	Blood pressure and anxiety	_____
	Confidence and anxiety	_____
	Self-concept and trust	_____
	Relaxation and stimuli	_____

Occasionally variables are measured in such a way that a low score indicates more of the attribute than a higher score does. In such instances the conclusion regarding direct or inverse relationships is exactly opposite to the usual; a negative correlation coefficient indicates a positive correlation relationship between the two variables, and a positive correlation coefficient indicates an inverse relationship between the two variables. This is illustrated in the example concerning Pearson's r, which is presented in the next section.

The strength of a correlation is revealed by its numerical size. A perfect correlation is represented by a correlation coefficient of 1.00—either positive or negative. As the magnitude of the association decreases, the numerical value of the correlation coefficient decreases until it reaches chance levels and finally zero, which represents no association.

If an investigator suspects that two variables are related to each other, she or he hypothesizes that a positive or negative nonchance relationship exists. The opposite of this research hypothesis is the null hypothesis. The null hypothesis (which the investigator usually expects to reject) merely states that no significant relationship exists between the two variables. Hays (1981) clarifies the nature of correlational analyses with elegant simplicity as follows:

> In some situations, the experimenter exercises no control whatsoever over the values of X that occur in the study, nor over the values of Y. Rather, in this sampling situation each individual included simply "brings along" a value of X and a value of Y. We will call this approach "a problem in correlation."*

Correlational analyses sometimes focus on studies designed to predict a value of a dependent variable based on its relationships with other (predictor) variables. For example, an attempt could be made to predict nursing students' grade point averages from selected predictors such as scores on college entrance examinations, scores on tests of psychomotor skills, and high school or prenursing grade point averages. Such problems are problems of regression and are beyond the scope of this book.

Pearson's product moment correlation coefficient

The most commonly used correlation coefficient is Pearson's product moment correlation coefficient, usually called simply Pearson's r. This statistic was introduced in the discussion of reliability in Chapter 4, and a problem for its calculation was presented. As shown in Table 7-1, it is represented simply as r. Pearson's r is a parametric statistic and requires the usual conditions for the use of parametric statistics: both variables must be normally distributed, variance is about equal in the samples, random sampling must have been used, both variables are at the interval (or ratio) level of measurement, and the data when plotted tend to follow a straight line rather than a curve such as a J or U shaped distribution. This last condition is referred to as an assumption of linearity.

A word about the first two assumptions. For a number of years parametric statistics were used only with datasets that were known to be normally distributed, and nonparametric statistics were used for analyzing data from skewed distributions. Nonparametric tests were also mandatory when homogeneity of variance could not be demonstrated. However, many studies have shown "that parametric tests are relatively insensitive to violation of these two assumptions

---

*From Hays W (1981). *Statistics*, 3rd ed. New York: Holt, Rinehart & Winston, p 444.

especially when only one occurs at a given time and the groups are nearly equal in size" (Shelley, 1984, p. 441). However, caution should be exercised when the distribution is highly skewed or multimodal and when samples are small. In such cases the use of parametric statistics can lead to seriously distorted results. Thus there are several considerations in selecting test statistics:

1. Is the test statistic appropriate for testing the hypothesis?
2. What is the sample size?
3. What are the distributions of the variables?
4. Can the conditions of the appropriate parametric test be met? Would more accurate results be obtained by using a nonparametric test?

For convenience the computational formula for Pearson's r is repeated below:

$$r_{xy} = \frac{n(\Sigma XY) - (\Sigma X)(\Sigma Y)}{\sqrt{[n(\Sigma X^2) - (\Sigma X)^2][n(\Sigma Y^2) - (\Sigma Y)^2]}}$$

where

$$
\begin{aligned}
r &= \text{correlation between variables } X \text{ and } Y \\
n &= \text{number of linked pairs of scores} \\
XY &= \text{product of paired scores } X \text{ and } Y \\
\Sigma X &= \text{sum of all } X \text{ scores} \\
(\Sigma X)^2 &= \text{sum of all } X \text{ scores, which is then squared} \\
\Sigma Y &= \text{sum of all } Y \text{ scores} \\
(\Sigma Y)^2 &= \text{sum of all } Y \text{ scores, which is then squared} \\
X^2 &= \text{an } X \text{ score squared} \\
\Sigma X^2 &= \text{sum of all squared } X \text{ scores} \\
Y^2 &= \text{a } Y \text{ score squared} \\
\Sigma Y^2 &= \text{sum of all squared } Y \text{ scores}
\end{aligned}
$$

A concrete example is presented to clarify the use of correlation analysis in nursing research. Rutledge (1987) used the health belief model (HBM) (Becker, 1974; Maiman, Becker, Kirscht, Haefner, and Drachman, 1977) in a study titled "Factors Related to Women's Practice of Breast Self-examination." The correlation section of this study report is used here.

Breast self-examination was the preventive health behavior for which various readiness factors were evaluated by means of Pearson's product moment correlation coefficients. The readiness factors related to perceived threat were perceived susceptibility to breast cancer (SUSC) and perceived seriousness of breast cancer (SER). Those related to perceived cost benefits were perceived barriers to breast self-examination (BAR) and perceived benefits of breast self-examination (BEN). Personal factors believed to modify this preventive health behavior included age (AGE), self-concept (TSCS), and social network and support—both total functional support (TLFUNCT) and total network support (TLNETWK). A crisis-coping response framework is frequently used for research on the HBM. For this study a framework is depicted in Fig. 7-1. The crisis is the threat of breast cancer. The mediating factors are the variables, which represent perceived threat, perceived cost benefit, and personal factors. The coping response is the likelihood of peforming breast self-examination. In assisting women to adopt

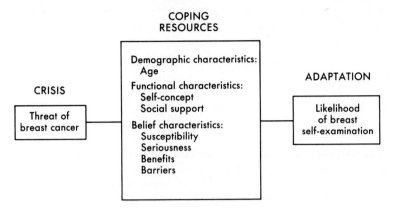

Fig. 7-1 Health belief model framework as crisis-adaptation model.

the practice of regular breast self-examination, it is useful to know what factors make a difference. In this case the question asked is: What factors are significantly (nonchance at a specified level of statistical significance) related to breast self-examination?

Champion's instrument (1984) was used to measure the aforementioned HBM variables of susceptibility (SUSC), seriousness (SER), benefits (BEN), and barriers (BAR). The higher the benefits, the lower the scores; therefore a direct relationship would be predicted by a negative correlation coefficient. Similarly, the lower the barriers, the higher the scores; therefore an inverse relationship would be predicted by a positive correlation coefficient. AGE was simply the reported age in years. (A negative relationship between age and likelihood of breast self-examination was predicted.) The Tennessee Self-Concept Scale (TSCS) was used to measure self-esteem, and the Norbeck Social Support Questionnaire (NSSQ; Norbeck, Lindsey, and Carrieri, 1981) was used to gather scores of total functional social support (TLFUNCT) and total network social support (TLNETWK). Postive relationships were predicted for these variables with the dependent variable. The dependent variable was represented by the number of breast self-examinations reported within the preceding year.

Rutledge (1987) reported the probabilities associated with each correlation coefficient:

SUSC	$r = .0662$	$p = .264$
SER	$r = .1613$	$p = .066$
BEN	$r = -.2231$	$p = .016$
BAR	$r = .4505$	$p = .001$
AGE	$r = -.0069$	$p = .474$
TSCS	$r = .2369$	$p = .015$
TLFUNCT	$r = .0519$	$p = .311$
TLNETWK	$r = -.0106$	$p = .460$

How many correlation coefficients have _p_ values less than .05? _____ Which variables are they?

We can say that these variables are significantly related to likelihood of peforming breast self-examination at a statistical significance level of .05—or an alpha value of .05. In a percentage, how sure are we that these factors are related to likelihood of performing breast self-examination? _____ %

What do the negative signs on the _r_'s for AGE and TLNETWK mean? Are they chance or real relationships?

Is the hypothesis that predicted a negative relationship between age and likelihood of breast self-examination supported?

Table 7-2   Significant values of the correlation coefficient levels of significance

df	.1	.05	.02	.01	.001
10	.4973	.5760	.6581	.7079	.8233
11	.4762	.5529	.6339	.6835	.8010
12	.4575	.5324	.6120	.6614	.7800
13	.4409	.5139	.5923	.6411	.7603
14	.4259	.4973	.5742	.6226	.7420
15	.4124	.4821	.5577	.6055	.7246
16	.4000	.4683	.5425	.5897	.7084
17	.3887	.4555	.5285	.5751	.6932
18	.3783	.4438	.5155	.5614	.6787
19	.3687	.4329	.5034	.5487	.6652
20	.3598	.4227	.4921	.5368	.6524
25	.3233	.3809	.4451	.4869	.5974
30	.2960	.3494	.4093	.4487	.5541
35	.2746	.3246	.3810	.4182	.5189
40	.2573	.3044	.3578	.3932	.4896
45	.2428	.2875	.3384	.3721	.4648

For many years investigators set a level of significance (for example, alpha = .05) in advance. The computed correlation coefficient was then compared with the critical value of the correlation coefficient at a given level of significance. If its value equaled or exceeded the table value, the result was considered to be statistically significant. To enter the table in Appendix A, one needs only to know the sample size. The degrees of freedom *(df)*, a value needed to enter the table, is simply the number of pairs of values minus 2. One needs merely to go down the left column to reach the correct *df* value and then go across the table to the column that corresponds to the selected significance level. To be statistically significant, the computed value of Pearson's *r* must be equal to or larger than the table value. Table 7-2 is a portion of the table in Appendix A and illustrates this process for an alpha of .05 and a computed *r* of .3884 with a sample of 20. Since the *df* is 18 (20 − 2 = 18), *r* must be equal to or greater than .4438 to be considered statistically significant. Since *r* is smaller than .4438, a real relationship between the two variables does not exist at a 95% confidence level.

Computer-based statistical programs generally report the probability level associated with the computed correlation coefficient and thus eliminate the need for consulting tables. However, students should understand the concept of critical values for given sample sizes and levels of significance.

Rutledge (1987) gathered data from 93 subjects. What was the *df* value for this study?

Are the following *r* values significant (S) or not significant (NS) at .05 for the given sample size (n)?	**n = 20, r = .4664**	_____
	n = 27, r = .2996	_____
	n = 32, r = .3778	_____
	n = 22, r = .4888	_____
	n = 18, r = .3441	_____

What if the *df* is not a table value? For example, a sample size of 28 produces a *df* of 26. In this case the process of interpolation is used to estimate the missing table value. The two table values on each side of 26 are:

df	Table value
25	.3809
30	.3494

The *df* value of 26 is one fifth of the way from 25 to 30. Thus one fifth of the difference between the two table values is subtracted from .3809:

.3809 − .3494 = .0315
.0315/5 = .0063
.3809 − .0063 = .3746

The process of interpolation can be used in any statistical table to estimate values associated with missing *df* values.

Problem 7-1

Correlates of children's immunization status

A nurse scientist, Juan Smart Kuki, is stimulated by the Rutledge study to look at mothers' behavior in keeping their children's immunizations up to date within the HBM framework. In the cases of mothers with more than one child, he gathered data about the youngest child in the family. Assume that he used data collection instruments of adequate validity and reliability in gathering data from 40 mothers regarding the following variables:

AGE   (age of mother in years)
NCH   (number of children)
SUSC (susceptibility ranging from 1 to 34)
SER   (seriousness ranging from 1 to 22)
BEN   (benefits ranging from 1 to 28; higher perceived benefits indicated by lower scores)
SE   (self-esteem ranging from 1 to 30)
BAR   (barriers ranging from 1 to 45; low perceived barriers indicated by higher scores)
SS   (a total social support measure ranging from 1 to 60)
LIKI (the dependent variable, likelihood of maintaining proper immunizations, ranging from 1 to 32)

Kuki's first null hypothesis is stated as follows: There is no significant relationship between mothers' ages and their likelihood to maintain proper immunizations for their youngest child. Hypotheses II to VII were worded similarly for the remaining variables: SUSC, SER, BEN, SE, BAR, and SS. For BEN and BAR, negative relationships provide support for rejecting the null hypotheses because of the way they were scored.

The data

ID	AGE	NCH	SUSC	SER	BEN	SE	BAR	SS	LIKI
01	32	1	22	14	12	25	28	44	26
02	28	2	20	21	25	22	10	50	30
03	30	3	17	12	23	14	20	52	31
04	34	1	21	21	09	20	12	37	32
05	33	2	18	16	23	20	38	29	16
06	38	2	20	17	16	26	21	48	29
07	32	3	21	14	26	18	37	33	15
08	28	1	19	12	12	24	22	42	26
09	29	2	26	18	06	22	32	40	29
10	33	3	26	14	17	19	22	34	25
11	31	2	23	18	13	21	29	30	21
12	31	3	13	12	24	26	24	23	12

Problem 7-1, cont'd

The data

ID	AGE	NCH	SUSC	SER	BEN	SE	BAR	SS	LIKI
13	29	1	23	19	15	19	22	36	19
14	26	2	28	22	06	19	36	54	32
15	24	2	25	20	09	23	34	50	30
16	28	3	28	18	17	22	33	33	28
17	25	1	29	20	10	28	40	40	29
18	30	2	14	10	27	28	24	45	24
19	34	2	27	18	11	22	26	34	28
20	29	1	12	13	22	26	12	26	09
21	31	3	23	11	14	22	27	43	24
22	27	2	24	20	24	23	11	52	32
23	28	3	14	15	26	13	22	50	30
24	30	1	26	20	08	21	13	38	30
25	23	3	18	17	22	22	36	27	14
26	31	2	25	17	16	26	21	40	19
27	26	1	21	13	24	18	33	30	13
28	31	2	18	13	13	22	23	40	23
29	48	1	24	18	09	23	30	41	26
30	39	2	26	15	18	20	22	33	25
31	41	1	22	19	15	23	30	42	27
32	37	3	14	10	22	27	25	27	11
33	39	2	25	20	17	17	20	33	17
34	26	1	20	13	26	19	16	34	12
35	23	2	20	14	09	23	14	20	10
36	25	2	27	17	15	20	23	27	20
37	26	1	19	14	19	28	20	26	19
38	31	3	14	12	26	27	22	46	22
39	36	1	22	13	11	24	28	30	20
40	38	2	10	15	21	25	14	25	07

Use a computer-based statistical program to complete the table below.

Ages and numbers of children of study participants (n = 40)

Variable	n	Range	$\overline{X}$	Standard deviation
Age				
Number of children				

Problem 7-1, cont'd

Correlates of children's immunization status

Use a computer-based statistical program to compute Pearson's correlation coefficients in order to test hypotheses I to VII. Construct a table to report the findings using the same format used by Rutledge (1987).

Pearson's correlations of selected variables with frequency of breast self-examination

Variable	$\bar{X}$	r	p
AGE			
SUSC			
SER			
BEN			
SE			
BAR			
SS			

Spearman's rank order correlation coefficient

The calculation of Spearman's rank order correlation coefficient (rho) was derived from Pearson's r. It is a nonparametric statistical test used when the assumption of normality cannot be met, the sample is small, and the data are ordinal. It has about 90% of the power of Pearson's r (Siegel, 1956). The formula and procedures for calculating Spearman's rho were adapted from Siegel (1956).

$$r_s = 1 - \frac{6\sum d^2}{N^3 - N}$$

where d is the difference between each subject's rank for the two variables involved and N is the total number of subjects.

Let's turn to an example of the use of rho. Ten hypertensive patients have scores for medication compliance (X) and dietary compliance (Y). This is a small sample and the data are only ordinal, so a rho rather than a Pearson's r will be computed to determine the relationship between the two measures of compliance.

Step 1. Make a table of the subjects' scores and ranks and determine d for each pair of ranks. Square each of these differences and add up the squared values.

Subject	X		Y		d	d²
	Score	Rank	Score	Rank		
01	46	4	32	3	1	1
02	51	6	40	9	−3	9
03	52	7	35	5	2	4
04	41	2	34	4	−2	4
05	54	8	38	7	1	1
06	43	3	29	2	1	1
07	55	9	39	8	1	1
08	57	10	42	10	0	0
09	35	1	22	1	0	0
10	49	5	36	6	−1	1

$$\sum d^2 = 22$$

Step 2. Substitute this $\sum d^2$ value in the formula and solve for rho.

$$r = 1 - \frac{6\sum d^2}{N^3 - N} = 1 - \frac{(6)\,(22)}{1000 - 10} = 0.867$$

Step 3. Consult Appendix B to see whether this value of rho is significant at either .05 or .01. The table values are .564 at .05 and .746 at .01. Therefore this computed rho is significant at .01.

Is the computed value of rho also significant at .05?

In this example there were no tied ranks. If only a few ties exist, this formula is still applicable. The tied ranks are simply assigned the average value of the two ranks that would be assigned them had there been no ties. For example, if two subjects both have X scores of 44 and their consecutive ranks would be 6 and 7, they are both assigned the rank of 6.5. No values are assigned the ranks of 6 and 7. If three tied scores occur, they are all assigned the rank of the middle rank. That is, if they would consecutively be given the ranks of 6, 7, and 8, all three subjects' scores are assigned the rank of 7. If the proportion of ties is high, Siegel (1956) can be consulted for a correction factor or Kendall's tau, another nonparametric statistic, described below can be used.

Kendall's tau

Kendall's tau (τ) is another nonparametric measure of association. Although it is numerically different from Spearman's rho, Kendall's tau has exactly the same power as rho in detecting statistically significant relationships. When relatively large numbers of ties exist in a set of ranking, Kendall's tau is preferred over

Spearman's rho. The formula and procedures for calculating it have been adapted from Siegel (1956):

$$\tau = \frac{\text{Actual score}}{\text{Maximum possible score}} = \frac{S}{(N/2)(N - 1)}$$

where S = sum (see below). The derivations of the actual score and the maximum possible score are illustrated in the example that follows. Two nursing instructors rank five students on their clinical performance. The two sets of rankings are as follows:

	Student				
	a	b	c	d	e
Instructor 1	3	4	1	2	5
Instructor 2	4	5	2	1	3

Step 1. Rearrange the data so that the first instructor's rankings fall in a natural (increasing) order and the second instructor's rankings are tabulated in that same order:

	Student				
	c	d	a	b	e
Instructor 1	1	2	3	4	5
Instructor 2	2	1	4	5	3

Step 2. Compare instructor 2's first ranking with every ranking to its right, assigning a $+1$ to every pair in which the order is natural and a -1 to every pair in which the order is unnatural:
Comparing 2 with 1 produces a -1
Comparing 2 with 4 produces a $+1$
Comparing 2 with 5 produces a $+1$
Comparing 2 with 3 produces a $+1$
Repeat for each of instructor 2's subsequent rankings:
Comparing 1 with 4 produces a $+1$
Comparing 1 with 5 produces a $+1$
Comparing 1 with 3 produces a $+1$
Comparing 4 with 5 produces a $+1$
Comparing 4 with 3 produces a -1
Comparing 5 with 3 produces a -1

Step 3. Add these measures of "disarray": Sum = 4 and substitute this sum in the formula above for S.

Step 4. Since N = 5, the formula becomes:

$$\tau = \frac{4}{(2.5)\ (4)} = .400$$

Step 5. The possible statistical significance can be determined by two procedures depending on sample size. If N is equal to or less than 10, use the table in Appendix C. In this example the value of tau is .400 and the table probability is .242; thus it would not be statistically significant at an alpha of .05. For problems in which N is greater than 10, a z must be computed for the tau obtained:

$$z = \frac{\tau}{\sqrt{\dfrac{2(2N + 5)}{9N(N - 1)}}}$$

Problem 7-2

Relationship of mothers' self-esteem to their social support

Use the immunization data (IMMUN) from Problem 7-1. Your research question is as follows: Is there a relationship between mothers' self-esteem and their total social support?

Use a computer-based statistical package program to compute a Spearman's rho and a Kendall's tau for the variables self-esteem (SE) and social support (SS) in your IMMUN data from Problem 7-1.

What is the value of Spearman's rho? _____
Is it statistically significant at .05?

What is the value of Kendall's tau? _____
Is it statistically significant at .05?

Chi-square test of independence and the contingency coefficient

The chi-square test of independence is a nonparametric test designed to determine whether two variables are independent or related. The value of chi square is computed when two variables are cross classified. Hypotheses are formulated concerning the proportion of cases that fall in each of the cells created in the cross-tabulation. Such tables are called contingency tables. Table 7-3 is a contingency table.

Table 7-3 displays the results of asking beginning and graduating nursing students whether research should be a part of every nurse's practice. The actual numbers agreeing that it should are 82 graduating nursing students and 30 beginning nursing students, whereas the numbers disagreeing with the statement are 12 and 66, respectively. The theoretical frequencies (shown in parentheses) are obtained from the total frequencies under the hypothesis that there is no real difference between the proportions of agree and disagree in the two samples.

Cross-tabulation and the computation of chi square can be made when the variables are nominal, as well as ordinal, interval, or ratio, and the chi-square

Table 7-3 Contingency table (responses to statement "Research should be a part of every nurse's practice")

	Agree	Disagree	
Graduating nursing students	82 (55.41)	12 (38.59)	94
Beginning nursing students	30 (56.54)	66 (39.41)	96
	112	78	

statistic is useful for discrete or continuous variables. However, it is assumed that data occur in every category; thus no cell may have an observed frequency of zero. Until recently the number of cells that could have expected frequencies less than 5 was restricted to 20%, but this requirement has been shown to be unnecessary.

The formula for the degrees of freedom for calculating chi square and the contingency coefficient is

$$df = (k - 1)(r - 1)$$

where k = number of columns in the contingency table and r = number of rows in the contingency table.

The formula and procedures for calculating chi square (χ^2) and the contingency coefficient (C) are as follows:

$$\chi^2 = \frac{\sum_{i=1}^{r}\sum_{j=1}^{k}(O_{ij} - E_{ij})^2}{E_{ij}} \qquad C = \sqrt{\frac{\chi^2}{N + \chi^2}}$$

where O_{ij} is the observed number of cases found in the ith row of the jth column and E_{ij} is the expected frequency obtained by multiplying the two marginal totals for each cell and dividing the product by N.

For example, a sample of nurses with different interests in management took a leadership potential test. The management interest scores were used to divide the group into high, medium, and low groups, and the leadership scores were used to label each student as being in a high or low group (by computing the median of the scores). The data are the frequency counts of scores falling in each cell.

Step 1. Cross-classify the data and compute the marginal totals:

	Low leader score	High leader score	Total
Low management interest score	(A) 21	(B) 17	38
Middle management interest score	(C) 19	(D) 12	31
High management interest score	(E) 20	(F) 24	44
TOTAL	60	53	113

Step 2. Compute the expected frequency (f) for each cell by dividing the product of the marginal totals for each cell by the total N, in this case, 113.

$$f_A = \frac{38 \times 60}{113} = 20.2$$

$$f_B = \frac{38 \times 53}{113} = 17.8$$

etc.

	Low leader score	High leader score	Total
Low management interest score	(A) 21 (20.2)	(B) 17 (17.8)	38
Middle management interest score	(C) 19 (16.5)	(D) 12 (14.5)	31
High management interest score	(E) 20 (23.4)	(F) 24 (20.6)	44
TOTAL	60	53	113

Step 3. Compute χ^2.

$$\chi^2 = \frac{\sum\limits_{i=1}^{r} \sum\limits_{j=1}^{k} (O_{ij} - E_{ij})}{E_{ij}} =$$

$$\frac{(21 - 20.2)}{20.2} + \frac{(17 - 17.8)}{17.8} + \frac{(19 - 16.5)}{16.5} + \frac{(12 - 14.5)}{14.5} +$$

$$\frac{(20 - 23.4)}{23.4} + \frac{(24 - 20.6)}{20.6} = 1.93$$

Step 4. Compute C.

$$C = \sqrt{\frac{1.93}{113 + 1.93}} = \sqrt{0.017} = .13$$

Step 5. Compute df and consult the χ^2 table (Appendix D) with this df to determine the level of significance of χ^2 and C.

$$df = (2 - 1)(3 - 1) = 2$$

The table value of χ^2 at .05 and $df = 2$ is 5.911, meaning that the computed χ^2 would have to be equal to or greater than 5.911 to be statistically significant at an alpha of .05.

The use of contingency tables and the chi-square statistic has important limitations. Although no association is indicated by a zero, a perfect association is *not* indicated by a 1.00. Moreover, the size of chi square is influenced by both the size of the contingency table and the size of the sample. It is easy to see that the addition of rows and columns as a table grows is accompanied by larger

and larger values of chi square—even when the association remains essentially
constant! Moreover, if the sample size is tripled, the value of chi square is tripled,
everything else remaining the same. Since degrees of freedom depend on the
number of rows and columns, not the sample size, inflated values of chi square
occur for large samples.

A number of alternatives to chi square as measures of association have been
developed to deal with these problems. One, the contingency coefficient, is
usually calculated along with chi square as it is in the preceding example. It
should be noted, however, that two contingency coefficients are not comparable
unless they have been computed from tables the same size. The statistic C is
not comparable to r, rho, or tau.

Problem 7-3

Relationship of number of children in a family and immunization status

Return to the IMMUN data you saved in Problems 7-1 and 7-2. To illustrate the
use of chi square and the contingency coefficient, your research question is: Is
there a significant relationship between the number of children a mother has
and her likelihood of maintaining a proper immunization schedule?
 Restate this question as a null hypothesis:

Before computing a chi square and contingency coefficient, you should put
the LIKI scores into categories. (Using LIKI as a continuous variable would
create too many cells, and some would have zero frequencies, thus violating
the conditions needed for computing a meaningful chi square.) Use a
computer-based statistical program to determine the median of the LIKI scores,
and recode that variable into high (median to maximum) and low (minimum to
the score just below the median) groups.
 Use the cross-tabulation program from your statistical package to produce a
contingency table, a chi-square value, and a value for the contingency
coefficient.
 What is the result of testing your null hypothesis?

Most statistical packages can produce a number of correlation coefficients
along with contingency tables and chi squares. The conditions for using each
one can be found in discussions of correlation in advanced statistics books. Brief
summaries of two of them follow; they were selected because of the way they

improve on chi square and the contingency coefficient in giving the investigator a clearer understanding of the magnitude of the relationships.

Phi. The correlation coefficient phi (∅) makes a correction for the size of the sample when the table size is 2 × 2. Its formula follows (Nie et al., 1975):

$$\emptyset = \sqrt{\left(\frac{\chi^2}{N}\right)}$$

Phi is zero when no relationship exists and 1 when variables are related perfectly. When tables are not 2 × 2, phi has no upper limit and is not a suitable statistic to use. The statistical significance of phi may be tested by calculating a corresponding chi-square value and assigning a *df* of 1 to it (Thorndike, 1976):

$$\chi^2 = N(phi)$$

Cramer's V. Cramer's V is an adjusted phi, modified so that it is suitable for tables larger than 2 × 2. The value of *V* is zero when no relationship exists and 1 when a perfect relationship exists. The formula for Cramer's V follows (Norusis, 1987):

$$V = \sqrt{\frac{\chi^2}{N(k-1)}}$$

Thus, when 2 × 2 tables are involved, phi gives a more useful measure of the relationship between the two variables than chi square provides. For tables larger than 2 × 2, Cramer's V is the statistic of choice.

SUMMARY OF THE USEFULNESS OF CORRELATIONS

All types of correlation coefficients do one thing—they tell the nature and extent of association between two variables. Each measure has conditions that must be met for its use to be appropriate. The first step in analyzing relationships is always selection of the proper measure of association based on the conditions of the study and the hypotheses to be tested.

Measures of association are useful for a variety of studies. Correlation coefficients are used in exploratory studies to determine relationships among variables in new study areas. The results of such studies allow investigators to formulate further research questions or hypotheses to delve more deeply into the study area. In some studies the hypotheses focus on associations between selected variables and the correlation coefficients serve to test these hypotheses. Similarly, hypotheses based on expected associations among variables make important contributions to theory building.

Finally, correlation coefficients are used to manage threats to validity in experimental and quasiexperimental studies. They can be used to test the credibility of findings wherein groups have been compared by checking on the association of independent and extraneous variables with the dependent variable. This is discussed further in Chapter 8.

REFERENCES

Becker M (1974). *The health belief model and personal health behavior.* Thorofare, NJ: Slack Inc.

Champion V (1984). Instrument development for health belief model constructs. *Advances in Nursing Science* 6:73-85.

Hays W (1981). *Statistics.* 3rd ed. New York: Holt, Rinehart & Winston Inc.

Maiman L, Becker M, Kirscht J, Haefner D, and Drachman R (1977). Scales for measuring health belief model dimensions. *Health Education Monographs* 5:214-231.

Nie N, Hull C, Jenkins J, Steinbrenner K, and Bent D, eds (1975). *SPSS.* 2nd ed. New York: McGraw-Hill Inc.

Norbeck J, Lindsey A, and Carrieri V (1981). The development of an instrument to measure social support. *Nursing Research* 30:264-269.

Norusis M (1987). *The SPSS guide to data analysis for SPSS-X.* Chicago: SPSS Inc.

Rutledge D (1987). Factors related to women's practice of breast self-examination. *Nursing Research* 36:117-121.

Shelley S (1984). *Research methods in nursing and health.* Boston: Little, Brown & Co.

Siegel S (1956). *Nonparametric statistics.* New York: McGraw-Hill Inc.

Thorndike R (1976). *Correlational procedures for research.* New York: Gardner Press Inc.

REFERENCES FOR FURTHER STUDY

Armstrong, G (1981). Parametric statistics and ordinal data: a pervasive misconception. *Nursing Research* 30:60-62.

Christman N, McConnell E, Pfeiffer C, Webster K, Schmitt M, and Ries J (1988). Uncertainty, coping and distress following myocardial infarction: transition from hospital to home. *Research in Nursing and Health* 11:71-82.

Devine E and Werley H (1988). Test of the nursing minimum data set: availability of data and reliability. *Research in Nursing and Health* 11:97-104.

Fridl G, Kopare T, Gaston-Johansson F, and Norvell K (1988). Factors associated with more intense labor pain. *Research in Nursing and Health* 11:117-124.

Guilford J (1978). *Fundamental statistics in psychology and education.* New York: McGraw-Hill Inc.

Haack B (1988). Stress and impairment among nursing students. *Research in Nursing and Health* 11:125-134.

Kendall M (1975). *Rank correlation methods.* London: Charles Griffin & Co Ltd.

Lusk S, Disch J, and Barkauskar V (1988). Interest of major corporations in expanded practice of occupational health nurses. *Research in Nursing and Health* 11:141-151.

Mercer R, Ferketich S, May K, DeJoseph J, and Sollid D (1988). Further exploration of maternal and paternal fetal attachment. *Research in Nursing and Health* 11:83-95.

Munro BH, Visitainer MA, and Page EB (1986). *Statistical methods for health care research.* Philadelphia: JB Lippincott Co.

Norbeck J, Lindsey A, and Carrieri V (1983). Further development of the Norbeck Social Support Questionnaire. *Nursing Research* 32:4-9.

Nunnally JC (1978). *Psychometric theory.* New York: McGraw-Hill Inc.

Popham WJ and Sirotnik KA (1973). *Educational statistics: use and interpretation.* New York: Harper & Row, Publishers Inc.

CHAPTER 8

Analyzing data to compare groups

Objectives

After completing this unit of study, students will be able to:

1. Explain the difference between independent and related group comparisons
2. Identify and describe common inferential statistics for comparing independent groups under varying conditions
3. Identify and describe common inferential statistics for comparing dependent groups under varying conditions
4. Explain the assumptions accompanying the statistics used for comparing groups
5. Select the appropriate statistic(s), given problems in nursing research
6. Use comparisons of groups to add credibility to the findings from experimental and ex post facto studies
7. Use a statistical package effectively and efficiently to compare groups
8. Interpret tables that report group comparisons
9. Interpret computer output from statistical programs used for group comparisons
10. Present results from comparative analyses effectively

Analysis of data to compare two or more groups regarding values of dependent variables is used commonly in both experimental (and quasiexperimental) and ex post facto designs. In experimental and quasiexperimental designs an independent variable is manipulated and outcomes comparing one or more experimental and control groups are assessed. The purpose of the experiment is to attribute differences in outcomes to the manipulation of the independent variable—the experimental treatment. In ex post facto designs the groups are constituted on some naturally occurring phenomenon among the study participants, such as age, gender, or personality traits. The investigator does not manipulate the grouping variable. Rather, the study participants sort themselves into groups depending on the nature of the research question(s).

This chapter is organized to present approaches to group comparisons when the groups are independent and when they are dependent. Independent samples are obtained by drawing subjects for experimental and control groups at random from the sampling frame (the study population), from assigning subjects at random from a pool of subjects obtained in either random or other than random sampling, and from constituting groups based on the value of some identified independent variable (such as age or gender). Dependent samples are obtained from using each subject as his or her own control or by pairing study participants on the basis of variables relevant to the study purpose and assigning one member of each pair to the two study groups.

In general, the use of dependent samples increases the precision of experiments because of the control exercised over extraneous variables that might affect results. For example, a teaching intervention used as an experimental intervention may be evaluated more precisely if the investigators can state that the experimental and control groups were matched. Otherwise, differences in outcomes might be due to uncontrolled variables such as age, gender, attitudes toward health behavior, or native intelligence. Matching is often used because random assignment to groups may or may not be effective in controlling for the influence of extraneous variables. The effectiveness of random sampling depends on the sample size; the larger the sample is, the more effectively random sampling equates comparison groups.

In research involving group comparisons, investigators often perform additional analyses to demonstrate that the groups were comparable on some important characteristics. Such analyses attempt to deal with threats to external and internal validity. This topic is addressed in the sections on comparing independent and dependent groups under various conditions.

COMPARING TWO INDEPENDENT GROUPS

Table 8-1 summarizes the statistical tests used for comparing two independent groups, which are presented in this section.

Student's *t* test

Independent *t* tests are used to compare the means of two groups from ex post facto, experimental, and quasiexperimental designs. The groups need not be equal in size. The *t* value is computed (usually with a computer package program), and the probability (alpha) associated with the computed *t* value is ex-

Table 8-1 Statistical tests used for comparing two independent groups

Test	Abbreviation	Conditions for use
t test	t	Random sampling; normally distributed data with equal variances; interval level data; questions about differences between population means
Mann-Whitney U test	U	Random sampling; distribution-free; ordinal level data; questions about differences between population rankings
Chi square	χ^2	Random sampling; distribution-free; nominal level data; data in contingency tables; no cells with value of zero; questions about differences between population proportions when N is greater than 20
Fisher's Exact test	D	Random sampling; distribution-free; nominal level data; data in 2 × 2 contingency tables; sample less than 20; may have cells with value of zero

amined. If the computer program does not provide probability levels for the t test, the value obtained is compared with a table value corresponding to the degrees of freedom (df) and the alpha level. It should be recalled that df, an important concept in statistics, is a measure of the number of independent observations in a file of data, that is, the number of observations that are free to vary around a value. Suppose that we have a sum of 10 numbers. Only nine of these are free to vary because one number must be the difference of the total sum and the sum of the other nine numbers. The df for an independent t test equals the sum of the two numbers (n) minus 2 because this is the sum of the df for the two samples:

$$df = (n_A - 1) + (n_B - 1)$$

or

$$df = n_A + n_B - 2$$

Referring to Appendix E, we see that two alpha levels are given, one for directional (one-tailed) hypotheses and one for nondirectional (two-tailed) hypotheses. Suppose we have two groups totaling 28. The $df = 26$, and we can enter the table at the alpha that has been set; in this case we will use a two-tailed test with an alpha set at .05. Going down the nondirectional column labeled .05 to the row labeled 26 gives us the value 2.056. A t test computed for these samples would have to be 2.056 or larger to be significant at .05. The computational formula for the independent t test is as follows:

$$t = \frac{\overline{X}_A - \overline{X}_B}{\sqrt{\frac{\Sigma x_A^2 + \Sigma x_B^2}{df}\left(\frac{1}{n_A} + \frac{1}{n_B}\right)}}$$

where
$\overline{X}_A$ = the mean of group A
$\overline{X}_B$ = the mean of group B
Σx_A^2 = the sum of the group A squared deviation scores
Σx_B^2 = the sum of the group B squared deviation scores
n_A = the number of subjects in group A
n_B = the number of subjects in group B

Turning to a concrete example, suppose that a survey study has been completed in which subjects' health practices scores are of interest. It is hypothesized that the scores of the younger group (group A) will differ from those of the older group (group B), and the alpha level is set at .05 ($\overline{X}_A > \overline{X}_B$).

Is this an experimental or ex post facto design? Why?

Each group has 10 subjects. Tabulating the scores as illustrated in the following is the easiest way to arrange the work. The first step is to calculate the mean for each set of scores so that the deviation scores for each subject can be computed. These deviation scores are then squared and summed. All values are substituted in the preceding equation, and the value obtained is checked against the table value for a df of 18 $(10 + 10 - 2)$ and a nondirectional alpha of .05. The computed t test must be equal to or larger than 2.101.

Group A			Group B		
X_A	x_A	x_A^2	X_B	x_B	x_B^2
25	−3	9	20	−2	4
31	3	9	27	5	25
27	−1	1	21	−1	1
24	−4	16	18	−4	16
29	1	1	23	−1	1
32	4	16	19	−3	9
30	2	4	20	−2	4
28	0	0	24	2	4
26	−2	4	26	4	16
31	3	9	17	−5	25

$\Sigma X_A = 283$ $\Sigma x_A^2 = 69$ $\Sigma X_B = 215$ $\Sigma x_B^2 = 105$
$\overline{X}_A = 28$ $\overline{X}_B = 22$

$$t = \frac{28 - 22}{\sqrt{\left(\frac{69 + 105}{18}\right)\left(\frac{1}{10} + \frac{1}{10}\right)}} = 1.22$$

Since this value for t is less than the table value, the results are not statistically significant. Thus the investigator concludes that there are no differences in health practices of the younger and older groups as measured by the research tool. The difference between the means (that is, 28 minus 22) can be attributed to chance.

This example is included to illustrate the variables used in computing an independent t test. In practice, computer programs make such calculations unnecessary.

Problem 8-1

The effects of bladder reconditioning on urinary dysfunction

Several investigators (Williamson, 1978, 1982; Oberst, Graham, Geller, Stearns, and Tiernan, 1981) have compared the effectiveness of two approaches to urinary catheter management in controlling postoperative urinary dysfunction. Bladder dysfunction can lead to such problems as discomfort from mucosal irritation, bladder distention, retention of residual urine, and bacteriuria. In most hospitals an indwelling (Foley) catheter is inserted at the time of surgery and remains in place for 6 to 14 days, with continual gravity drainage used to keep the bladder decompressed until the catheter is removed. The alternative approach used by Williamson and by Oberst and co-workers involved an attempt to restore bladder muscle tone by a systematic program of clamping and drainage. The bladder was allowed to fill and empty in an approximation of a normal pattern by use of periodic clamping and release. This experimental treatment was called bladder reconditioning.

In this problem, a replication, a sample of women patients who had indwelling catheter durations of at least 36 hours was studied. Excluded were patients who had a history of urinary tract infections or urinary incontinence or who had had indwelling catheters within the previous 12 months. Also excluded were patients whose admission urinalysis revealed bacteriuria. Patients with spinal cord injuries or muscular degenerative disorders were not considered for the study, nor were patients with baseline residual urine volumes (RUVs) of more than 25 ml, measured at the time of catheter insertion. Women who agreed to participate during the 18-week study period were randomly assigned to the experimental and control groups. A total sample of 32 patients, aged 24 to 45 years, was obtained.

Is this a quasiexperimental study or an experimental study? Why?

Problem 8-1, cont'd

The effects of bladder reconditioning on urinary dysfunction

For the purpose of this study, bladder dysfunction was defined in terms of time lapse before resumption of normal micturition and in terms of postvoiding RUVs. The hypothesis to be tested is that patients who receive bladder reconditioning will have less bladder dysfunction after catheter removal than patients who do not receive reconditioning.

State a null hypothesis for each outcome variable:

The 16 subjects randomly assigned to the experimental group received bladder reconditioning before removal of their Foley catheters. Reconditioning followed the protocol nurses most commonly use: the catheter was clamped in 3-hour cycles to prevent drainage of urine, and at the end of each 3-hour period the catheter tubing was unclamped for 5 minutes to allow complete emptying of the bladder, simulating voiding. This was repeated three times. Thus reconditioning required 9 hours and 15 minutes before the indwelling catheter removal for each experimental group subject. The 16 subjects assigned to the control group received standard nursing care, which did not include reconditioning.

After catheter removal each subject in both groups maintained a minimum fluid intake of 100 ml per hour and was instructed to empty her bladder as soon as she became aware of an urge to void. The length of time each subject required to reestablish normal voiding was recorded, and the first voided volume was measured, immediately after which a straight in-and-out catheterization yielded the RUV, furnishing one indication of the degree of dysfunction. The table on p. 213 gives data for the 16 experimental group patients followed by the 16 control group patients.

Problem 8-1, cont'd

The data

ID	Age	Baseline RUV (ml)	Time of catheter in place (hr)	Fluid intake during 3 hr (ml)	Time from catheter out to first void (hr)	Volume voided (ml)	Postcatheter RUV (ml)
03	22	23	76.5	375	2.25	160	34
04	38	22	71.0	375	1.80	150	50
05	36	21	38.3	375	1.90	200	40
06	28	22	48.6	370	2.33	180	40
07	38	11	82.3	375	2.10	150	24
08	35	22	66.5	375	1.60	200	20
09	40	14	72.0	375	1.10	170	34
10	42	21	56.8	375	2.00	180	28
11	40	22	63.2	300	1.75	210	22
12	41	20	78.3	375	1.50	180	42
13	29	18	59.5	375	2.20	170	20
14	25	12	61.6	375	1.75	165	24
15	33	23	65.5	375	2.33	180	26
16	34	14	58.8	375	1.88	165	25
17	32	20	71.2	375	3.22	170	38
18	28	22	66.5	375	2.75	150	29
19	43	23	88.5	375	3.20	176	33
20	40	24	55.8	370	2.10	158	29
21	35	21	58.8	375	3.20	180	41
22	38	17	64.5	375	3.00	160	38
23	32	12	58.6	375	1.80	170	42
24	31	17	76.6	375	3.40	146	38
25	25	21	66.5	375	2.80	154	32
26	29	22	59.6	375	3.10	144	36
27	37	22	60.7	375	2.40	156	30
28	34	20	58.8	370	1.90	158	34
29	42	14	66.4	375	3.25	178	39
30	44	24	74.5	375	2.75	165	28
31	34	22	76.6	275	3.20	154	32
32	43	20	80.0	375	3.20	140	29

In this problem you should enter the data so that several analyses will be easy to do. First, use independent t tests to compare the time lapse from removal of the Foley catheter to the first voiding of the experimental and control groups. Second, test the second hypothesis by comparing the post–Foley catheter RUVs of the two groups. Third, check the influence of other variables by comparing the two groups on such variables as age and baseline RUVs.

Problem 8-1, cont'd

The effects of bladder reconditioning on urinary dysfunction

The hypotheses predict that the experimental group will have a shorter time lapse and smaller post–Foley catheterization RUVs than the control group. Should you use one-tailed or two-tailed tests?

Comparison of time lapse to first voiding and post–Foley catheterization RUVs: experimental versus control groups (n = 32)

Variable	Experimental		Control		
	$\bar{X}$	SD	$\bar{X}$	SD	t
Time lapse					
Post–Foley catheterization RUVs					

SD, Standard deviation.

You may wish to examine other variables that might account for the results. For example, one group might on average be significantly older than the other, or the baseline RUVs might differ significantly. It is good practice to investigate whether other variables differ between the two groups. If they do, these differences might need to be cited as limitations of the study, or a statistical method of controlling for the variables might be used. (You may wish to consult a book on statistics to learn about analysis of covariance.) If the groups do not differ in any of these other variables, the credibility of your findings is enhanced. Conduct additional t tests to complete the table below.

Comparisons of extraneous variables: experimental versus control (n = 32)

Variable	Experimental		Control		
	$\bar{X}$	SD	$\bar{X}$	SD	t
Age					
Baseline RUVs					
Time Foley catheter in place					
Fluid intake					
Volume voided					

SD, Standard deviation.

Problem 8-1, cont'd

Write a paragraph or two to report the results of this study.

Mann-Whitney U test

The purpose of the Mann-Whitney U test is to compare two independent groups when variables are at least ordinal level and the assumption of a normal distribution cannot be made confidently. Tests may be one or two tailed. For example, data are derived from samples drawn from populations A and B. For a one-tailed test the null hypothesis is:

H_1: distribution$_A$ > distribution$_B$, and p $(a>b)$ > 1/2

or

H_2: distribution$_B$ > distribution$_A$, and p $(b>a)$ > 1/2

For a two-tailed test the null hypothesis is:

H_0: distribution$_A$ = distribution$_B$, and p $(a>b)$ = 1/2

We start with two groups: (A) n_A = number of cases of smaller group, and (B) n_B = number of cases of larger group. Then:

$$N = n_A + n_B$$

The procedure for obtaining the value U is as follows:

Step 1: Rank the entire set of scores, assigning 1 to the lowest score. Assign tied scores the average of the tied ranks.

Step 2: Compute U by the counting or computational method. In the counting method the scores from both groups must be combined and ranked in order of increasing values. For example:

Group A: n = 3   8, 10, 14
Group B: n = 4   5, 7, 9, 12
Combined and ranked:

```
5   7   8   9   10   12   14
B   B   A   B   A    B    A
```

Step 3: Consider B, and count the number of A scores that precede each B
score:
0   0   1   2
Step 4: Add these values to obtain the value of U:
U = 0 = 0 = 1 = 2 = 3
Step 5: Go to the table in Appendix F, choosing the subtable that corresponds
to the smaller group.

For this problem the probability associated with this value of U for a one-
tailed test is $p = .200$. For a two-tailed test it is .400, both nonsignificant if the
usual alpha level of .05 has been used. Note that *smaller* values of U are associated
with more stringent probabilities.

When the alternative computational method is used, the sums of the ranks
are obtained and substituted in the following formulas:

$$U = n_A n_B + \frac{n_A(n_A + 1)}{2} - R_A$$

$$U = n_A n_B + \frac{n_B(n_B + 1)}{2} - R_B$$

where R_A = sum of ranks assigned to A group
R_B = sum of ranks assigned to B group

Since the smaller value of U is always used, only the first formula needs to
be calculated. To check that the smaller value is actually the one that has been
obtained, it is easier to calculate U as follows:

$$U = n_A n_B - U$$

An example follows:

n_A	Rank (n_A)	n_B	Rank (n_B)
124	9	75	7
68	5	60	4
49	3	71	4
46	2	42	6
		91	8
$R_A = 19$		$R_B = 26$	

$$U_B = (4)(5) + \frac{5(5 + 1)}{2} - 26 = 9 \text{ (Group B produces the smaller } U).$$

For relatively large samples (if $n > 20$), compute z by the following formula
and use Appendix A in the book by Siegel (1956) to determine the probability
of the value of U.

$$z = \frac{U - \frac{n_A n_B}{2}}{\sqrt{\frac{(n_A)(n_B)(n_A + n_B + 1)}{12}}}$$

Some investigators wrongly assume that their data are interval merely because they have a large sample, and therefore they use the *t* test instead of the Mann-Whitney U test. Even with large samples the Mann-Whitney U test is the test of choice when data are ordinal. For example, Lawrence and Lawrence (1989) examined the knowledge and attitudes toward acquired immunodeficiency syndrome in two samples: nursing (n = 110) and nonnursing (n = 72) groups. They assumed that the scores from the knowledge and attitude scores were interval and used independent *t* tests to answer their research questions. A more conservative approach would have involved the use of the Mann-Whitney U test with very little loss of power.

Chi-square test for independent samples

In Chapter 7 contingency tables were devised and chi squares were computed to see whether two groups were independent or associated. Obviously the chi-square test can be used to determine whether two or more groups differ with respect to some variable. The proportions of cases from one group in the various cells must be compared with the proportions of cases from the other group. For convenience the formula for computing chi square is repeated, but the example of calculating chi square from this formula is provided in Chapter 7 and should be reviewed:

$$\chi^2 = \frac{\sum_{i=1}^{r} \sum_{j=1}^{k} (O_{ij} - E_{ij})^2}{E_{ij}}$$

For 2 × 2 contingency tables the formula can be simplified:

$$\chi^2 = \sum \frac{(|O_i - E_i| - 0.5)^2}{E_i}$$

The *df* for chi square is always the number of rows minus 1 times the number of columns minus 1. However, the use of computer statistical packages makes these calculations unnecessary.

Problem 8-2

Continuing education needs of geriatric nurses

Educators and directors of nursing in Idaho's long-term care facilities were asked what continuing nursing education topics were needed for nurses who work with elderly patients. The list of topics is an arbitrary one, selected from an actual study completed by Thomas and Price in 1985. Your task is to investigate whether the ratings given by the educators and the directors of nursing differ significantly (at an alpha or *p* value of .05) for any of the topics listed on p. 218.

Problem 8-2, cont'd

Continuing education needs of geriatric nurses

The following scale was used for rating importance of the topics:
0 = no importance
1 = slight importance
2 = moderate importance
3 = great importance
However, the sample for this problem is not large enough to allow computation of chi squares based on the eight cells that would be created if all four ratings were used. (The problem is that cells containing expected frequencies of zero would likely be included, invalidating the meaning of the chi-square statistic.) Thus the categories are "collapsed" into two classes: 1 = no or slight importance and 2 = moderate or great importance.
The list of topics follows:
General physical assessment
Oral health
Functional status
Vision and hearing problems
Nutritional status
Depression
Potential for falls
Misuse of drugs
Hypothermia
Sleep disturbances
Mobility problems
Incontinence
The coding guide for the data is as follows:

Column	Variable
1	ID
2	Group: 1 = nurse educators (NEs), 2 = directors of nursing (DONs)
3-14	Responses to the 12 items (in order): 1 = no or slight importance, 2 = moderate or great importance

The data

ID	Group	IT1	IT2	IT3	IT4	IT5	IT6	IT7	IT8	IT9	IT10	IT11	IT12
01	1	1	2	2	1	2	2	2	2	2	2	2	1
02	1	2	1	1	1	1	2	2	1	2	2	2	2
03	1	1	1	2	2	2	2	2	2	2	2	2	1
04	1	1	1	2	2	1	2	2	1	1	2	1	2
05	1	2	1	1	1	1	1	2	1	1	2	1	2
06	1	2	1	2	2	2	2	1	2	2	1	2	1
07	1	1	1	1	1	2	1	2	1	1	2	1	2
08	1	2	2	2	2	2	2	2	1	2	2	2	1
09	1	1	1	1	1	2	2	2	1	2	1	1	2

Problem 8-2, cont'd

The data

ID	Group	IT1	IT2	IT3	IT4	IT5	IT6	IT7	IT8	IT9	IT10	IT11	IT12
10	1	1	2	2	1	2	2	1	2	1	1	1	1
11	1	1	2	2	2	2	1	2	1	1	1	1	2
12	1	1	2	1	1	2	1	2	2	2	1	1	2
13	1	2	1	2	2	2	1	2	2	1	1	1	2
14	1	2	1	2	2	2	1	2	1	2	2	2	1
15	1	1	2	1	1	2	1	2	1	1	2	2	1
16	1	2	2	2	1	1	2	1	2	2	1	2	1
17	2	1	2	2	2	1	2	1	2	2	1	2	1
18	2	1	1	1	1	1	1	2	2	2	1	1	1
19	2	1	1	2	2	1	2	1	1	2	2	1	2
20	2	2	2	2	1	1	1	1	2	1	1	2	2
21	2	1	2	2	1	1	2	2	1	2	2	1	1
22	2	2	2	1	1	2	2	1	1	2	1	2	1
23	2	1	1	1	1	1	1	1	2	2	2	1	2
24	2	2	1	2	1	1	2	2	1	2	2	1	1
25	2	1	2	2	2	1	2	2	1	1	2	1	2
26	2	1	1	2	1	1	2	1	2	1	2	2	1
27	2	1	2	2	1	1	1	2	2	1	1	2	1
28	2	1	2	2	2	1	2	2	1	2	1	2	2
29	2	2	1	1	2	2	2	1	1	2	1	1	2
30	2	1	2	2	2	1	2	1	2	1	2	2	1
31	2	1	2	2	1	2	2	1	1	2	1	2	1
32	2	2	1	1	1	1	1	1	2	2	2	1	2

Comparisons of ratings of continuing education topics for directors of nursing and for nurse educators (frequencies and chi squares)

Topic	NEs		DONs		
	1	2	1	2	χ^2
General physical assessment					
Oral health					
Functional status					
Vision/hearing problems					
Nutritional status					
Depression					
Potential for falls					
Misuse of drugs					
Hypothermia					
Sleep disturbances					
Mobility problems					
Incontinence					

Continuing education needs of geriatric nurses

Summarize your results in a brief paragraph.

Groups may sometimes be compared to bolster the scientific rigor of a study. For example, Gennaro (1988) used chi squares and t tests for some post hoc analyses when she experienced severe sample attrition, that is, loss of subjects during the course of a study. The question of whether dropouts differ in significant ways from subjects who remain in the study is an important factor in judging the study's validity.

In her study of postpartal anxiety and depression among mothers of preterm and term infants, Gennaro (1988) first recruited mothers of preterm infants who met several criteria (infant admitted to newborn intensive care unit during study period, no congenital anomalies in infant, infant less than 37 weeks' gestational age, and infant weight between 1000 and 2500 g). Her next step was to match each of these subjects with mothers of term infants on the basis of race, parity, type of delivery, and age. Forty-one pairs completed the data collection instruments the first week, but only 10 mothers of term infants and 16 mothers of preterm infants completed all seven questionnaires during the 7 weeks of the study, for a completion rate of only 32%. Gennaro (1988) used chi-square analyses to test for differences between full participants and dropouts in the variables race, type of delivery, type of baby (term or preterm), and parity. No significant differences were found. Thus she demonstrated that no statistically significant differences existed between full participants and dropouts in relation to race, type of delivery, type of baby, and parity. She used t tests to examine the possibility of differences in age, socioeconomic status (SES), and first-week anxiety and depression scores. No significant differences were found in any of these comparisons. Thus any differences between the full participants and the dropouts in the variables age, SES, and first-week anxiety and depression scores were only at a chance level. These analyses supported the investigator's conclusion that the high attrition rate resulted from the burden of weekly data collection rather than from any systematic differences between the continuing participants and the dropouts. Thus she demonstrated that the attrition was unlikely to have affected the results of her study.

Fisher's Exact test

Fisher's Exact test is the test of choice when samples are too small to use chi-square analysis, when the contingency table is 2 × 2, and when one or more cells contain a zero.

The steps used in comparing groups with Fisher's Exact test are as follows:

Step 1: Cast the frequencies for each group in a 2 × 2 contingency table such as that illustrated in Fig. 8-1. Enter the marginal totals for the rows and columns and the grand total.

Step 2: Use the table of factorials (!) (Fig. 8-2) to substitute proper values in the formula that follows:

$$p = \frac{(A + B)!\,(C + D)!\,(A + C)!\,(B + D)!}{N!\,A!\,B!\,C!\,D!}$$

NOTE: Calculating a factorial (!) involves multiplying every number up to and including the stated number together. For example, (6!) is

N	N!
1	1
2	2
3	6
4	24
5	120
6	720
7	5040
8	40320
9	362880
10	3628800
11	39916800
12	479001600
13	6227020800
14	87178291200
15	1307674368000
16	20922789888000
17	355687428096000
18	6402373705728000
19	121645100408832000
20	2432902008176640000

	Agree	Disagree	
Group 1	10	15	25
Group 2	24	11	35
	34	26	60
	68	52	

Fig. 8-1 A 2 × 2 contingency table.

Fig. 8-2 Table of factorials.

obtained by multiplying $1 \times 2 \times 3 \times 4 \times 5 \times 6$. When a fraction is used as it is here, cancellation of like members should precede calculation of the products.

Step 3: This is the exact probability associated with the distribution of frequencies displayed in the 2×2 contingency table. Compare this value with the preset alpha level. If it is equal to or smaller than alpha, the results are statistically significant at that level.

Siegel (1956) describes a method of using tables with the cell frequencies to determine significance level (not exact probabilities). However, for small samples the use of the table of factorials makes computation by the preceding formula relatively simple.

COMPARING TWO DEPENDENT GROUPS

Table 8-2 summarizes the tests commonly used to compare two related or dependent groups, which are presented in this section.

Table 8-2 Statistical tests used for comparing two dependent groups

Statistic	Abbreviation	Conditions for use
t test	t	Random sampling; normally distributed data with equal variances; interval level data; questions about differences between means of matched samples
Sign test		Random sampling; distribution-free, ordinal level, continuous data; different procedures for samples under and over n = 25; questions about differences of medians of matched samples
McNemar test	χ^2	Random sampling; distribution-free, nominal or ordinal data from a pretest, posttest design that can be cast in a four-cell table; questions about differences in the magnitude of change from pretest to posttest

Paired t tests

As noted earlier, some investigators exercise careful control in their studies by comparing two matched samples. In some cases data are obtained twice from the same subjects, as in the case of pretests and posttests. In other cases subjects are matched on one or more relevant variables and one member of the pair is assigned to each group.

The df for a paired t test is $n - 1$ where n is the number of pairs being examined, and the formula for t is:

$$t = \frac{\overline{D}_{X-Y}}{\sqrt{\dfrac{\Sigma d^2}{n(n-1)}}}$$

where X and Y = pairs of scores
$\overline{D}_{X-Y}$ = the mean difference between paired scores
d^2 = the sum of squared deviation difference scores
n = the number of pairs of scores

Computation of paired t tests is commonly available in computer statistical programs, but an example of calculating this statistic illustrates its meaning more clearly.

Subject	X	Y	D(X − Y)	d	d²
1	94	102	−8	−4	16
2	101	108	−7	−3	9
3	98	100	−2	2	4
4	100	110	−10	−6	36
5	87	92	−5	−1	1
6	101	94	7	11	121
7	86	92	−6	−2	4
8	91	98	−7	−3	9
9	107	110	−3	1	1
10	105	104	1	5	25

$\overline{D}_{X-Y} = -40/10 = -4$ $\Sigma D_{X-Y} = -40$ $\Sigma d^2 = 226$

$$t = \frac{-4}{\sqrt{226/10(10-1)}} = -1.59$$

Consulting the table in Appendix E, we see that for this n and an alpha of .05 the t value must equal or exceed 2.262 to be statistically significant. Note that the same table used for the independent t test is used, but the df dictates that it be entered differently. The computed t test is not significant at .05. The negative sign indicates that the Y scores were larger than the X scores, but in this case the difference was due only to chance.

How does use of matched pairs affect the ease of obtaining statistical significance?

Probably the most common use of the paired *t* test is for pretesting and posttesting subjects in experimental studies. In a study of the affective states of mothers of preterm infants, Brooten and colleagues (1988) used Zuckerman and Lubin's Multiple Affect Adjective Checklist, Revised (MAACL) (1965) to measure anxiety, depression, and hostility at two times: when the infant was discharged and when the infant was 9 months old. In a sample of 47 subjects the investigators found that the anxiety and depression measures were significantly higher at discharge than at 9 months. There was no significant difference in the hostility scores. In addition, a subset of 12 mothers was tested shortly after the births of their perterm infants. There were no significant differences on any of the scores compared with the discharge scores. Paired *t* tests were used for all of these analyses.

The investigators also checked for possible differences on the three scores (anxiety, depression, and hostility) based on marital status, maternal age, education, parity, socioeconomic status, and length of the infant's hospital stay. Parity and length of hospital stay showed differences at the point of infant discharge. Multiparas were significantly more depressed than primiparas; however, there were no differences in anxiety and hostility. (There were no differences at all when the infants were 9 months old.) Mothers whose infants remained in the hospital longer than the mean of 51 days were significantly less depressed at discharge than mothers whose babies had shorter hospital stays. There were no other differences at discharge and no differences at 9 months.

Would the investigators use independent or paired *t* tests for these last analyses? Why?

Are the comparisons for marital status, age, education, parity, socioeconomic status, and length of the infant's hospital stay an experimental or ex post facto design? Why?

Comparisons of anxiety, depression, and hostility in mothers of preterm infants over time

A team of nurse clinicians decided to replicate the study about mothers of preterm infants described above except that these nurses omitted the comparisons based on age, marital status, parity, and so forth. They collected data after the birth, at the time of the infants' discharges, and when the infants were 9 months old. Complete data were obtained for 28 mothers. The research questions were as follows:

1. Is there a significant difference in (a) anxiety scores, (b) depression scores, and (c) hostility scores for mothers of preterm infants at birth and at the time of discharge of the infants?
2. Is there a significant difference in (a) anxiety scores, (b) depression scores, and (c) hostility scores for mothers of preterm infants at birth and at the age of 9 months?
3. Is there a significant difference in (a) anxiety scores, (b) depression scores, and (c) hostility scores for mothers of preterm infants at the time of each infant's discharge and at the age of 9 months?

Possible scores for anxiety (A) range from 1 to 28. Depression scores (D) range from 1 to 40, and hostility scores (H) range from 1 to 28. In all cases, the higher the score, the stronger the characteristic. Data for the 28 mothers are tabulated below.

The data

	Birth			Discharge			9 months		
Subject	A	D	H	A	D	H	A	D	H
01	14	24	16	12	20	13	13	22	15
02	10	18	12	18	22	14	14	17	11
03	15	32	16	16	18	16	15	14	15
04	20	34	23	18	28	24	19	19	17
05	11	12	10	15	15	09	12	13	11
06	13	22	12	23	29	11	14	20	12
07	19	37	23	15	30	20	13	23	15
08	12	10	08	16	12	10	11	10	10
09	18	09	06	20	10	08	14	07	08
10	15	15	11	19	17	10	15	14	11
11	09	09	05	12	13	06	08	08	05
12	17	13	03	19	17	04	16	14	05
13	14	16	10	18	19	10	14	15	09
14	18	19	12	22	16	11	16	14	10
15	15	28	12	20	22	10	13	15	10
16	12	10	14	17	11	13	15	10	11
17	17	17	13	19	22	11	12	18	09
18	20	12	03	20	11	04	16	10	03

Comparisons of anxiety, depression, and hostility in mothers of preterm infants over time

The data

Subject	Birth			Discharge			9 months		
	A	D	H	A	D	H	A	D	H
19	13	19	10	16	24	11	14	18	09
20	14	20	12	18	28	13	16	22	13
21	19	33	12	21	27	13	12	21	12
22	15	19	08	19	29	10	14	19	09
23	13	20	12	19	26	11	15	22	10
24	18	22	10	20	28	11	17	22	10
25	11	12	07	17	19	10	15	12	09
26	18	27	17	20	29	16	12	21	14
27	16	21	11	19	28	10	17	25	11
28	12	27	09	19	31	10	16	23	09

Compute descriptive statistics and paired t tests to complete the tables below from your computer output.

Comparisons of anxiety, depression, and hostility scores for mothers of preterm infants at three points in time (n = 28)

Variable	Birth		Discharge		9 Months	
	$\bar{X}$	SD	$\bar{X}$	SD	$\bar{X}$	SD
Anxiety						
Depression						
Hostility						

SD, Standard deviation.

What do these results mean?

In the following table, use asterisks to denote any t values that are statistically significant at an alpha of .05. Add a footnote to your table if you use any asterisks.

Paired t tests for anxiety, depression, and hostility scores

	t value		
Variable	**1**	**2**	**3**
Anxiety			
Depression			
Hostility			

1, Birth versus discharge; *2*, birth versus 9 months; *3*, discharge versus 9 months.

How can you interpret these results?

Sign test

The sign test is a nonparametric test useful for comparing the scores of two dependent groups when the level of measurement is at least ordinal and when no assumptions about the distribution are made. The variable being examined must have a continuous distribution. The power of the test is quite high for small samples but declines as the sample size increases. This discussion applies only to samples of less than 25. It tests the null hypothesis:

$$p(X_A > X_B) = p(X_A < X_B) = 1/2$$

where X_A and X_B are the pairs of scores. If this null hypothesis were true, about half the differences between the X_A and X_B would be positive and half would be negative; the null hypothesis is rejected if either the positive or the negative differences are dominant at a nonchance level.

The data are tabulated as pairs of scores, and the sign of the difference between each pair is recorded. The value of N is the number of pairs whose differences show a sign. The value of x is the number of fewer signs. Use the table in Appendix G using the N and x to determine the one-tailed probability for the sign test.

Since the sign test is relatively simple to calculate for small samples, a concrete illustration is included. Suppose that parents of children scheduled for appendectomies were asked to rate their children on prehospitalization anxiety. The

ratings ranged from 1 = little anxiety to 5 = great anxiety. It was hypothesized
that mothers' ratings would be higher than fathers' ratings.

Couple	Mother's rating	Father's rating	Difference	Sign
1	4	2	2	+
2	3	3	0	0
3	5	4	1	+
4	3	4	−1	−
5	4	2	2	+
6	5	2	3	+
7	2	2	0	0
8	4	3	1	+
9	3	1	2	+
10	4	5	−1	−
11	3	1	2	+
12	3	4	−1	−
13	3	3	0	0
14	2	3	−1	−
15	5	4	1	+

The value of N (the number of couples whose ratings differed) is 12. The value
of x (the number of fewer signs) is 4 (negative signs for couples No. 4, 10, 12,
and 14). Entering the table in Appendix G with these values, we find the probability of this one-tailed test to be .194; thus the research hypothesis that the
mothers' ratings would be higher than those of the fathers was not supported.

Problem 8-4

Ratings of interventions by parents of children with Down syndrome

In an attempt to gain a better understanding of how parents deal with the birth
and rearing of handicapped children, Damrosch and Perry (1989) compared
selected variables of mothers and fathers in families having a child with Down
syndrome. Their review of the literature revealed a paucity of studies
regarding fathers. However, they cited studies that showed the following: (1)
fathers focus more on instrumental concerns (such as financial concerns)
whereas mothers are more concerned with emotional strains, (2) fathers
typically maintain a low level of caregiving of handicapped children, (3) a
father's most important role may lie in the support he provides for the mother,
and (4) mothers report more ups and downs, as well as more negative
consequences, than fathers do.

There were three distinct phases in this study. In phase 1 the investigators
asked parents to choose one of two graphs as more nearly representing their
own responses to the birth of a child with Down syndrome. One graph
started with a high point (before diagnosis of Down syndrome) when the

parents felt "just great," followed by a sharp dip representing "awful" feelings when they learned that their child had Down syndrome. This low point was followed by a steady rise representing a slow, gradual recovery from the crisis. The second graph depicted the same first two points—high before the diagnosis and low after it. Instead of a steady recovery, however, the low point was followed by a series of moderate peaks and deep valleys, representing periods of moderately positive feelings interspersed with lows of awful feelings. Content and concurrent validities were established for use of these graphs. Results revealed that 83% of the fathers selected the steady improvement graph and 68% of the mothers selected the chronic periodic crises graph.

Damrosch and Perry (1989) also gathered data from both parents on a Parental Coping Scale, adapted from Folkman and Lazarus' Ways of Coping Scale (1980). High scores indicate a high frequency of using the coping strategies and are not related to the strategies' success or failure. Mothers scored significantly higher than fathers on four of the measure's eight subscales: expression of negative affect, self-blaming, communication of feelings, and special feelings (such as feeling embarrassed in public). The subscales that showed no significant differences were cognitive restructuring, wish-fulfilling fantasy, information-seeking, and minimization of threat.

The investigators used t tests. Would independent or paired t tests be more appropriate? Why?

In phase 3 of their study, Damrosch and Perry (1989) used a scale listing seven professional approaches to be evaluated by each parent on a scale of 1 (not useful) to 5 (extremely useful). Using paired t tests, they found the mothers' means to be higher than the fathers' means on the following approaches: 3, encouraging expression of sadness; 5, allowing parents to be weak; and 7, giving parents positive feedback. There were no differences for the remaining four items: 1, assuming cheerful attitude toward parents; 2, encouraging parents not to dwell on the negative; 4, encouraging parents to be strong; and 6, giving parents chances to escape the situation temporarily.

For this problem you are to partially replicate *only phase 3 regarding approaches 3, 5, and 7 of the study, using a somewhat modified approach.* You will use the scale of 1 to 5, but you view these data as no better than ordinal data. Since the data are paired, you decide to use the sign test. The parents' ratings are tabulated on p. 230. Complete the table and use the sign test to determine whether any significant differences exist.

Problem 8-4, cont'd

Ratings of interventions by parents of children with Down syndrome

Parents' ratings of professional approaches used to assist parents of handicapped children (n = 16)

Sub-ject pair	Approach 3				Approach 5				Approach 7			
	Mother	Father	Differ-ence	Sign	Mother	Father	Differ-ence	Sign	Mother	Father	Differ-ence	Sign
01	5	3			4	4			3	3		
02	4	3			4	2			4	1		
03	3	3			5	3			4	2		
04	5	5			4	1			3	2		
05	3	1			5	5			4	2		
06	4	4			4	3			3	3		
07	3	1			2	2			4	2		
08	2	2			5	3			3	4		
09	2	4			2	3			2	4		
10	4	3			4	4			5	4		
11	5	4			2	1			3	2		
12	3	5			2	2			3	2		
13	4	4			3	5			4	5		
14	3	1			2	2			3	4		
15	4	3			5	4			3	3		
16	3	3			4	3			4	3		

Complete the table to determine the sign test results for each approach. Use the directional hypothesis that the mothers' scores are higher for each approach.

What are your results?

Approach 3

Approach 5

Approach 7

Problem 8-4, cont'd

What conclusions can you draw?

McNemar test for significance of changes

When an experiment is designed to use each subject as his or her own control and the data are nominal or ordinal, the McNemar test is a useful choice. Suppose that we are dealing with an experimental treatment that changes some subjects' opinions from "agree" to "disagree" and vice versa. Fig. 8-3 illustrates the possibilities, showing that the subjects in cells *B* and *C* retained their original opinions whereas those in cells *A* and *D* changed their opinions. In a totally chance situation (that is, in the case that the null hypothesis is supported), we would expect 1/2 (*A* + *D*) to change in one direction, and 1/2 (*A* + *D*) to change in the other direction. This is parallel to computing a chi square using only data from cells *A* and *D*:

$$\chi^2 = \sum_{A,D} \frac{(O - E)^2}{E}$$

	Disagree	Agree
Agree	A	B
Disagree	C	D

Fig. 8-3 Contingency table for McNemar test.

Simplifying this expression produces the following:

$$\chi^2 = \frac{(A - D)^2}{A + D}$$

The *df* for this statistic is 1. However, this use of chi square, which is a continuous distribution, must be corrected for use with a discrete distribution. Yates (1934) provided such a correction:

$$\chi^2 = \frac{(|A - D| - 1)^2}{A + D}$$

The *df* remains 1, and the chi-square table in Appendix D is used to check for significance.

COMPARING THREE OR MORE INDEPENDENT GROUPS

Different statistics must be used when three or more independent groups are to be compared. Table 8-3 summarizes the tests and the conditions for their use, which are presented in this section.

One-way analysis of variance (ANOVA)

To compare variables of three or more groups where the dependent variable(s) are at least interval, the distribution is normal, the variance among groups is equal, and random sampling has been used, the simplest approach is a one-way analysis of variance (ANOVA). The test statistic is called the F ratio. It compares systematic variance with nonsystematic variance as a way of determining whether differences among groups can be attributed to chance. The research question is whether the variance from the independent variable contributes a significant portion of the variance, which also includes variance re-

Table 8-3 Statistics used in comparing three or more independent groups

Statistical test	Abbreviation	Conditions for proper use
Analysis of variance	F ratio	Random sampling; interval level data; normal distribution; homogeneity of variance
Kruskal-Wallis one-way analysis of variance	H	Random sampling, ordinal level data; distribution-free; continuous data
Chi square	χ^2	Random sampling; nominal level data; distribution-free; questions about discrete categories; same as test for two groups

sulting from measurement error, fatigue, mood, and so forth. The null hypothesis states that the population means for three or more groups will be the same or will differ at only a chance level. The research hypothesis states that these means will differ at a nonchance level.

Step 1: Calculate the sum of squares for between groups $(SS)_B$, which represents the sum of squared deviations of the individual group means from the grand mean. The grand mean is the mean of all scores disregarding group membership.

$$SS_B = \frac{(\Sigma X_A)^2}{n_A} + \frac{(\Sigma X_B)^2}{n_B} + \frac{(\Sigma X_C)^2}{n_C} + \ldots - \frac{(\Sigma X)^2}{N}$$

Step 2: Calculate the sum of squares within groups $(SS)_W$, which is derived from the sum of squared deviations of each individual score from its own group mean.

$$SS_W = \left[\Sigma X_A^2 - \frac{(\Sigma X_A)^2}{n_A} \right] + \left[\Sigma X_B^2 - \frac{(\Sigma X_B)^2}{n_B} \right] + \left[\Sigma X_C^2 - \frac{(\Sigma X_C)^2}{n_C} \right] + \ldots$$

Step 3: Divide each sum of squares by its degrees of freedom. For between-groups, this df is the number of groups minus 1. For the mean squares calculation, divide the sums of squares by the respective degrees of freedom.

$$MS_B = \frac{SS_B}{df_B} \qquad MS_W = \frac{SS_W}{df_W}$$

where

$$df_B = \frac{SS_B}{k-1}$$

$$df_W = \frac{SS_W}{N-k}$$

Step 4: Divide the MS_B by the MS_W to obtain the F ratio.

$$\frac{MS_B}{MS_W} = F$$

Step 5: Compare this F ratio with the values in Appendix H by locating the column headed by df_B and finding the row corresponding to the df_W. If you set the alpha at .05 and the df_B were 3 and the df_W were 24, the computed F ratio would have to equal or exceed 3.01 to be statistically significant at .05.

Suppose a control group *(A)* were compared with two experimental groups *(B* and *C)* to test the efficacy of two different nursing interventions in improving compliance with medication regimens among epileptic patients at a large university medical center. A small portion of the data will be used to illustrate the computation of the F ratio.

Group A		Group B		Group C	
X_A	X_A^2	X_B	X_B^2	X_C	X_C^2
17	289	23	529	27	729
22	484	26	676	24	576
16	256	31	961	23	529
23	529	25	625	21	441
20	400	21	441	29	841
13	169	22	484	27	729
26	676	29	841	33	1089
15	225	23	529	30	900
25	625	28	784	22	484
21	441	19	361	20	400

$\Sigma X_A = 198$ $\Sigma X_A^2 = 4094$ $\Sigma X_B = 247$ $\Sigma X_B^2 = 6672$ $\Sigma X_C = 256$ $\Sigma X_C^2 = 6718$

$\overline{X}_A = 19.8$ $\overline{X}_B = 24.7$ $\overline{X}_C = 25.6$

Sum of all scores $\Sigma X = 701$
Grand mean $\Sigma X/30 = 23.37$
Sum of squared scores $\Sigma X^2 = 17484$
Sum of scores squared $(\Sigma X)^2 = 491,401$

$$SS_B = \frac{198^2}{10} + \frac{247^2}{10} + \frac{256^2}{10} - \frac{491,401}{30} = 194.90$$

$$SS_W = 4094 - \frac{(198)^2}{10} + 6672 - \frac{(247)^2}{10} + 6718 - \frac{(256)^2}{10} = 909.1$$

$MS_B = 194.90/2 = 97.45$
$MS_w = 909.1/27 = 33.67$
F ratio $= 97.45/33.67 = 2.89$

Consulting the table in Appendix H, we find that at $df = 2,27$, the F ratio must equal or exceed 3.35 to be statistically significant at .05. Since our computed F ratio is smaller than this number, it is not significant at .05.

Analysis of variance can establish only that some differences exist in the data and does not point to the source of the differences. Several post hoc tests have been designed for exploring the source of differences once a significant F ratio has been obtained. Scheffe (1959) devised a simple approach that is applicable under a wide variety of conditions. It can be used when there are groups of unequal sizes and even when there are departures from the requirements of a normal distribution and homogeneity of variance (Hays, 1981). Scheffe's test is a systematic way of comparing all pairs of means. The formula for Scheffe's test is as follows (Shelley, 1984):

$$S = \sqrt{(k - 1)F}\sqrt{\frac{2\,MS_w}{n}}$$

Since computer programs that produce analyses of variance can also produce values for Scheffe's test, there is no need to learn the computational procedures.

An example of using Scheffe's test is illustrated in Fig. 8-4. In this example

SOURCE	D.F.	SUM OF SQUARES	MEAN SQUARES	F RATIO	F PROB.
BETWEEN GROUPS	2	260.6409	130.3204	4.2607	.0280
WITHIN GROUPS	21	642.3175	30.5865		
TOTAL	23	902.9583			

GROUP	COUNT	MEAN	STANDARD DEVIATION	STANDARD ERROR	MINIMUM	MAXIMUM	95 PCT CONF INT FOR MEAN
Grp 1	8	34.5000	7.9102	2.7967	21.0000	46.0000	27.8869 TO 41.1131
Grp 2	9	42.1111	2.9345	.9782	38.0000	47.0000	39.8555 TO 44.3667
Grp 3	7	40.2857	4.7509	1.7957	33.0000	48.0000	35.8919 TO 44.6796
TOTAL	24	39.0417	6.2657	1.2790	21.0000	48.0000	36.3959 TO 41.6874

ANOVA

-----------------------------ONEWAY-----------------------------

Variable DM2
By Variable TRT
MULTIPLE RANGE TEST

1 'CONTROL' 2 'EXPER1' 3 'EXPER2'

SCHEFFE PROCEDURE
RANGES FOR THE 0.050 LEVEL -
  3.72   3.72

THE RANGES ABOVE ARE TABLE RANGES.
THE VALUE ACTUALLY COMPARED WITH MEAN(J)-MEAN(I) IS..
  3.9107 * RANGE * DSQRT (1/N(I) + 1/J(J))
(*) DENOTES PAIRS OF GROUPS SIGNIFICANTLY DIFFERENT AT THE 0.050 LEVEL

```
           G G G
           r r r
           p p p

           1 3 2
Mean     Group
34.5000   Grp 1
40.2857   Grp 3
42.1111   Grp 2   *
```

Fig. 8-4 Illustration of SPSS-X output for ANOVA and Scheffe test.

three groups were compared on a single outcome measure. Here the ANOVA table indicates significant differences among the three groups because the F ratio of 4.26 (*df* = 2,21) has a probability level of .0280. The investigator has information about the means: group 1's mean was 34.50; group 2's mean was 42.11; group 3's mean was 40.28. This information suggests that the difference among the three groups is probably due to the difference between the means of groups 1 and 2. This is only speculation, and Scheffe's test is required to furnish evidence to this effect.

Problem 8-5

Retirement attitudes and health status

This problem was suggested by a study conducted by Daly and Futrell (1989) titled "Retirement Attitudes and Health Status." They studied the extent to which retirement attitudes influenced selected health status variables among preretired and retired men and women. Atchley's 20-item semantic differential (1974) was used to measure retirement attitudes. This tool consists of 20 bipolar adjectives such as "idle-busy." The possible range of scores is 20 to 100, with higher scores indicating more positive attitudes toward retirement. For health status the Duke–University of North Carolina Health Profile (Parkerson, Gehlbach, Wagner, and James, 1981) was used. It consists of four subscales: symptom status scale (26 items), physical scale (9 items), emotion scale (23 items), and social health scale (5 items); higher scores on each of these subscales indicate better health status.

In this problem the focus is on retired men, 50 to 70 years of age, who are not institutionalized and have agreed to participate in the study. The men are divided into three equal-sized groups (low, middle, and high) based on their scores on the attitudes toward retirement instrument. Since the health status scores are regarded as interval data, the test statistic will be the F ratio obtained from performing an analysis of variance.

Data on the ages and the social status of subjects in prior studies were also gathered to check on the possible influence these variables might have on health status variables.

The coding guide for this problem is as follows:

Column	Variable
1	ID
2	Age in years (AGE)
3	Social status of job before retirement (SSJ): 1 = low, 2 = middle, 3 = high
4	Retirement attitude group (RET): 1 = low, 2 = middle, 3 = high
5	Symptom status scale (SSS) scores (0-26)
6	Physical scale (PHS) (0-9)
7	Emotion scale (ESS) (0-23)
8	Social health scale (SHS) (0-5)
9	Total health status (THS) scale scores (0-63)

Problem 8-5, cont'd

The data

					Column			
1 ID	2 AGE	3 SSJ	4 RET	5 SSS	6 PHS	7 ESS	8 SHS	9 THS
01	64	3	1	12	5	13	2	32
02	70	2	1	10	5	11	4	30
03	68	1	1	20	6	15	3	44
04	57	3	1	12	6	14	1	33
05	62	2	1	21	4	19	5	49
06	68	2	1	22	6	16	4	48
07	67	2	1	16	2	10	2	30
08	59	3	1	22	7	12	3	44
09	54	2	1	14	4	19	3	40
10	66	2	1	18	6	15	4	43
11	59	2	2	19	7	17	4	47
12	61	3	2	22	4	12	5	43
13	70	2	2	21	4	15	3	43
14	67	2	2	17	6	14	4	41
15	60	3	2	18	7	19	4	48
16	54	3	2	19	6	17	3	45
17	58	3	2	20	7	15	4	46
18	57	2	2	18	6	17	4	45
19	69	2	2	17	4	16	3	40
20	63	2	2	18	6	15	4	43
21	65	1	3	21	5	17	5	48
22	60	2	3	19	7	18	3	47
23	67	2	3	21	7	19	4	51
24	51	3	3	19	5	19	4	47
25	63	1	3	21	5	20	5	51
26	58	3	3	18	8	17	5	48
27	55	3	3	16	4	15	3	38
28	65	3	3	22	5	13	4	44
29	61	2	3	20	7	16	4	47
30	55	2	3	18	8	20	5	51

For this problem a one-way analysis of variance should be computed for each subscale score and for the total score with retirement attitude group used as the grouping variable. Use an alpha of .05, and construct ANOVA tables to report findings from these analyses. The form of the first table is shown on p. 238.

Problem 8-5, cont'd

Retirement attitudes and health status

ANOVA for the symptom status scale scores by level of attitude toward retirement

Source	df	Sum of squares	Mean squares	F
Between groups				
Within groups				
TOTAL				

Kruskal-Wallis one-way analysis of variance

When the level of measurement of dependent variables is only ordinal, the Kruskal-Wallis test is used as a nonparametric alternative to the F ratio. It is distribution-free but requires that the dependent variable(s) be continuously distributed. This test has a power efficiency of about 95% of the F ratio. The numbers in the groups need not be equal. The formula for computing H, the test statistic, is as follows (Siegel, 1956):

$$H = \frac{12}{N(N + 1)} \sum_{j=1}^{K} \frac{R_j^2}{n_j^2} - 3(N + 1)$$

where k = the number of groups
   n_j = the number of subjects in the jth group
   N = the total number of subjects
   R_j = the sum of ranks in the jth group (column)

This test statistic is distributed as chi square when the group sizes are five or more. In such a case, $df = k - 1$ where k is the number of groups and Appendix D is used. If H equals or exceeds the table value at a given alpha, it is significant at that level. If five or fewer subjects are in each group, Appendix I is used. Siegel (1956) describes procedures to use when ties are a factor; however, the example below contains no ties.

Step 1: Combine scores from all groups and assign a rank to each. Tabulate scores and ranks of each group in separate columns.

Step 2: Add the ranks in each column, assigning R_A to the first set, R_B to the second set, and so on.

Step 3: Square the sum of ranks for each group and divide each R by its n. Add these quotients.

Step 4: Use the formula above, substituting your answer from step 3 in the equation for $\Sigma R_j^2/n_j^2$ to compute the value of H.

Step 5: Compare the computed value of H with the appropriate table value.

Group A scores	Rank order of scores	Group B scores	Rank order of scores	Group C scores	Rank order of scores
34	4	42	11	36	6
45	12	41	10	37	7
46	13	48	14	51	15
39	8	33	3	40	9
35	5	32	2	30	1

$\Sigma R_A = 42$ $\Sigma R_B = 40$ $\Sigma R_C = 38$

$\Sigma R_A^2/n_A = 352.8$ $\Sigma R_B^2/n_B = 320$ $\Sigma R_C^2/n_C = 288.8$

$\Sigma R_j^2/n_j = 961.6$

$$H = \frac{12}{(15)(16)} (961.8) - 3(16) = 0.09$$

Consulting Appendix I, we see that our H would have to equal or exceed 5.66 to be statistically significant at .05. Since the value of H was only 0.09, we must conclude that there are only chance differences among the groups.

Chi-square test for three or more independent groups
The approach used with chi square for three or more independent groups is exactly the same as that for two independent groups. The data are cast into a contingency table, and the test statistic is computed from the observed and expected frequencies.

COMPARING THREE OR MORE DEPENDENT GROUPS
Table 8-4 summarizes the tests commonly used to compare data from three or more dependent groups.

Table 8-4 Statistical tests used for comparing three or more dependent groups

Statistic	Abbreviation	Conditions for proper use
Analysis of variance by repeated measures	F ratio	Random sampling; interval level data; homogeneity of variance; normal distribution
Friedman two-way analysis of variance	Σ_r^2	Random sampling; ordinal level data; distribution-free
Cochran's Q	Q	Random sampling; nominal level data; distribution-free

Analysis of variance by repeated measures
We have seen that matching subjects and using subjects as their own controls are methods that reduce error and increase the precision of research. When there are three or more matched groups or when three or more measures have been gathered from the same subjects, analysis of variance by repeated measures may be used. The only difference in the computation of the F ratio from the ANOVA discussed earlier is that the sum of squares within is reduced. A sum of squares for subjects is calculated, and this value is subtracted from the sum of squares within. The sum of squares of subjects is calculated as follows (Shelley, 1984):

$$SS = \frac{(X + X + \ldots X)^2 + (Y + Y + \ldots Y)^2 + (Z + Z + \ldots Z)^2}{k} - \left(\frac{\Sigma X,Y,Z}{N}\right)^2$$

where $(X_1 + X_2 + \ldots X)^2$ = squared sum of all subject one's scores
$(Y_1 + Y_2 + \ldots Y)^2$ = squared sum of all subject two's scores
$(Z_1 + Z_2 + \ldots Z)^2$ = squared sum of all subject three's scores
k = number of repeated measures per subject
$(\Sigma X,Y,Z)^2$ = sum of all scores across subjects and measures, squared
N = total number of observations
$df = N - 1$

Table 8-5 Two-way table representing the scores of 30 adolescent subjects for Friedman two-way analysis of variance

| | Teaching treatment | | |
Set	A	B	C
01	2	3	1
02	6	4	5
03	7	8	9
04	11	10	12
05	14	13	15
06	16	18	17
07	20	19	21
08	22	24	23
09	27	25	26
10	28	29	30

Friedman two-way analysis of variance

The Friedman two-way analysis of variance is a useful alternative to analysis of repeated measures when the data are only ordinal. The matching may be achieved by using subjects as their own controls or by matching subjects on relevant variables. Suppose we wish to study the differences in adolescents' health promotion attitudes achieved by three different teaching methods, A, B, and C. We might obtain 10 sets of three adolescents each, matched for gender, age, and educational development scores. One adolescent from each of the 10 sets is randomly assigned to each of the three groups. In Table 8-5 we see that the rows represent the matched sets of subjects and the columns represent the three teaching treatments.

After subjects are randomly assigned to the three teaching treatments, the interventions are implemented and the subjects are tested on an Attitudes Toward Health Promotion instrument. Imagine that each subject's number is now replaced with his or her score in Table 8-5. For example, the first three sets might have the following scores:

Set 01	17	22	26
Set 02	22	19	25
Set 03	27	23	24

Step 1: Rank each row *separately*; the lowest score in each row is given a rank of 1, the middle score is given a rank of 2, and the highest score in each row is given a rank of 3. (The test could be done as well by ranking from highest to lowest.)

Step 2: Add the ranks for each column, ΣR_x, as shown in Table 8-6.

Step 3: Compute the test statistic χ^2, using the following formula (Siegel, 1956):

$$\chi_r^2 = \frac{12}{Nk\,(k+1)} \sum_{j=1}^{k} (R_j)^2 - 3N(k+1)$$

Table 8-6 Ranks of adolescent subjects' scores by row

	Ranks		
Set	A	B	C
01	2	1	3
02	1	2	3
03	1	3	2
04	2	1	3
05	3	1	2
06	2	3	1
07	2	1	3
08	1	2	3
09	3	2	1
10	2	1	3
SUMS $\Sigma(R_x)$	19	17	24

where N = the number of rows
  k = the number of columns
  ΣR_j = the sum of ranks in the jth column

$$\chi_r^2 = \frac{12}{30(4)} [(19)^2 + (17)^2 + (24)^2] - (3)(10)(4) = 2.6$$

This value of χ_r^2 has a probability larger than the alpha of .05; therefore the hypothesis of no differences must be accepted.

For samples of 10 and more, the $df = (k - 1)$, and the test statistic is compared with the value of chi square at that df in Appendix D. For smaller samples, special tables for χ_r^2 in statistics books such as Siegel's (1956) can be consulted.

Cochran's Q

Cochran's Q test permits a determination of whether the frequencies or proportions of three or more related samples differ significantly among themselves. It is most useful for nominal data or dichotomized ordinal data such as yes or no responses. The computational formula for Cochran's Q is as follows (Siegel, 1956):

$$Q = \frac{(k - 1) \left\{ k \sum_{j=1}^{k} G_j^2 - \left(\sum_{j=1}^{k} G_j \right)^2 \right\}}{k \sum_{i=1}^{k} L_i - \sum_{i=1}^{N} L_i^2}$$

where G_j = total number of positive responses in the jth column
  $\overline{G}$ = the mean of G
  L_i = total number of positive responses in the ith row

Since the sampling distribution of Q can be represented by the chi-square distribution, the significance of Q is determined by checking the computed value with a chi-square table (Appendix D).

Step 1: Assign a 1 to each yes or success and 0 to each no or failure. Tabulate these scores in a $k \times N$ table where k is the number of columns and N is the number of cases in each of the k groups.

Step 2: Substitute the observed values in the formula above and compute Q.

Step 3: Use $df = k - 1$ and compare the Q with the table value in a chi-square table at the predetermined level of significance.

Suppose a nurse wants to investigate the effects of talking through the labor experience with new mothers within 2 days of the birth. Criteria are set up for the study (first baby, normal vaginal delivery, intent to keep baby, full-term, and so forth) so that three matched groups of 10 each are to be interviewed and tested 3 weeks later with the question, "Are you satisfied with the way you handled labor and delivery?" For one group the nurse interviewed each mother warmly with questions designed to elicit the full account of her childbirth experience. For the second group she interviewed the mothers by asking in a matter-of-fact way how the childbirth went. No further attempts were made to elicit a recollection of their experiences. For the third group the interviewer merely asked each new mother how she was getting along with the new baby. Three weeks later yes (1) and no (0) responses were tabulated as follows. The L column lists the number of yes responses. Each of these values must be squared and summed.

ID (set)	Group 1	Group 2	Group 3	L	L^2
1	0	0	0	0	0
2	1	1	0	2	4
3	1	0	0	1	1
4	1	1	0	2	4
5	1	0	0	1	1
6	1	1	1	3	9
7	1	1	0	2	4
8	1	0	0	1	1
9	1	1	0	2	4
10	1	0	0	1	1

$$\Sigma G_1 = 9 \qquad \Sigma G_2 = 5 \qquad \Sigma G_3 = 1 \qquad \Sigma L = 15 \qquad \Sigma L^2 = 29$$

Substituting these values in the formula, we solve for Q:

$$Q = \frac{(3 - 1)\ 3\{(9)^2 + (5)^2 + (1)^2\} - (15)^2}{(3)(15) - 29} = 26.06$$

The probability of a Q of 26.06 occurring by chance is less than .001 according to table values of chi square with df of 2. Thus the researcher concludes that the frequencies (or proportions) of the three related groups do differ at a nonchance level. There is a statistically significant difference in the proportions of yes and no responses in the three groups.

REFERENCES

Atchley R (1974). The meaning of retirement. *Journal of Communication* 24:97-101.

Brooten D, Gennaro S, Brown L, Butts P, Gibbons A, Bakewell-Sachs S, and Kunar S (1988). Anxiety, depression and hostility in mothers of preterm infants. *Nursing Research* 37:213-216.

Daly E and Futrel M (1989). Retirement attitudes and health status. *Journal of Gerontological Nursing* 15:29-32.

Damrosch S and Perry L (1989). Self-reported adjustment, chronic sorrow, and coping of parents of children with Down syndrome. *Nursing Research* 38:25-30.

Folkman S and Lazarus R (1980). An analysis of coping in a middle-aged community sample. *Journal of Health and Social Behavior* 21:219-239.

Gennaro S (1988). Postpartal anxiety and depression in mothers of term and preterm infants. *Nursing Research* 38:82-85.

Hays W (1981). *Statistics*, 3rd ed. New York: Holt, Rinehart & Winston.

Lawrence S and Lawrence R (1989). Knowledge and attitudes about acquired immunodeficiency syndrome in nursing and nonnursing groups. *Journal of Professional Nursing* 5:92-101.

Oberst M, Graham D, Geller N, Stearns M, and Tiernan E (1981). Catheter management programs and postoperative urinary dysfunction. *Research in Nursing and Health* 4:175-181.

Parkerson G, Gehlbach S, Wagner E, and James S (1981). The Duke-UNC health profile: an adult health status instrument for primary care. *Medical Care* 19:806-828.

Scheffe H (1959). *The analysis of variance.* New York: John Wiley & Sons.

Shelley S (1984). *Research in nursing and health.* Boston: Little, Brown & Company.

Siegel S (1956). *Nonparametric statistics.* New York: McGraw-Hill Book Co.

Thomas B and Price M (1985). *Continuing education needs of nurses in long-term care facilities.* Unpublished paper, Iowa City: University of Iowa.

Williamson M (1978). *Reducing post-catheterization bladder dysfunction by reconditioning.* Unpublished master's thesis, Lexington: University of Kentucky.

Williamson M (1982). Reducing post-catheterization bladder dysfunction by reconditioning. *Nursing Research* 31:26-28.

Zuckerman M and Lubin B (1965). *Manual for the Multiple Affect Adjective Checklist.* San Diego: Educational and Industrial Testing Service.

REFERENCES FOR FURTHER STUDY

Hays W (1981). *Statistics*, 3rd ed. New York: Holt, Rinehart & Winston.

Hogg R and Tanis E (1977). *Probability and statistical inference.* New York: Macmillan, Inc.

Kachigan S (1982). *Statistical analysis.* New York: Radius Press.

Munro B, Visintainer M, and Page E (1986). *Statistical methods for health care research.* Philadelphia: JB Lippincott Co.

Scheffe H (1959). *The analysis of variance.* New York: John Wiley & Sons.

Shelley S (1984). *Research in nursing and health.* Boston: Little, Brown & Co.

Siegel S (1956). *Nonparametric statistics.* New York: McGraw-Hill Book Co.

Winer B (1962). *Statistical principles in experimental design*, 2nd ed. New York: McGraw-Hill Book Co.

CHAPTER 9

Problems in nursing research

Objectives

After completing this unit of study, students will be able to:

1. Perform preliminary data analyses used to select appropriate statistical tests for problems in nursing research

2. Select appropriate descriptive statistics for completing problems such as description of samples or summaries of surveys

3. Select appropriate inferential statistics for completing problems involving examination of relationships or comparisons of groups

4. Perform data analysis using one or more statistical packages

5. Interpret results from hand calculations or computer printouts

6. Present results in narrative form, in tables, and in graphs

7. Identify assumptions and limitations in simulated studies

8. Identify practice and research implications of research findings

I n many ways data analysis is the most exciting stage of the research process. Research is the treasure hunt, and the data analysis stage is the point at which the treasure is located. Chapters 6 to 8 explain the processes involved in data analysis, identify appropriate kinds of statistical tests to use, and provide examples and problems employing these tests. In each problem in these chapters the nature of the statistical test explained points to the appropriate tests to employ.

This chapter is different. There are no additional statistical procedures outlined or explained, nor is there much guidance as to the direction one should take in solving the problems. Instead the chapter presents simulated problems in nursing research that require use of the data analysis techniques studied in Chapters 6 through 8. The basic task is to develop plans for data analysis, carry them out, interpret the results, and present findings. Special questions are asked for different problems. Narrative accounts, tables, and graphs should be used to complete the problems. You are on your own!

Problem 9-1

Registered nurses' return for baccalaureate study

A nurse decided to investigate the factors that influence registered nurses (RNs) to return for baccalaureate study. She developed a questionnaire to collect data from two samples: RNs who had returned and completed baccalaureate degrees (BSNs) within the past 5 years and RNs who had not completed BSNs.

The first group was obtained from records at baccalaureate programs in New Jersey; the second group was obtained from sampling New Jersey Board of Nursing data, that is, RNs sorted to produce a sampling frame of RNs without baccalaureate degrees.

The research hypotheses were as follows:
1. There will be a significant difference between the ages of these groups.
2. There will be a significant difference between the groups in the social support as measured by the Social Support Scale (SSS).
3. There will be a significant difference between these groups in their achievement orientation as measured by the Achievement Orientation Scale (AOS).

The data were coded as follows:

No.	Variable
1	ID
2	1 = returned, 2 = not returned
3	Age in years
4	Years since became an RN
5	Distance (miles) to nearest BSN program
6	SSS scores
7	AOS scores

Problem 9-1, cont'd

The data

1	2	3	4	5	6	7
01	1	23	3	34	33	23
02	1	33	12	54	27	26
03	1	26	5	44	20	29
04	1	22	2	17	29	27
05	1	27	7	28	24	21
06	1	30	10	30	34	26
07	1	24	3	23	34	22
08	1	28	8	12	29	23
09	1	25	4	31	32	26
10	1	40	19	24	29	22
11	1	37	16	40	36	28
12	1	26	5	39	29	27
13	1	20	0	26	26	24
14	1	33	12	24	20	18
15	1	23	3	55	35	28
16	1	28	7	32	29	25
17	1	34	12	26	34	27
18	1	26	5	8	32	24
19	1	31	11	15	28	28
20	1	27	6	28	25	23
21	1	30	9	26	32	26
22	1	32	12	27	28	25
23	1	34	13	65	33	27
24	1	24	3	42	30	20
25	1	27	6	86	27	29
26	1	25	4	18	24	23
27	1	21	1	22	32	22
28	1	36	15	43	27	25
29	1	29	8	22	26	26
30	1	32	11	46	35	24
31	2	26	6	23	17	25
32	2	28	7	43	26	22
33	2	26	5	38	30	14
34	2	37	16	17	17	20
35	2	25	4	65	27	20
36	2	43	22	28	29	19
37	2	33	12	37	22	21
38	2	24	4	40	25	12
39	2	37	17	28	17	18
40	2	35	14	88	27	28
41	2	28	7	40	24	21
42	2	24	3	34	21	20
43	2	40	12	45	33	26

Problem 9-1, cont'd

Registered nurses' return for baccalaureate study

The data

1	2	3	4	5	6	7
44	2	28	7	27	20	14
45	2	26	5	35	19	24
46	2	27	6	42	20	13
47	2	28	6	17	31	16
48	2	40	18	44	19	18
49	2	34	9	60	28	23
50	2	27	6	32	22	20
51	2	37	16	56	30	22
52	2	33	12	28	22	18
53	2	28	7	30	24	20
54	2	32	11	15	17	15
55	2	24	3	39	27	23
56	2	31	9	42	22	16
57	2	26	5	15	26	19
58	2	25	4	36	22	26
59	2	37	16	20	22	13
60	2	22	1	55	24	24

Test the hypotheses, using an alpha level of .05, and report findings, using both tables and narrative accounts to describe your results.

Problem 9-1, cont'd

Describe ways in which variables 4 and 5 influence the results, if they do.

Outline additional data you would like to gather if you decided to do a partial replication of this study.

Problem 9-2

Improving outcomes of intramuscular injections

Intramuscular injections, a common therapeutic technique nurses use, can cause various degrees of discomfort and lesions in patients receiving frequent injections. Roberts' master's degree research (1975) demonstrated that both pain and injection site lesions occur among patients who receive frequent injections as part of their medical regimen. She found that 20 of 60 patients reported pain, burning, numbness, or other discomfort after 15 minutes from the injection. Of the 60 patients, 53 (88%) had at least one visible injection site lesion. Two factors that have been suggested as causing the lesions are the deposition of the injected fluid into subcutaneous tissue rather than the intended musculature and leakage of the fluid into the subcutaneous tissue after withdrawal of the needle. Use of a broken injection pathway, the Z-track technique, has been recommended as a way of dealing with these problems, but it has not been tested or adopted widely.

Keen (1986) studied the incidence of discomfort and lesions associated with standard and Z-track injection techniques by using each subject as his or her own control. One group received Z-track injections in the left ventrogluteal site and standard injections in the right ventrogluteal site; the procedure was reversed in the other group. These sites had not been used for at least 1 month before the study and were used exclusively in the study.

The patients in Keen's study had pancreatitis or sickle cell anemia. Patients with both diseases received prescribed doses of intramuscular meperidine at frequent intervals.

For this partial replication of Keen's study, you are to focus only on the discomfort variable, operationally defined as the score achieved on an orally administered questionnaire 15 minutes after the injection. Each of five items was scored 0 for no discomfort, 1 for mild discomfort, 2 for moderate discomfort, or 3 for severe discomfort; thus the possible total ranged from 0 to 15. The standard and Z-track discomfort scores (n = 6 for each) were summed to represent the dependent variable, providing ranges of two scores from 0 to 90 for each patient.

Are these scores independent or related measures?

Assume that these data can be treated as interval data, and test the following research hypothesis: Among patients receiving intramuscular injections of meperidine (alone or in conjunction with promethazine) every 3 to 4 hours, there will be less discomfort associated with the use of the Z-track technique than with the standard technique.

Is this a directional or a nondirectional hypothesis? Use .05 as your significance level.

Problem 9-2, cont'd

The data

Subject	Age	Standard						Z-track					
		1	2	3	4	5	6	1	2	3	4	5	6
01	32	9	7	5	7	3	11	12	4	7	8	3	4
02	46	11	12	9	6	8	9	9	4	5	9	10	8
03	22	13	6	8	7	5	10	3	7	8	11	4	6
04	28	8	11	7	9	10	14	4	9	9	7	12	7
05	39	12	6	9	8	4	12	5	7	11	8	6	5
06	54	13	8	7	7	7	9	6	7	8	4	3	8
07	58	12	11	6	9	13	11	11	9	9	6	10	7
08	61	7	8	10	7	11	11	12	8	5	10	5	8
09	46	13	12	11	9	10	10	10	7	12	9	9	6
10	37	11	8	6	9	11	8	9	5	11	8	7	7
11	29	5	8	8	11	8	9	6	6	9	10	4	5
12	36	10	9	7	7	9	12	10	9	7	11	3	7
13	41	8	8	10	12	8	5	7	7	12	4	4	3
14	52	14	9	8	12	10	9	11	8	8	10	6	6
15	59	7	8	9	4	6	8	8	8	4	6	7	6
16	28	9	7	10	7	9	9	8	9	5	5	11	5
17	24	8	7	5	9	11	12	10	8	8	5	9	6
18	29	11	9	3	7	6	9	8	8	8	9	5	10
19	30	14	11	12	10	9	8	10	9	12	11	7	5
20	43	9	8	8	7	5	10	11	3	7	4	8	7

What did you call your data file?

What statistical test(s) did you use? Why?

Restate the research hypothesis as a null hypothesis:

Did your results reject this null hypothesis?

Improving outcomes of intramuscular injections

Make a table to report the primary results.

Both men and women were used in the study, but gender was not studied. However, age was recorded and checked as a possible intervening variable. It ranged from 22 to 61 years. What is the mean age for the study group?

The standard deviation of ages?

Is there a significant relationship between age and the dependent variables at an alpha of .05?

How did you find the answers to this question?

Problem 9-2, cont'd

How would you improve on the design and analyses if you were to do another partial replication of this study?

Problem 9-3

Patterns of infant crying during air travel

This problem is a replication of a study, "Infant Crying during Aircraft Descent," reported by Byers (1986). The abstract of her study follows:

The phenomenon of infant crying during aircraft descent is described, based on in-flight observations of 37 infant-mother pairs and mother interviews. The hallmark was crying during descent that was not alleviated by mothers' strategies that had been effective prior to descent. A significant relationship was found between bottle feeding and crying during descent; 18 (78%) of the nonfeeding infants cried, compared with 4 (29%) of the bottle feeders. All infants with colds cried during descent, and descent crying always occurred more than 9 minutes after adults perceived the need to clear their ears. Only 4 of the 22 mothers (18%) with crying infants attributed the crying to ear pain, yet the findings support the explanation of otalgia due to inadequate middle ear ventilation. Developmental factors that put airborne infants at risk for otic barotrauma, educational implications, and directions for future research are discussed.*

In this replication two groups of infant-mother pairs were studied: those who gave their infants a bottle or pacifier during descent, and those who did not give either bottle or pacifier during descent. Variables kept constant were as follows: all flights were nonstop and lasted between 2.5 and 3.8 hours, all infant-mother pairs were seated in the first five rows of the aircraft, the cruising altitude of the flights was between 31,000 and 33,000 feet, and all flights terminated at O'Hare International Airport in Chicago.

The purpose of the study was strictly descriptive—to describe infants' crying behavior during descent and the reasons given by mothers and aircraft

*From Byers, P (1986). Infant crying during aircraft descent. *Nursing Research* 35:260-262.

Problem 9-3, cont'd

Patterns of infant crying during air travel

cabin personnel for each infant's crying and to evaluate the possibility that otalgia occurs when ventilation of the middle ear fails to compensate for the increase in cabin pressure during descent.

The research questions are these:

1. What patterns of infant crying occur during the flight and during the descent of the aircraft?
2. What strategies do mothers use to calm their crying infants?
3. What reasons do mothers and flight attendants give for infant crying during aircraft descent?
4. Do the data support the notion that otalgia is a major factor in infant crying during aircraft descent?

Data were gathered from 42 mother-infant pairs and 24 cabin staff members during 21 nonstop flights. The data gathered are tabulated as follows.

The data

No.	Infant's age (mo)	Cold?	Bottle?	Time cried/ flight (sec)	Time cried/ descent (min)	Adults' need* (min)	Adults' clear† (min)
1	4.2	No	No	46	5.5	10.2	21.5
2	6.5	No	Yes	57	3.5	12.4	24.5
3	6.8	Yes	Yes	22	4.8	14.2	27.0
4	3.0	No	Yes	0	0	11.5	20.2
5	4.2	No	No	38	3.5	9.0	22.5
6	4.8	No	Yes	79	5.8	12.2	24.2
7	5.5	No	Yes	29	0	10.8	28.8
8	7.0	No	No	82	9.8	11.2	20.5
9	5.0	No	Yes	93	0	9.8	19.5
10	7.8	Yes	No	118	10.5	9.6	22.4
11	5.4	Yes	Yes	128	5.7	10.4	21.5
12	6.2	No	Yes	95	0	12.4	22.8
13	2.8	No	Yes	22	0	11.6	20.5
14	4.5	No	Yes	192	4.2	12.4	23.4
15	4.8	Yes	No	223	11.4	13.5	24.0
16	5.2	Yes	No	54	8.6	8.8	28.2
17	5.4	No	Yes	0	0	11.5	26.2
18	6.2	No	Yes	0	4.3	10.8	20.4
19	3.6	No	Yes	0	0	9.8	19.5
20	3.8	No	Yes	48	3.1	10.4	21.4
21	5.0	No	No	38	6.8	11.5	23.2
22	5.2	No	Yes	122	0	12.2	22.5

*Time from the moment the mother felt ear discomfort until the time any infants started to cry.
†Total time adults (the mothers) needed to clear their ears.

Problem 9-3, cont'd

The data

No.	Infant's age (mo)	Cold?	Bottle?	Time cried/ flight (sec)	Time cried/ descent (min)	Adults' need* (min)	Adults' clear† (min)
23	4.0	Yes	No	88	7.8	14.4	21.0
24	3.6	No	Yes	54	2.5	11.2	22.4
25	5.8	Yes	No	34	8.9	9.8	20.5
26	4.2	Yes	No	123	4.8	9.8	18.3
27	4.2	No	Yes	56	0	9.9	22.2
28	6.1	No	No	0	6.5	10.6	21.2
29	5.0	No	Yes	32	0	11.2	18.8
30	3.8	No	Yes	49	5.4	9.8	20.2
31	4.5	Yes	Yes	111	3.7	9.4	19.8
32	2.0	No	Yes	22	0	10.6	21.2
33	6.1	Yes	No	132	6.9	11.2	19.8
34	5.8	No	No	43	8.9	12.0	19.6
35	4.0	No	Yes	28	4.4	11.2	22.4
36	5.1	Yes	No	122	9.4	12.2	23.1
37	4.2	No	Yes	156	2.1	9.8	19.8
38	3.6	No	Yes	87	1.4	10.5	21.4
39	1.8	No	Yes	0	0	11.2	22.4
40	2.4	No	No	0	9.8	10.2	24.1
41	5.6	No	No	24	6.6	9.8	22.1
42	3.5	No	Yes	198	3.2	9.5	18.5

Reasons given for descent crying

Reason	Mothers (n)	Staff (n)
I don't know	19	11
Fussy baby	3	6
Ear pain	18	7
Infant upset about something	2	0

Strategies used during descent crying

Strategy	Mothers (n)
Offering a bottle	26
Shifting infant's position	34
Rocking	12
Back patting	14
Talking to infant	28
Offering a pacifier	3

Problem 9-3, cont'd

Patterns of infant crying during air travel

Answer the four research questions in narrative form.

(If necessary continue your answer on separate page.)

Prepare a pie graph to illustrate the strategies mothers used.

Problem 9-4

Parents' adjustment to childhood epilepsy

This problem was suggested by a study reported by Austin, McBride, and Davis (1984), "Parental Attitude and Adjustment to Childhood Epilepsy." These investigators, noting the paucity of research on parenting children with epilepsy, stated that the majority of nursing articles on epilepsy in children focus on types of seizures, nursing care, treatment, and psychosocial problems associated with epilepsy. A few studies that describe parents' attitudes were summarized. Reported were a positive relationship between parents' positive attitudes and children's social maturity, strong correlations between negative parental attitudes and behavior disorders among their children, and greater dependency of children with recently diagnosed epilepsy than of children with recent tonsillectomies or cystic fibrosis.

Austin, McBride, and Davis noted that, although the literature points to the association of negative parental attitudes with negative parental adjustment, there were methodological flaws in prior studies, including a failure to distinguish between attitudes and adjustment. The purpose of their study was to describe parenting attitudes and adjustment and examine the relationship between the two variables and among selected additional variables. They used multiple regression to see how much of the parents' adjustment could be explained by each of the variables they selected for study.

The purpose of the study in this problem is to investigate the attitudes and adjustment of parents whose children have epilepsy and to determine whether these attitudes and adjustment patterns are similar for fathers and mothers. In addition, the impact of age of onset, length of time since diagnosis of epilepsy, seizure control, number of anticonvulsant medications taken, and self-reported compliance with medication regimens will be investigated. The specific research questions are as follows:

1. Among mothers of children with epilepsy, what is the relationship between adjustment and
   a. Attitudes toward the disease?
   b. Age of onset?
   c. Length of time since seizures began?
   d. Seizure control?
   e. Number of anticonvulsant medications taken?
   f. Compliance with the medication regimen?
2. Among fathers of children with epilepsy, what is the relationship between adjustment and
   a. Attitudes toward the disease?
   b. Age of onset?
   c. Length of time since seizures began?
   d. Seizure control?
   e. Number of anticonvulsant medications taken?
   f. Compliance with the medication regimen?
3. Do mothers and fathers differ in (a) their attitudes? (b) their adjustment?

Parents' adjustment to childhood epilepsy

Research subjects are 50 pairs of parents whose children have a diagnosis of epilepsy, uncomplicated by any other medical problems, and who are of normal intelligence. Excluded were parents who have epilepsy themselves or are single parents.

It is assumed that the measures used for all variables have been adequately tested and refined so that valid, reliable measures comprise the variables. The attitude scale measures anxiety, distress, and so forth, so that the higher the score, the more negative the attitude. The adjustment scale, however, is in the positive direction; the higher the score, the better the adjustment. Complete data were obtained from the 50 couples.

The data were coded as follows:

Column or field	Variable
1	ID
2	Seizures prior month: 0 = 1, 1-4 = 2, 5-10 = 3, 11+ = 4
3	Sex: female = 1, male = 2
4	Number of anticonvulsants taken
5	Medication compliance
6	Age at onset: birth = 0, age in years for others
7	Present age
8	Mother's attitude score (higher more negative)
9	Father's attitude score (higher more negative)
10	Mother's adjustment score (higher positive)
11	Father's adjustment score (higher positive)

The data

1	2	3	4	5	6	7	8	9	10	11
01	1	1	1	31	5	8	90	94	31	36
02	2	1	1	33	4	6	85	96	42	30
03	4	2	2	29	4	5	110	104	23	27
04	3	2	1	24	3	10	88	77	32	40
05	2	2	2	28	6	11	72	39	55	60
06	4	1	1	19	0	5	100	96	22	26
07	2	1	3	29	10	12	84	95	31	30
08	3	2	1	33	0	3	118	91	23	32
09	4	1	1	19	4	8	94	76	26	44
10	4	2	1	27	4	8	98	102	22	20
11	3	2	1	24	9	11	94	64	36	40
12	2	1	2	41	8	10	54	58	31	43
13	2	2	1	37	7	12	50	53	36	34
14	1	1	3	44	6	10	69	82	43	52
15	2	1	3	29	7	10	88	70	51	50

Problem 9-4, cont'd

The data

1	2	3	4	5	6	7	8	9	10	11
16	1			07		09		12		11
17	1			12		14		17		15
18	1			11		08		17		18
19	1			05		09		09		13
20	1			09		11		11		15
21	1			10		10		15		17
22	1			04		06		09		11
23	2			08		09		12		14
24	2			04		06		13		17
25	2			11		12		18		21
26	2			06		08		12		12
27	2			08		10		13		17
28	2			12		14		18		20
29	2			10		11		16		18
30	2			06		10		11		15
31	2			09		08		15		14
32	2			10		09		18		17
33	2			05		07		17		15
34	2			12		16		19		23
35	2			07		09		15		17
36	2			11		13		18		19
37	2			08		09		15		17
38	2			10		10		16		17
39	2			08		09		16		14
40	2			07		05		11		12
41	2			09		13		16		18
42	2			11		11		14		16
43	2			12		11		12		15
44	2			11		10		17		18
45	2			09		07		12		12
46	2			06		09		14		16
47	2			11		10		18		22
48	2			07		03		14		14
49	2			11		12		18		20
50	2			07		10		11		16

You may wish to recode some of these data or perform other operations to create data transformations.

Parents' adjustment to childhood epilepsy

Answer the research questions, using both narrative accounts and tables.

(If necessary, continue your answer on separate page.)

Identify implications for nursing practice and nursing research.

Identify any assumptions or limitations of this study.

Ethical dilemmas and nurses' decisions

This project was suggested by an article by Swider, McElmurry, and Yarling (1985), "Ethical Decision Making in a Bureaucratic Context by Senior Nursing Students," although it differs from that study in significant ways.

A team of investigators was interested in examining the decisions nurses make about ethical dilemmas confronted in clinical situations. They hypothesized that associate degree– and diploma-prepared nurses would make decisions based on institutional considerations more often than baccalaureate-prepared nurses, who would refer to values of professionalism in nursing as a basis for reaching autonomous decisions.

Ten vignettes were prepared that gave nurses choices of actions to take; each respondent could mark one action or more than one action for each situation. The items were scaled so that two scores were produced: institution-centered (IC) choices and professionalism-centered (PC) choices. The possible scores for each scale ranged from 10 to 50.

Test these hypotheses at an alpha level of .05:

H1: There will be no significant differences among the three groups of nurses, associate degree, diploma, and baccalaureate prepared, on the IC and PC scores.

H2: There will be no significant difference in the IC and PC scores of two groups: the associate degree– and diploma-prepared nurses versus the baccalaureate degree nurses.

H3: There is no significant relationship between the ages of the nurses and the IC or PC scores.

The team gathered data from three hospitals, all having between 300 and 500 beds. Assume that a random sample was selected and that human subjects review guidelines for participation were properly handled.

The coding guide for the data is as follows:

Column	Variable
1-2	Age
3	1 = associate degree, 2 = diploma, 3 = BSN
4-5	IC scores
6-7	PC scores

Problem 9-5, cont'd

Ethical dilemmas and nurses' decisions

The data

Column				Column			
1-2	3	4-5	6-7	1-2	3	4-5	6-7
36	1	24	28	23	3	35	36
24	2	36	14	29	3	25	32
28	2	41	12	34	2	33	28
25	3	33	46	54	2	47	23
28	3	23	34	36	2	19	27
24	1	34	27	33	3	25	38
24	1	28	25	37	3	29	28
28	2	36	23	33	2	31	31
22	2	33	34	60	2	35	31
44	2	47	26	43	3	16	24
37	3	31	36	36	1	37	22
24	2	38	29	28	1	33	34
39	2	33	32	26	2	29	15
56	2	22	17	24	3	25	44
33	3	26	44	33	3	34	26
32	3	32	29	42	2	47	19
33	2	42	15	55	2	43	35
47	3	22	39	44	2	27	19
23	2	33	34	49	2	41	33
51	2	41	21	26	3	22	43
46	2	33	29	34	2	34	33
34	2	31	21	25	1	40	29
30	3	24	40	27	1	33	34
31	3	23	42	25	1	25	22
49	1	29	22	28	3	23	41
43	2	34	21	37	3	30	31
19	1	24	21	26	3	29	36
28	3	33	47	24	1	33	24
34	3	14	33	42	2	50	16
37	2	42	36	44	2	36	30
41	3	30	43	48	2	22	18
26	1	30	31	34	1	33	23
25	1	44	18	26	3	28	33
33	2	13	45	47	2	42	33
27	1	41	25	28	1	35	23
25	1	34	22	24	3	21	34
22	2	32	29	33	2	17	36
44	2	44	23	43	2	42	19
36	1	34	28	33	3	27	33
34	1	22	38	56	2	29	24
51	2	27	29				

How many associate degree–prepared nurses are there in
   sample? ————
Diploma? ————
BSN? ————
Report the results of testing the three hypotheses.

Identify assumptions and limitations.

Teaching patients undergoing angioplasty

This problem is a replication of a study by Murphy, Fishman, and Shaw (1989) titled, "Education of Patients Undergoing Angioplasty: Factors Affecting Learning during a Structured Educational Program."

The incidence of percutaneous transluminal coronary angioplasty (PTCA), the inflation of a balloon catheter in a coronary artery stenosis, has increased rapidly since its introduction in 1977. Since patients are hospitalized for this procedure only an average of 3 days, nurses must meet patients' needs for knowledge and support quickly. Murphy, Fishman, and Shaw (1989) developed an educational program for such patients. The program consisted of a slide-tape presentation, an angioplasty booklet, and a nurse-patient consultation. Both the slide-tape presentation and the booklet included information about cardiac anatomy and physiology, coronary artery disease, risk factors, PTCA procedures, permitted activities, emergency coronary bypass surgery, the recovery room–telemetry unit, the cardiac care unit, and after-procedure protocol. Questions frequently asked after PTCA (such as about exercise, diet, medications, follow-up, and return to work) were also addressed.

To assess the effectiveness of the educational program, the investigators developed parallel forms of a knowledge test, which they called the Coronary Angioplasty Risk Factor Inventory (CARFI). You have decided to use the two forms of the CARFI as a pretest and a posttest for each of two groups of patients. The CARFI consists of two subscales: one on the procedure and the other on risk factors. Both the subscales and the total scales are to be analyzed.

You have set the following criteria for admission to the study: coronary artery occlusion documented by angiographic study, no prior PTCA procedures attempted, English speaking, age between 30 and 70 years, and willingness to participate and sign an informed consent form. You have collected baseline data from 22 patients who agreed to participate in the study. That is, these patients were pretested and tested again at discharge before the special educational program was introduced. After collection of these data, you plan to recruit 28 additional patients for the study. These patients will receive the educational program as an experimental intervention between their pretests and posttests.

An alpha of .05 is adopted to test the following research hypotheses:

H1-H6: The posttest scores of both subscales and the total CARFI measure will be higher than the corresponding pretest scores for both groups of patients.

H7: The posttest scores of the experimental group will be higher than the posttest scores of the control group.

Data are coded as follows:

ID	Identification number
GRP	1 = control, 2 = experimental
PRO-PRE	Pretest procedures
RIS-PRE	Pretest risk factors
PRO-POST	Posttest procedures
RIS-POST	Posttest risk factors

Problem 9-6, cont'd

The data

ID	GRP	PRO-PRE	RIS-PRE	PRO-POST	RIS-POST
01	1	09	08	11	12
02	1	12	10	14	13
03	1	13	14	15	15
04	1	07	08	12	11
05	1	09	10	12	16
06	1	10	11	13	14
07	1	04	07	11	09
08	1	05	11	11	13
09	1	06	10	10	14
10	1	12	13	17	17
11	1	09	11	13	13
12	1	06	10	10	15
13	1	16	18	18	22
14	1	12	11	13	14
15	1	08	07	10	11
16	1	07	09	12	11
17	1	12	14	17	15
18	1	11	08	17	18
19	1	05	09	09	13
20	1	09	11	11	15
21	1	10	10	15	17
22	1	04	06	09	11
23	2	08	09	12	14
24	2	04	06	13	17
25	2	11	12	18	21
26	2	06	08	12	12
27	2	08	10	13	17
28	2	12	14	18	20
29	2	10	11	16	18
30	2	06	10	11	15
31	2	09	08	15	14
32	2	10	09	18	17
33	2	05	07	17	15
34	2	12	16	19	23
35	2	07	09	15	17
36	2	11	13	18	19
37	2	08	09	15	17
38	2	10	10	16	17
39	2	08	09	16	14
40	2	07	05	11	12
41	2	09	13	16	18
42	2	11	11	14	16
43	2	12	11	12	15

Problem 9-6, cont'd

Teaching patients undergoing angioplasty

The data

ID	GRP	PRO-PRE	RIS-PRE	PRO-POST	RIS-POST
44	2	11	10	17	18
45	2	09	07	12	12
46	2	06	09	14	16
47	2	11	10	18	22
48	2	07	03	14	14
49	2	11	12	18	20
50	2	07	10	11	16

Report the results of testing the seven hypotheses.

Problem 9-6, cont'd

Did you use one-tailed or two-tailed tests? Why?

As far as you can tell, were the two groups comparable on the pretests?

What additional data might you have wanted to gather to bolster the credibility of your findings?

Problem 9-7

Temperature recording in the neonate

Kunnell, O'Brien, Munro, and Medoff-Cooper (1988) compared four sites for temperature recording in the neonate—rectal, femoral, axillary, and skin-to-mattress—to find out whether accurate temperature recordings could be made at various sites and to determine optimal thermometer placement times at the sites. One reason for the study was to examine alternatives to rectal temperature taking because of the risks involved, particularly rectal perforation. Another factor to be considered was the necessity of obtaining accurate temperature readings from neonates during their extrauterine adjustment period and first few weeks of life.

Because infants have a relatively large body surface for their weight, poor thermal insulation because of their lack of fatty covering, and a small mass to retain heat, they are vulnerable to changes in environmental temperatures. Moreover, a change in temperature may be the only indication of an important systemic disease. Kunnel and co-workers (1988) describe prior research in this area as sparse and flawed and note the importance of evaluating body

Problem 9-7, cont'd

Temperature recording in the neonate

temperature in the newborn. Both accuracy and optimal measurement time are essential in providing high-quality nursing care.

Results of the study by Kunnel and co-workers showed that placement times varied from a mean of 2.66 minutes for the rectal site to 8.52 minutes for the skin-to-mattress site, in marked contrast to placement times reported earlier by Mayfield and associates (1984). These investigators concluded that "femoral and axillary sites are the most efficient routes for optimum temperature measurement with minimal concerns for safety" (Kunnell, O'Brien, Munro, and Medoff-Cooper, 1988, p. 164).

This replication is designed to examine the conflict in findings regarding placement times of the thermometers. To eliminate a major risk factor (perforation from rectal temperature measurement), you decide to compare only the femoral, axillary, and skin-to-mattress sites.

The research questions are as follows:
1. What is the optimal placement time for measuring neonates' temperature in each of three sites?
2. Is there a significant relationship between optimal temperature times and (a) gender, (b) birth weight, and (c) activity level?

You should assume that optimal placement times and birth weights are interval level data, activity levels are ordinal level data, and gender is nominal level data. You elect to use the same design used by Kunnell and co-workers; that is, each subject serves as his or her own control. Femoral, axillary, and skin-to-mattress temperatures were taken simultaneously on 38 full-term neonates after informed parental consent was obtained. All infants were in stable condition with no known abnormalities. Measurements were taken when the infants were 1 to 4 days old. The mercury was shaken down below 94° F before each measurement, and all thermometers were left in place for 15 minutes with the temperatures from all three sites recorded each minute. Only the times necessary to register the optimal temperature at the three sites are included in the data tabulated below. Three additional variables are tabulated: gender (1 = female and 2 = male), birth weight in grams, and activity level (1 = sleeping, 2 = awake and quiet, 3 = awake and fussing slightly, 4 = awake and crying lustily).

Problem 9-7, cont'd

The data

ID	Time (min) Femoral	Axillary	Skin-to-mattress	Sex	Birth weight	Activity level
01	5.20	5.90	9.20	1	3240	1
02	4.10	4.80	8.50	1	2990	2
03	5.75	6.30	9.30	1	2886	2
04	7.10	8.00	10.55	2	3348	2
05	4.60	4.90	7.50	2	3630	3
06	5.20	7.40	9.00	1	3188	4
07	6.30	7.20	8.80	2	3668	4
08	5.75	6.25	7.88	1	3076	3
09	5.20	5.30	6.80	2	2886	4
10	7.22	7.80	10.44	1	2684	1
11	6.88	8.85	9.40	2	2997	2
12	6.10	8.50	8.80	1	3124	1
13	7.40	7.30	9.90	1	3444	2
14	5.50	6.05	8.40	2	3556	1
15	5.60	7.20	9.40	2	3220	1
16	4.30	5.20	8.10	1	3088	2
17	6.08	6.04	7.30	2	2698	1
18	5.20	6.16	8.96	2	2985	1
19	4.86	7.32	9.56	1	3128	3
20	5.50	7.04	8.04	2	3558	2
21	7.10	7.80	9.80	1	3218	2
22	5.50	6.20	8.60	2	3446	4
23	6.08	7.64	9.10	2	2875	3
24	4.30	7.50	8.20	1	3065	2
25	5.08	6.38	7.88	1	2887	2
26	6.22	7.34	8.68	2	3242	1
27	7.34	8.88	9.45	2	3876	4
28	3.56	6.10	8.74	1	3093	1
29	5.40	5.88	8.20	2	2899	2
30	7.20	8.86	10.44	1	3142	3
31	8.21	8.68	9.54	2	3417	2
32	6.20	6.44	9.10	1	2997	1
33	5.74	6.24	8.08	2	3122	3
34	5.04	6.78	7.42	1	3086	4
35	3.75	4.66	7.08	2	3446	3
36	4.12	7.22	8.75	2	3049	2
37	5.22	6.77	8.50	1	2987	4
38	6.78	7.21	7.98	2	3450	3

Temperature recording in the neonate

Write a paragraph describing the sample in terms of gender, birth weight, and activity level.

Answer the research questions. Use both narrative accounts and tables to report your findings.

Problem 9-7, cont'd

Prepare a bar graph to illustrate the mean times of placement for the different sites.

Problem 9-8

Stress and coping in renal transplant recipients

Sutton and Murphy (1989) recruited a sample of 40 renal transplant recipients to determine the incidence and severity of selected stressors and coping strategies used and to explore the influence of time on stress and coping patterns. To examine the time factor, they divided their sample into patients who had undergone the transplant up to 23 months before and 24 to 48 months before data collection.

In their review of the literature, Sutton and Murphy noted that transplantation is generally preferred to continual hemodialysis but noted also that "transplantation is not a panacea" (Sutton and Murphy, 1989, p. 46). They outlined the problems transplant patients face: dietary restrictions, blood pressure problems, weak bones, continued sexual dysfunction, and unpleasant side effects associated with immunosuppressive protocols.

Stress and coping in renal transplant recipients

Two data collection instruments were used: an adaptation of the End-Stage Renal Disease (ESRD) Stressor Scale developed by Baldree, Murphy, and Powers (1982) and the Jawoliec Coping Scale (Jawoliec and Powers, 1981). On the first scale (35 items) each stressor was rated on a five-point Likert Scale ranging from 1 = not at all to 5 = a great deal; thus, the higher the stress, the higher the score. The second tool consisted of 40 coping behaviors to be rated on a five-point scale (1 = never use to 5 = always use). This measure also produces a problem-oriented coping (PC) score and an affective-oriented coping (AC) score.

In this partial replication you will analyze data from 40 renal transplant outpatients who underwent their transplants from 6 to 48 months before data collection. The research questions are as follows:
1. What stressors to renal transplant patients report as most stressful? Least stressful?
2. Are there differences in impact of selected stressors based on gender? On time elapsed since the transplant?
3. Are there differences in coping patterns based on gender? On time elapsed since the transplant?

There is no need to handle the massive amount of data created in the original study to gain valuable experience in data analysis. Therefore this study focuses on only 10 stressors and only the PC and AC scores of the 40 subjects are analyzed, not the individual coping responses. The data are coded as follows:

Column	Variable
1	ID
2	Gender: 1 = female, 2 = male
3	Time lapse following transplant in months
4	Group according to time lapse: 1 = short, 2 = long
5-14	Responses to 10 stressor items: 1 = not at all, 2 = a slight amount, 3 = a moderate amount, 4 = a great deal
15	Stressor score
16	PC score
17	AC score

The 10 stressor items are as follows:
1. Fear of kidney rejection
2. Nausea and vomiting
3. Cost factors
4. Weight gain
5. Limitation of fluid
6. Limitation of physical activities
7. Reversal in family roles with children
8. Number of medications
9. Uncertainty concerning the future
10. Lack of information and understanding

Problem 9-8, cont'd

The data

ID	GEN	TIME	TGRP	IT1	IT2	IT3	IT4	IT5	IT6	IT7	IT8	IT9	IT10	SS	PC	AC
01	2	8	1	2	3	3	3	2	4	3	2	2	1	25	42	63
02	1	14	1	3	3	3	3	3	2	3	1	1	3	25	55	44
03	2	29	2	1	1	2	2	2	1	1	2	1	2	15	68	50
04	2	36	2	2	2	3	2	1	1	2	2	3	4	22	31	84
05	2	34	2	3	1	2	1	2	2	3	3	4	3	24	39	95
06	1	22	1	1	2	1	1	3	3	4	4	4	2	25	47	82
07	2	23	1	4	4	4	4	4	3	3	4	3	4	37	65	98
08	2	14	1	3	3	4	4	4	2	3	3	2	3	31	58	40
09	1	18	1	1	1	1	1	2	1	3	4	4	1	19	51	78
10	2	38	2	2	2	2	4	4	4	4	4	3	4	35	27	88
11	2	42	2	4	4	3	4	3	2	4	2	2	3	31	47	42
12	2	45	2	4	4	4	2	2	4	3	3	3	4	35	19	46
13	2	40	2	2	2	3	4	4	3	2	3	2	2	27	32	92
14	1	20	1	3	3	3	4	4	3	2	2	4	3	31	44	60
15	2	16	1	4	3	2	2	3	2	3	4	4	2	29	30	86
16	2	9	1	1	2	2	1	2	1	1	3	3	3	19	73	74
17	1	7	1	4	3	2	3	3	3	2	2	2	3	27	58	81
18	2	12	1	3	3	4	4	1	2	2	3	1	4	27	70	32
19	2	33	2	2	2	3	3	2	2	3	1	1	1	20	28	54
20	2	38	2	3	3	2	1	1	2	3	1	3	2	21	47	86
21	1	42	2	2	1	1	2	3	3	1	2	1	1	17	52	34
22	1	23	1	3	2	1	1	2	1	2	3	3	3	21	33	56
23	2	21	1	2	3	3	3	3	3	2	2	1	3	25	60	72

Problem 9-8, cont'd

Stress and coping in renal transplant recipients

The data

ID	GEN	TIME	TGRP	IT1	IT2	IT3	IT4	IT5	IT6	IT7	IT8	IT9	IT10	SS	PC	AC
24	2	34	2	2	2	1	1	1	2	2	1	4	3	19	28	72
25	1	33	2	3	1	2	3	2	2	2	4	2	4	25	37	66
26	2	13	1	4	4	3	2	3	4	3	4	3	3	33	52	94
27	2	17	1	3	3	2	2	3	3	4	3	2	3	28	24	98
28	2	34	2	4	1	1	1	2	1	3	2	2	1	18	31	77
29	1	32	2	3	3	3	4	4	4	4	4	3	4	36	56	42
30	2	28	2	4	4	4	3	2	3	3	1	4	2	30	20	65
31	2	33	2	3	3	3	2	4	3	3	2	3	2	27	31	79
32	1	39	2	2	3	4	4	2	2	2	4	2	3	29	58	36
33	1	21	1	1	1	2	1	1	1	1	1	4	1	14	24	44
34	2	22	1	2	3	4	4	3	3	2	2	2	2	27	26	67
35	2	28	2	4	4	4	3	4	4	4	4	4	4	39	39	98
36	2	15	1	3	4	3	4	4	4	1	2	3	4	32	32	86
37	1	13	1	2	2	4	2	3	3	3	3	1	1	22	62	56
38	2	34	2	4	3	1	1	1	4	4	1	1	1	23	53	76
39	2	42	2	2	2	3	2	3	1	1	2	2	3	19	21	83
40	2	28	2	1	1	4	4	4	1	4	4	4	4	31	30	98

Problem 9-8, cont'd

How many men are in the sample? How many women are in the sample?

How many subjects are in the short-time lapse group? The long-time lapse group?

Answer the research questions, using both narrative accounts and tables to present your findings.

(If necessary continue your answers on separate page.)

REFERENCES

Austin J, McBride A, and Davis H (1984). Parental attitude and adjustment to childhood epilepsy. *Nursing Research* 33:92-96.

Baldree K, Murphy S, and Powers M (1982). Stress identification and coping patterns in patients on hemodialysis. *Nursing Research* 31:107-112.

Byers P (1986). Infant crying during aircraft descent. *Nursing Research* 35:260-262.

Jawoliec A and Powers M (1981). Stress and coping in hypertensive and emergency room patients. *Nursing Research* 30:10-15.

Keen MF (1986). Comparison of intramuscular injection techniques to reduce site discomfort and lesions. *Nursing Research* 35:207-210.

Kunnell M, O'Brien C, Munro B, and Medoff-Cooper B (1988). Comparisons of rectal, femoral, axillary, and skin-to-mattress temperatures in stable neonates. *Nursing Research* 37:162-164, 189.

Mayfield S, Bhatia J, Nakamura K, Rios G, and Bell E (1984). Temperature measurement in term and preterm neonates. *Journal of Pediatrics* 104:2712-2715.

Murphy M, Fishman J, and Shaw R (1989). Education of patients undergoing coronary angioplasty: factors affecting learning during a structured educational program. *Heart and Lung* 18:36-45.

Roberts RA (1975). *Frequency of discomfort and skin reactions from intramuscular injections.* Unpublished master's thesis. Cleveland: Case Western Reserve University.

Sutton T, and Murphy S (1989). Stressors and patterns of coping in renal transplant patients. *Nursing Research* 38:46-49.

Swider S, McElmurry B, and Yarling R (1985). Ethical decision-making in a bureaucratic context by senior nursing students. *Nursing Research* 34:108-112.

CHAPTER 10

Evaluating nursing studies critically

Objectives

After completing this unit of study, students will be able to:

1. Explain the importance of critical appraisal of nursing research to nursing practice

2. Identify standards for evaluating the scientific merit of nursing studies in general

3. Identify standards for evaluating the scientific merit of nursing studies specific to the type of design employed.

4. Describe a systematic approach to the critical evaluation of nursing research.

5. Write evaluations of different kinds of nursing studies

Most nurses agree that the primary purpose of nursing research is to improve nursing practice. However, nurses in all settings are often unsure about what research findings are sound enough to merit changes in nursing practice. Haller, Reynolds, and Horsely (1979) listed four criteria for assessing the adequacy of research findings for practice: evaluation of scientific merit, assessment of the extent to which findings have been replicated, evaluation of the clinical relevance of the nursing study, and evaluation of the outcomes of clinical use of the study findings. Nurses without research experience must somehow learn to understand the research process or rely on others to interpret findings reported in nursing studies for them. In recent years investigators have been encouraged to include in their reports a section about implications for nursing practice. Indeed, a current standard for judging research reports is whether nursing implications are a part of the interpretation of findings. All nurse investigators have a responsibility to inform the profession about the implications of their research findings for nursing practice. If a study is a replication of earlier work, this fact should be cited and the prior studies should be summarized. Investigator's responsibilities also include placing research reports where they will be most accessible to practicing nurses—in basic nonresearch journals such as the *American Journal of Nursing* and in specialty journals such as *Pediatric Nursing,* as well as in the mainline nursing research journals. All nurses can judge clinical merit; the question is simply whether the research addresses an important clinical practice problem. Nurses must also determine the feasibility of implementing the innovation. What resources will be needed? How much time will it take to learn and implement the innovation? What will the costs be?

The problems associated with utilization of relevant research results are described briefly in Chapter 1. Barriers to the use of research findings have been difficulties in dissemination of information (Walker, 1969; Fawcett, 1982; Rogers, 1983) and resistance to change, as explained by change theory (Lewin, 1951; Lippitt, 1966; Havelock and Havelock, 1973). The utilization process must begin with judging research findings to identify those that should be ignored or rejected, those that merit further study, and those that are established firmly enough to warrant integration into nursing practice and nursing education.

Two areas of expertise are needed to evaluate research findings: an understanding of the research process and in-depth knowledge of the substantive area of the research. The philosophy of this book is aimed at the former. To evaluate research findings critically and skillfully, nurses must have experience with the research process. Reading about research is not enough! To gain and maintain an in-depth knowledge about a substantive area, nurses must establish a lifelong habit of continued study. They should read at least two professional journals regularly. Hospitals and other health care agencies should maintain libraries of nursing journals. Other nurses' organizations should follow the lead of the Association of Operating Room Nurses (AORN); the research committee of the AORN submits quarterly reviews of studies relevant to operating room nursing, and these are published in the *AORN Journal* (Kleinbeck 1988).

GENERAL CONSIDERATIONS IN READING RESEARCH REPORTS

When reading a research report, the nurse should first consider the title, abstract, and statement of purpose. Are they accurate, clear, and informative? Is the purpose stated in the title and described promptly in the introduction? Readers should not have to study several pages before learning what a report is about. The abstract if present should provide the reader with an accurate overview of the study. Both the abstract and the introduction to the study should alert the reader to the importance of the topic area and its significance to nursing. Does the investigator give readers a rationale for undertaking the study, based on either theoretical or practical concerns?

The review of the literature is generally hard to judge unless the reader is familiar with the literature on the study topic. Without in-depth knowledge of the study area, it is difficult to know whether an investigator has omitted classic studies and important references. Similarly, it is hard to know whether studies that challenge the investigator's point of view have been omitted. This is a primary reason that reputable nursing journals have experts in various fields to serve as referees for submitted manuscripts. Publication of research in a refereed journal indicates that qualified experts reviewed the paper and found it worthy of publication. Publication in a nonrefereed journal indicates that the paper was accepted by the editor or an editorial board; acceptance may or may not be based on experts' opinions about the quality of the paper.

Although the literature on a topic may not be well known to all readers, everyone can judge the logic and organization of the literature review and can check the list of references for currency and use of both primary and secondary sources. The review of the literature should establish the rationale for the study. The investigator should analyze and evaluate the studies reviewed; mere summaries of prior work are inadequate. When critiquing the literature review, the reader should understand that journal editors have become more restrictive as to the length of the review. A good review is concise and tight in providing the reader with background information. It establishes the study's context. Every citation should have direct relevance to the study.

The clarity and precision of the problem statement are its most important considerations. The focus and scope of the research problem should be readily apparent. The study variables should be identified clearly. Although operational as well as conceptual definitions of variables are important parts of a problem statement, this is another area that has been shortened in many recent journal publications. The conceptual definitions are often part of the literature review and may not be repeated in the problem statement. The operational definitions are often identified only in terms of the data collection instruments used for the study, and these may be found in the methodology section rather than the problem statement.

Five aspects of the research should be clearly described in the methodology section: the general approach (design), the population or sample, the design and procedures, data collection (including strengths and its limitations), and data analysis. The design selected for the study should be described clearly and justified. A problem can usually be studied in several ways; reasons for employing the selected approach should be stated explicitly.

The target population and the sampling plan should be clearly described. These aspects of research methodology determine the generalizability of study findings and must be clearly identified. If random sampling was not possible, reasons for using convenience samples should be explained. Nonprobability samples should be clearly identified as convenience, systematic, quota, or purposive samples, as appropriate.

The procedures section should be detailed enough to allow readers to replicate the study. If the study employed interviews to collect data, the introductory remarks and probes used by the interviewer should be described.

If the investigator developed a new measure for a study, the development of the measure and its psychometric characteristics must be reported in detail. Psychometric properties include such factors as the stability and consistency of the instrument (its reliability) and its validity or focus on the topic of interest. If existing data collection instruments were used, the investigator must explain how the tools fit the research purpose and study sample. Psychometric properties of existing tools should be described fully. If an existing tool was adapted for a study population that differed radically from the study population of the research, the psychometric properties of the existing tool should be reestablished for this new population.

Provisions for ethical treatment of human subjects must be spelled out. An explanation of how subjects were recruited and informed about the study purpose is a strict requirement. Often provisions for voluntary participation in a study play havoc with plans for random sampling. However, the number of subjects who refused to participate should be reported. If possible their characteristics should be compared with those of the actual participants.

Approaches to data analysis are determined by the research purpose. Methods of data analysis, descriptive and inferential statistics used, and how the data meet the necessary assumptions for the selected tests must be described. Procedures for handling missing data should be explained.

In the results section, accuracy and parsimony are desired. Research questions and/or hypotheses should be answered in the order they were posed. Have the research problems been answered systematically and objectively? Has the investigator used tables and graphs judiciously to clarify and emphasize important findings? Is there a narrative account for each table and graph to clarify and augment what the table or graph reports? Have limitations been identified?

Often the conclusions and discussion section is separate from the results section. Are the conclusions thoughtful, comprehensive, and objective? Have the results been related to the theoretical or conceptual framework contained in the literature review? Has the investigator answered the question, "So what?" Has the investigator been careful not to go beyond the findings in discussing implications of the study? Have areas of agreement and disagreement been discussed? Is the significance of the work to theory, practice, administration, or education explicitly stated? Have suggestions for further research been made?

The reader should keep some general concerns in mind when reviewing the entire report. Is there evidence of originality in the formulation of the problem or in carrying out the study? Has a tone of objectivity been maintained throughout? Is the report concise, readable, interesting, and geared to its appropriate audience? After the paper has been read carefully with each of these questions addressed systematically, it is time to look again at the abstract. Does it summarize the major points of the study—both the problem and major findings—concisely? Is it an accurate overview of the article?

Systematic evaluation of each section of a research report increases the like-

	POOR	FAIR	GOOD
Purpose			
Clarity	P	F	G
Promptness of statement	P	F	G
Theoretical significance	P	F	G
Practical significance	P	F	G
Review of the literature			
Inclusion of current citations	P	F	G
Inclusion of classic studies	P	F	G
Citation of primary sources	P	F	G
Relevance	P	F	G
Organization (analysis and synthesis)	P	F	G
Statement of the problem			
Clarity	P	F	G
Precision	P	F	G
Conceptual definitions	P	F	G
Operational definitions	P	F	G
Identifications of assumptions	P	F	G
Methodology			
Definition of population	P	F	G
Adequacy of sampling	P	F	G
Representativeness of sampling	P	F	G
Clarity of procedures	P	F	G
Replicability of procedures	P	F	G
Data collection: validity	P	F	G
Data collection : reliability	P	F	G
Data collection: sensitivity	P	F	G
Data analysis: appropriateness	P	F	G
Data analysis: completeness	P	F	G
Data anlaysis: clarity of description	P	F	G
Results and conclusions			
Accuracy	P	F	G
Focus on questions/hypotheses	P	F	G
Significance to nursing	P	F	G
Use of tables, graphs, and figures	P	F	G
Idetification of limitations	P	F	G
Overall concerns			
Objectivity	P	F	G
Conciseness	P	F	G
Ethical considerations	P	F	G
Originality	P	F	G
Style, readability	P	F	G

Fig. 10-1 Guide to critiquing research reports.

lihood of reaching conclusions based on a balanced appraisal. Flaws or exceptionally innovative aspects of the research in one section should not overshadow other considerations. Fig. 10-1 illustrates a form that enables the user to take a systematic approach to critiquing. This rating form has been generalized for use with all research reports, and certain items may be more important for some reports than for others.

SPECIAL CONSIDERATIONS IN READING RESEARCH REPORTS
Qualitative research reports

Because qualitative research is inherently more subjective than quantitative research, readers must rely more on the investigator's expertise. The report almost never includes raw data, and readers are left to assume that the investigator has maintained objectivity in handling these data, including developing coding categories, coding data, and interpreting results. Therefore the investigator's credentials should be examined. There should also be evidence that the approach used was related properly to a parent discipline such as anthropology. If a report is said to employ an "ethnographic" approach, the author should convince the reader that the study was carried out with an in-depth understanding of ethnographic methods.

Chapter 5 noted that qualitative studies may be carried out for a variety of purposes. The research report must be evaluated in terms of the stated purpose (Knafl and Howard, 1984). Qualitative studies are sometimes conducted to develop a new data collection instrument. The first aspect to assess is the importance of the instrument. Does it address a theoretical or practical need in nursing research? Measurement represents the technology needed to advance nursing science. Have sound principles of measurement been followed? Does the investigator provide evidence that validity beyond face validity has been sought? Is there information about the reliability of the instrument? Has it been pretested? If subscales are claimed in the tool, have sufficient numbers of subjects been tested?

In studies that include qualitative data to illustrate quantitative results, the space devoted to the qualitative aspects of the study will be smaller than in a study describing phenomena based primarily on qualitative data. In the former case a brief description of the qualitative data collection procedures and data analyses is sufficient. In the latter case the report should include a convincing rationale for selecting a qualitative approach. The introduction or "background of the study" section should demonstrate that the topic area has received little study. There should also be evidence that the sample studied provided representative information about the study population. Information attesting to the validity and reliability of the data collection measures and an adequate description of data anlaysis procedures should be present to enable the reader to judge the study's objectivity. Especially important is a description of the process by which results and conclusions were derived from the coded data.

In qualitative studies aimed at testing theory, investigators must provide readers with a clear description of the theoretical framework for the study. The reason for using the qualitative approach to test the theory should be stated.

Scientific rigor must be examined as in any experimental/quasiexperimental report. If an ex post facto design was employed, the reader should look for caution concerning statements about causality. As Kerlinger (1986) noted, an investigation of alternative hypotheses should always be part of an ex post facto study.

Qualitative studies designed to generate theory—usually termed "grounded theory"—are often difficult to evaluate. They are generally based on massive amounts of data, and the reader can gain little feel for the raw data. Such reports must provide sufficient detail about the methodology to explain data collection procedures at the beginning of the study and the rationale for changing them during the course of the study if this occurred. Changes in data collection queries are not flaws in grounded theory studies. As such studies proceed, the data and emerging theory commonly dictate that new questions be addressed. The quantity of data collected and the time span for its collection should be described. Information about the processing of the data, such as organization, coding, and memoing, should be explained clearly.

As with all nursing research, implications of study findings should be stated explicitly. Was the study worth doing? Did the insights and information generated from the study further the status of nursing science? Limitations of the data should be noted in relation to implications for practice, nursing education, and further research. The investigator should answer the "so what?" question about the findings in all three realms.

Quantitative, nonexperimental research reports

The purpose of exploratory studies and descriptive surveys is to identify relevant variables in specific settings and situations and describe phenomena of interest to the nursing profession. Thus the purpose of the research should focus on important concerns: significance to nursing is a primary consideration. This is true for all research, of course, but it is especially pertinent in evaluating nonexperimental studies.

Since the purpose of description is not limited to the sample at hand but is intended to be generalized to a target population, the sampling plan is also an important aspect of the research. Is the target or study population identified clearly? Given realistic limitations on resources, is the target population appropriate and is the sample size adequate? Is the sample representative? Are comparison groups used? Should they have been used? If comparison groups are involved, were adequate steps taken to ensure that they are reasonably equivalent?

In a correlational survey, have measures of association been used properly? Are conditions necessary for the use of certain test statistics met? Does the investigator maintain a focus on relationships without drifting into suggestions of causality?

Experimental and quasiexperimental research reports

Experimental and quasiexperimental studies must be examined for special attributes related to the scientific rigor of the research. The first aspect to examine is the construct validity of the experiment. This has to do with how well the measures employed to operationalize the independent and dependent variables represent the causal constructs being tested and how appropriate the methodology is to the experiment's aims (Shelley, 1984). Experiments always involve the manipulation of an independent variable to assess the effects of the manipulation on a dependent variable. The reader should be informed of the nature and strength of the experimental treatment. Was the independent variable manipulated in such a way as to maximize its impact on the experimental subjects? Is the investigator's description of the experimental treatment detailed enough to allow replication of the experiment by other investigators? Does the treatment appear robust enough to cause measurable differences in the dependent variable? Is there evidence of separation of treatments? Is it clear that all of the experimental subjects and none of the control subjects received the experimental treatment?

In assessing a study's internal validity, the reader must assess how well the investigator has managed the potential effects of extraneous variables. Campbell and Stanley (1963) identified eight classes of extraneous variables that can affect experimental outcomes: history, maturation, selection, mortality, the Hawthorne effect, testing, instrumentation, and regression. Some of these threats to internal validity are discussed in Chapter 4. Different emphasis may be placed on certain sources of error depending on the design of the experiment. For example, history and maturation are especially important factors in a one-group, pretest, posttest design. Selection bias can occur in any design, and the explanation of how experimental and control groups were constituted is an important focus in the evaluation of experimental studies. Similarly, the Hawthorne effect can cause problems in any design. Has the investigator made a realistic attempt to minimize this effect? The importance of mortality testing and instrumentation depends on the design employed, the number of data collection procedures used, and the duration of the experiment. Evaluation of these aspects of the research report focuses on examining the investigator's awareness of the problems and the provisions made to enhance the study's credibility. There is no perfect experiment. However, we can expect nurse scientists to make reasonable efforts to control for the effects of extraneous variables.

Examination of external validity (generalizability) requires the reader to assess the sampling plan used and the method of obtaining experimental and control groups. Was the pool of subjects obtained by random sampling procedures? Was assignment to the groups random or random/matched?

Problem 10-1

Critiquing a research report

Choose one of the following articles and use the guidelines from Fig. 10-1 to write a brief critique of the report. Limit yourself to one or two pages handwritten or typed double spaced. Evaluate the report; do not summarize it.

Hall L and Farel A (1988). Maternal stresses and depressive symptoms: correlates of behavior problems in young children. *Nursing Research* 37:156-161.

Megel M, Langston N, and Creswell J (1988). Scholarly productivity: a survey of nursing faculty researchers. *Journal of Professional Nursing* 4:45-54.

Brown B, Roberts J, Browne G, Byrne C, Love B, and Streiner D (1988). Gender differences in variables associated with psychosocial adjustment to a burn injury. *Research in Nursing and Health* 11:23-30.

REFERENCES

Campbell D and Stanley J (1963). *Experimental and quasi-experimental designs for research.* Chicago: Rand McNally.

Fawcett J (1982). Utilization of nursing research findings. *Image* 14:57-59.

Haller K, Reynolds M, and Horsley J (1979). Developing research-based innovation protocols. *Research in Nursing and Health* 2:45-51.

Havelock R and Havelock M (1973). *Training for change agents: a guide to the design of training programs in education and other fields.* Ann Arbor: University of Michigan Press.

Kerlinger F (1986). *Foundations of behavioral research.* New York: Holt, Rinehart & Winston, Inc.

Kleinbeck S (1988). Poster sessions bring research to the OR. *AORN Journal* 47:1299-1304.

Knafl K and Howard M (1984). Interpreting and reporting qualitative research. *Research in Nursing and Health* 7:17-24.

Lewin K (1951). *Field theory in social science.* New York: Harper & Brothers.

Lippitt R (1966). The process of utilization of social research to improve social practice. In Shostak A (ed). *Sociology in action: case studies in social problems and directed social change.* Homewood, Ill: Dorsey Press.

Rogers E (1983). *Diffusion of innovations,* 3rd ed. New York: The Free Press.

Shelley S (1984). *Research methods in nursing and health.* Boston: Little, Brown & Co., Inc.

Walker J (1969). The diffusion of innovation among the American states. *American Political Science Review* 63:880-899.

REFERENCES FOR FURTHER STUDY

Cobb A and Hagemaster J (1987). Ten criteria for evaluating qualitative research proposals. *Journal of Nursing Education* 26:138-143.

Fawcett J (1986). Analysis of research reports. *Journal of Nurse-Midwifery* 31:279-284.

Fleming J and Hayter J (1974). Reading research reports critically. *Nursing Outlook* 22:172-175.

Knafl K and Howard M (1984). Interpreting and reporting qualitative research. *Research in Nursing and Health* 7:17-24.

Leininger M (1968). The research critique: nature, function and art. *Nursing Research* 17:444-449.

Norbeck J (1979). The research critique. *Western Journal of Nursing Research* 1:296-306.

Scandlyn J (1987). How to read a research article. *Orthopaedic Nursing* 6:21-27.

Stetler C and Marram G (1976). Evaluation of research findings for applicability in practice. *Nursing Outlook* 24:559-563.

Stevenson P (1985). Reading a research report. *Intensive Care Nursing* 1:102-106.

Tanner C (1987). Evaluating research for use in practice. *Heart and Lung* 16:424-431.

Ward MJ and Felter ME (1978). What guidelines should be followed in critically evaluating research reports? *Nursing Research* 27:120-126.

Glossary

abscissa Horizontal (x) axis of a graph.

abstract Brief summary of a research proposal or report.

accidental sampling Selection of subjects based on convenience; a nonprobability sampling technique.

adequacy Desirable attribute of sampling whereby sufficient numbers of subjects (or objects) have been sampled to represent the population accurately.

alpha Greek letter that represents the probability of type I error in research.

analysis of variance Statistical procedure for comparing the effects of one or more treatments on two or more groups.

applied research Studies designed to seek answers to practical problems.

assumptions Basic ideas or concepts that are accepted as being true without empirical verification.

attrition Loss of subjects in a study. This can introduce bias, the direction or magnitude of which is unfortunately unknown. It can destroy random sampling provisions.

bar graph Display of frequencies as bars, either vertically or horizontally.

basic research Studies designed to produce new knowledge used to test or develop theory.

batch data processing Procedure whereby a job-stream consisting of commands and data is submitted all at once to a computer for processing.

behavioral measures Data collection techniques that rely on observation or measurement of human behavior.

beta Greek letter that represents the probability of type II error in research.

bias Phenomenon that distorts research data and results.

bibliography List of published and unpublished written work relating to a particular subject.

biophysiological measures Data collection techniques that produce measures of physiological status.

bracketing In qualitative data analysis, the process of putting aside what is known about a study topic to allow the data to convey undistorted information.

case study Research approach that relies on a comprehensive, in-depth analysis of a single entity: a patient, group, agency, or other social entity.

causal relationship Association between two or more variables so that the influence of one variable acts as a "cause" and the other acts as an "effect."

central tendency Descriptive statistical index used to describe some sort of center of a set of scores—usually the mean, median, or mode.

chi square Nonparametric statistical test used to determine the independence of variables, which is particularly useful for nominal level data.

clinical research Study designed to improve the practice of one of the health or helping professions.

cluster sampling Multistage procedure in which selection of units, such as hospitals, is followed by selection of subunits, such as patients.

Cochran's Q Nonparametric test designed to analyze variables consisting of dichotomous responses from related groups.

coding Procedure used to transform raw data into forms appropriate for computer-based data processing.

computer Electronic machine that can follow programmed instructions to perform mathematical operations with great accuracy and speed.

concept Abstract idea derived from empirical or logical evidence.

conceptual definition Accepted definition of a

phenomenon; the dictionary or authoritative definition of a concept.

conceptual framework Interrelated information derived from logical or empirical evidence that serves as a coherent scheme for studying relevant phenomena.

concurrent validity Attribute of a data collection instrument whereby the performance on the instrument is logically related to another measure.

confidence interval Range of values, derived from a statistical test, that is estimated to contain a population parameter.

confidence level In inferential statistics, the estimated probability that a population parameter lies within the computed confidence interval.

confidentiality Protection of the identities of research participants so that their names will not be linked to the data they provide.

construct Abstraction consisting of interrelated concepts.

construct validity Degree to which a data collection tool measures the attribute it was designed to measure.

content analysis Procedure for analyzing data produced by some sort of communication so that it can be described and summarized; data reduction.

content validity Attribute of a data collection instrument that indicates that the items represent the scope of the topic adequately.

contingency coefficient Inferential statistic computed with a chi square to express the degree of relationship between two nominal level variables.

contingency table Two-dimensional table constructed to cross-classify two categorical variables.

control group Research participants who are not exposed to the experimental treatment.

convenience sampling Nonprobability method of selecting research subjects based on their availabiliity and ease of recruitment.

correlation Relationship between two or more variables.

correlation coefficient Statistic that represents the degree of relationship between two variables.

correlation survey design Investigations that employ self-report data from research subjects to examine relationships among variables of interest.

Cramer's V Also known as Cramer's phi; a statistic used to represent the relationship between two nominal level variables.

criterion variable Outcome measure used to represent the effects of an independent variable; the dependent variable.

critical incident technique Method of data collection in which subjects are asked to describe specific occurrences that are related to the study purposes.

critique Analytical examination of a research report or proposal that involves a systematic assessment based on accepted standards of inquiry and communication.

Cronbach's alpha Statistic calculated to estimate the internal consistency or homogeneity of a data collection instrument.

cross-sectional study Research conducted at a single point in time based on data gathered from groups that differ on some variable of interest, such as age.

data Information collected in research.

degrees of freedom Statistical concept that refers to the number of sample values that cannot be calculated from information about other sample values and a computed statistic.

Delphi technique Procedure developed in management science for obtaining judgments from an expert panel through a series of questionnaires that pose questions and summarize group ideas.

dependent variable Outcome measure hypothesized to represent the effects of another (the independent) variable.

descriptive statistics Measures used to portray and summarize phenomena of interest in research.

descriptive study Research designed to portray the attributes of persons, groups, or situations accurately and objectively.

design Plan or blueprint for obtaining accurate information to answer research questions or test research hypotheses.

diary Record of events, opinions, or feelings that a person keeps over time.

dichotomous variable Characteristic or attribute that has only two values.

difficulty index Statistic, used in measurement, that represents the proportion of persons who answer a particular item correctly.

direct relationship Positive association between two variables.

directional hypothesis Educated guess that makes a statement concerning the direction of the relationship between two variables (that is, positive or negative relationship, or one group's attributes being greater than another's).

discrimination index Technique for describing relationships between items and total score.

dispersion Measure of the scatter of values of a variable.

effect size Statistical value that represents the magnitude of the results of a statistical analysis—for example, either a relationship between two variables or a comparison of groups.

empirical Reliance on information gained through use of the senses, such as observation.

empirical indicator Operational definition of a variable.

error of measurement Difference between the true scores and the obtained scores in measuring a variable.

ethics Respect for the rights of potential research participants in relation to professional, social, and legal responsibilities.

ex post facto study Research in which the independent variable is some naturally occurring attribute, such as gender or age; groups are constituted "after the fact."

experiment Study in which the investigator obtains and assigns research subjects randomly and manipulates an independent variable to examine its effects.

experimental group Research subjects who receive the experimental treatment.

exploratory research Study designed to identify relevant variables and examine relationships among variables in a preliminary way; a study devised to examine "new territory."

external validity Accuracy of generalizing results from an experimental study to the population.

extraneous variable Factors that may distort research results by their influence on study variables.

face validity Measurement attribute obtained by experts' review of a data collection instrument; the instrument appears to measure what it should measure "on the face of it."

factorial design Experimental design in which the effects of two or more independent variables are studied simultaneously; generally both main effects and interaction effects are analyzed.

Fisher's Exact test Nonparametric statistical test designed to determine whether two dichotomous variables are related.

fixed format Method of coding and entering data so that the same columns are used for the study variables for each case.

freefield format Method of data entry that places variable values in the same sequential order but not necessarily in the same columns for each case.

frequency distribution Tabular way of summarizing raw data.

frequency polygon Line graph constructed from a frequency distribution to show the number of times each value occurs in a set of data.

Friedman's two-way ANOVA Nonparametric statistical test designed to detect differences attributable to three or more treatments among dependent samples.

generalizability Degree to which research results can justifiably be stated to represent phenomena in the population.

graph Pictorial representation of data.

grounded theory Systematic treatment of qualitative data that leads to categories of information, related concepts, and ultimately "theory grounded in the data."

hardware Computer equipment.

Hawthorne effect Changes that occur in study subjects' behavior as a consequence of their awareness that they are being studied.

heterogeneity Degree of dissimilarity among subjects' attributes.

histogram Graphic representation of frequency distribution data.

homogeneity Degree of similarity among subjects' attributes.

hypothesis Statement of predicted relationships or differences among variables.

independent variable In experimental research, the manipulated variable; generally, the input rather than the output variable.

index Alphabetical list of terms or topics, appended to a written work, that gives numbers of pages containing information about the topic.

inferential statistics Mathematical procedures that permit investigators to infer whether relationships or differences occur at non-chance levels.

informed consent Agreement of potential research subjects to participate in a study with full understanding of its possible benefits and risks.

institutional review Process of peer review of a study design for ethical considerations.

instrument validity Degree to which a measurement technique measures what it purports to measure.

internal consistency Form of reliability that represents the degree to which all parts of a data collection instrument are measuring the same attribute.

internal validity Degree to which the outcomes of an experiment can be attributed to the manipulated variable(s) rather than to uncontrolled, extraneous factors.

interval measure Precise scale in which the distance between values is the same everywhere on the scale.

interview Data collection technique based on oral questions.

jobstream Set of statements consisting of (1) authorization to use the computer, (2) programming instructions for manipulating the data, (3) data, and (4) programming instructions for ending the job.

Kendall's tau Nonparametric measure of association used when one or both variables are measured at the ordinal level.

Kruskal-Wallis ANOVA Nonparametric statistical test for comparing the variance of variables at the ordinal level.

Kuder Richardson formulas Techniques for estimating internal consistency of a data collection instrument.

kurtosis Peakedness of a curve that represents the distribution of numerical data.

latent level Approach to content analysis that attempts to infer underlying motives or meaning of communications.

leptokurtic Tall, narrow curve that represents a distribution of numbers.

level of significance Represented by alpha; the probability of rejecting a null hypothesis when it is true.

Likert scale Commonly a measure of attitudes or opinions in which respondents indicate their degree of agreement or disagreement on an ordinal scale.

limitation Information that prevents study findings from being totally acceptable, such as a methodological flaw.

line graph Visual representation of information in which data points, determined by their values on the x and y axes, are connected.

literature review Systematic search of published works to gain information about a research topic.

logging on Procedure for signing onto a computer in which authorization codes—usually identification numbers and pass-

words—are entered at the beginning of a computer session.

longitudinal study Research in which data are collected from or about a group of subjects over time.

mainframe Enormous, time-sharing computer; also, a maxicomputer.

manifest level Approach to content analysis that relies only on the surface meaning of the communication.

Mann-Whitney U test Nonparametric statistical test designed to determine whether the medians of two groups are significantly different.

McNemar test Nonparametric statistical test for analyzing the significance of changes between dichotomous variables.

mean Arithmetic average of a set of numbers.

measurement Procedure of assigning numbers to attributes of objects according to accepted rules.

median Midpoint of a set of numbers.

mesokurtic Symmetrical curve representing a distribution of numbers.

microcomputer Stand-alone computer designed primarily for the personal use of one person.

minicomputer Large, time-sharing computer—smaller than a mainframe but many times larger than a microcomputer.

mode most frequently occurring value in a set of numbers.

model Symbolic representation of a theoretical or conceptual framework.

multimodal distribution Curve representing a distribution of numbers that has more than one peak.

multitrait multimethod matrix approach Procedure for establishing construct validity of a data collection instrument in which a strong relationship is demonstrated between the new measure and an existing measure known to be similar to the new measure, and a weak, nonexistent, or negative relationship is demonstrated between the new measure and an existing tool known to measure dissimilar attribute(s).

negative relationship Association between two variables in which higher values of one variable are associated with lower values of the other variable; as one variable increases, the other variable decreases.

negatively skewed distribution Curve whose tail is toward the low end of the abscissa.

nominal measure Categorical variables, such as

religion, that have no meaningful, numerical relationships among their classes.

nondirectional hypothesis Statement that predicts a difference or association between two variables but does not specify whether the association will be positive or negative or which group will have a larger mean or median than the other.

nonexperimental research Studies in which investigators do not manipulate an independent variable to examine its effects; rather, variables are identified, phenomena are described, or relationships are sought.

nonparametric statistics Mathematical approaches to data analysis that are distribution free and generally pertain to ordinal or nominal level variables.

nonprobability sampling Selection of research participants from a study population by nonrandom procedures—specifically called convenience, accidental, judgmental, quota, and systematic sampling.

normal curve Symmetrical, bell-shaped curve based on an exact mathematical equation that results in 68% of all values falling within two standard deviations of the mean (one above and one below) and 95% of all values falling in the area defined by two standard deviations above and two below the mean.

null hypothesis Statement that asserts there is no relationship or no difference between study variables. It is used with statistical tests as the statement to be rejected if support is demonstrated for the research hypothesis.

objectivity Unbiased examination of phenomena—a desirable attribute of scientific methods.

observational measures Data collection techniques that rely on the direct observation of research subjects' behavior.

one-tailed statistical test Type of procedure used when the research hypothesis specifies direction—for example, that one group's measure of central tendency will be greater than another's.

operational definition Definition of a variable that specifies how it will be measured.

ordinal measure Level of measurement that can be ordered or ranked.

ordinate Vertical (y) axis of a graph.

outcome measure Another term for dependent variable.

outlier Value for a variable that lies outside the normal range of values for the variable.

paired t test Parametric statistical test designed to determine whether the means of two dependent variables are significantly different.

parameter Population characteristic.

parametric statistic Mathematical procedure designed to make inferences about data; generally depends on assumptions regarding the distribution of the data, the level of measurement, and homogeneity of variance.

Pearson's correlation coefficient Parametric statistical test widely used to determine the relationships between variables.

phi Greek letter used to represent the relationship between two dichotomous variables.

pie graph Circle in which the percentages of a variable are represented as segments of the circle.

pilot study Preliminary research conducted to test elements of design before an actual full-scale study begins.

platykurtic Flat curve that represents a distribution of numbers.

population Universe for a study—all possible units that have the specified characteristic.

positive relationship Association between two variables in which higher values of one variable are associated with higher values of the other variable; as one variable increases, the other variables also increases.

positively skewed distribution Curve whose tail is toward the high end of the abscissa.

posttest Procedure in which data are collected after the administration of an experimental treatment.

power Ability of a research design to test relationships or differences among variables when those relationships or differences actually exist.

power analysis Procedure for estimating the likelihood that a type II error has been committed in a reported study; procedure for examining power prospectively for the purpose of determining the necessary sample size.

predictive validity Attribute of a data collection instrument that describes how well performance on the instrument predicts a future event or value on another data collection instrument.

pretest Collection of data before administration of an experimental treatment; also, preliminary trials with data collection instruments.

primary sources Firsthand information; in a literature review, the reports of the actual investigator's research.

principle Statement of the relationships between two or more concepts; a proposition.

probability sampling Random selection of subjects from a population so that all units of the population have an equal opportunity for being selected.

projective technique Approach to data collection that relies on the psychological evaluation of research subjects' responses to stimuli.

prospective study Research designed to examine variables of interest, going forward in time to examine changes that may have occurred.

psychometric characteristics Attributes of measurement of a data collection instrument or technique.

purposive sampling Nonprobability procedure for selecting study units based on certain relevant criteria.

Q sort Data collection method in which the subject sorts statements into specified piles based on the investigator's instructions—for example, agree, neither agree nor disagree, and disagree.

qualitative analysis Organization, summarization, and interpretation of communications that by nature are not numerical.

qualitative data Information from communication.

quantitative analysis Manipulation of data through various mathematical procedures designed to produce descriptive or inferential information.

quasiexperiment Study that does not meet all of the requirements of a true experiment—for example, the subjects may not have been randomly selected or randomly assigned to treatment groups.

questionnaire Method of data collection by means of paper-and-pencil, self-report data.

quota sampling Nonprobability procedure in which certain subject types are selected in predetermined numbers of proportions.

random assignment Placing research subjects into treatment groups so that each subject has an equal opportunity to be assigned to each group.

random sampling Probability procedure in which each potential unit has an equal opportunity of being selected.

range Difference between the highest score and the lowest score in a set of values, sometimes reported as the lowest to the highest instead of the difference.

ratio measure Level of measurement that has a zero value in addition to having all of the attributes of interval level measurement.

reactivity Distortion of research results that occurs because subjects change their behavior as a result of being exposed to some element of the experiment.

relationship Association between two or more variables.

reliability Consistency or stability of measurement in research.

replication Duplication of research procedures with a new sample to see whether the original results can be verified.

representativeness Desirable attribute of sampling in which the sample is like the population in relevant characteristics.

research Systematic use of scientific methods to find answers to questions.

research design Blueprint or plan for a study.

response rate Rate of participation in a study.

retrospective study Study that begins with an effect in the present and moves backward in search of trends or causal elements.

sample Portion of a population.

sampling Process of selecting units for study from a population.

sampling error Difference between a sample statistic and a population parameter.

scale Device for measuring variables.

secondary source Reference that quotes or summarizes information from original (primary) sources.

semantic differential Data collection instrument that consists of sets of bipolar adjectives separated by a scale for subjects' selection.

sensitivity Capability of a data collection technique for determining differences among individuals or groups or recognizing changes when they do occur.

sign test Nonparametric statistical test designed to analyze differences in directions of change scores between matched pairs of subjects.

simple random sample Study group derived by probability processes from a study population.

simple survey design Basic nonexperimental investigation that seeks to describe phenomena of interest.

skewness Property of asymmetry.

software Computer programs that control the actions of the computer; a computer's instructions.

Spearman's rank order coefficient Nonparametric statistical test used to determine the relationship between variables when measurement of one or both of them is at the ordinal level.

split half reliability Estimate of the internal consistency of a data collection instrument, obtained by correlating scores on one half of the measure with scores on the other half of the measure.

standard deviation Measure of dispersion; the square root of the variance.

statistics Applied mathematical science that permits investigators to estimate population parameters from sample data or determine whether a difference or relationship might occur at a nonchance level.

stratified random sample Aggregate obtained from dividing a population into subgroups and drawing units from each of the subgroups in a systematic manner.

subject Participant in a study.

survey Study conducted by means of questionnaires or interviews.

systematic sampling Procedure that commences with a random start, followed by the selection of every nth unit.

t **test** Parametric statistical test designed to determine whether the means of two variables differ significantly.

target population Universe from which a sample is selected.

test-retest reliability Estimate of the stability of a data collection instrument obtained by correlating the scores from successive administrations of the instrument to the same subjects.

text editor Computer program that allows the user to create, edit, and store documents or data.

theoretical framework Theory-based model for studying a problem.

time sharing Computer system large enough to accommodate many users simultaneously.

universe Total class of whatever is measured or observed in a study.

validity Extent to which a data collection instrument or procedure actually reflects the variable being studied.

variable Characteristic of persons or things under study.

variance Measure of dispersion; the square of the standard deviation.

vignette Short story or descriptive passage; in nursing research, a way of presenting hypothetical situations to research subjects for the purpose of obtaining their reactions.

Appendix A Critical values of Pearson's *r* for five significance levels

n − 2	.10	.05	.02	.01	.001
1	.98769	.99692	.999507	.999877	.9999988
2	.90000	.95000	.98000	.990000	.99900
3	.8054	.8783	.93433	.95873	.99116
4	.7293	.8114	.8822	.91720	.97406
5	.6694	.7545	.8329	.8745	.95074
6	.6215	.7067	.7887	.8343	.92493
7	.5822	.6664	.7498	.7977	.8982
8	.5494	.6319	.7155	.7646	.8721
9	.5214	.6021	.6851	.7348	.8471
10	.4973	.5760	.6581	.7079	.8233
11	.4762	.5529	.6339	.6835	.8010
12	.4575	.5324	.6120	.6614	.7800
13	.4409	.5139	.5923	.6411	.7603
14	.4259	.4973	.5742	.6226	.7420
15	.4124	.4821	.5577	.6055	.7246
16	.4000	.4683	.5425	.5897	.7084
17	.3887	.4555	.5285	.5751	.6932
18	.3783	.4438	.5155	.5614	.6787
19	.3687	.4329	.5034	.5487	.6652
20	.3598	.4227	.4921	.5368	.6524
25	.3233	.3809	.4451	.4869	.5974
30	.2960	.3494	.4093	.4487	.5541
35	.2746	.3246	.3810	.4182	.5189
40	.2573	.3044	.3578	.3932	.4896
45	.2428	.2875	.3384	.3721	.4648
50	.2306	.2732	.3218	.3541	.4433
60	.2108	.2500	.2948	.3248	.4078
70	.1954	.2319	.2737	.3017	.3799
80	.1829	.2172	.2565	.2830	.3568
90	.1726	.2050	.2422	.2673	.3375
100	.1638	.1946	.2301	.2540	.3211

From Fisher RA and Yates F (1978). *Statistical tables for biological, agricultural and medical research.* London: Longman Group Ltd. (previously published by Oliver & Boyd Ltd., Edinburgh). By permission of the authors and publishers.

Appendix B Critical values of τ_S, the Spearman rank correlation coefficient

| N | Significance level (one-tailed test) | |
	.05	.01
4	1.000	
5	.900	1.000
6	.829	.943
7	.714	.893
8	.643	.833
9	.600	.783
10	.564	.746
12	.506	.712
14	.456	.645
16	.425	.601
18	.399	.564
20	.377	.534
22	.359	.508
24	.343	.485
26	.329	.465
28	.317	.448
30	.306	.432

Adapted from Olds EG (1938). Distributions of sums of squares of rank differences for small numbers of individuals. *Annals of Mathematical Statistics* 9:133-148; and from Olds EG (1949). The 5% significance levels for sums of squares of rank differences and a correction. *Annals of Mathematical Statistics* 20:117-118. In Siegel S (1956). Nonparametric statistics for the behavioral sciences. New York: McGraw-Hill Book Co Inc.

Appendix C Probabilities associated with values as large as observed values of S in the Kendall rank correlation coefficient

	Values of N					Values of N		
S	4	5	8	9	S	6	7	10
0	.625	.592	.548	.540	1	.500	.500	.500
2	.375	.408	.452	.460	3	.360	.386	.431
4	.167	.242	.360	.381	5	.235	.281	.364
6	.042	.117	.274	.306	7	.136	.191	.300
8		.042	.199	.238	9	.068	.119	.242
10		.0083	.138	.179	11	.028	.068	.190
12			.089	.130	13	.0083	.035	.146
14			.054	.090	15	.0014	.015	.108
16			.031	.060	17		.0054	.078
18			.016	.038	19		.0014	.054
20			.0071	.022	21		.00020	.036
22			.0028	.012	23			.023
24			.00087	.0063	25			.014
26			.00019	.0029	27			.0083
28			.000025	.0012	29			.0046
30				.00043	31			.0023
32				.00012	33			.0011
34				.000025	35			.00047
36				.0000028	37			.00018
					39			.000058
					41			.000015
					43			.0000028
					45			.00000028

Adapted from Kendall MG (1948). *Rank correlation methods*. London: Charles Griffin & Co, Ltd. In Siegel S (1956). *Nonparametric statistics for the behavioral sciences*. New York: McGraw-Hill Book Co Inc.

295

Appendix D   Distribution of chi-square probability

df	Level of significance				
	.10	.05	.02	.01	.001
1	2.71	3.84	5.41	6.63	10.83
2	4.61	5.99	7.82	9.21	13.82
3	6.25	7.82	9.84	11.34	16.27
4	7.78	9.49	11.67	13.28	18.46
5	9.24	11.07	13.39	15.09	20.52
6	10.64	12.59	15.03	16.81	22.46
7	12.02	14.07	16.62	18.48	24.32
8	13.36	15.51	18.17	20.09	26.12
9	14.68	16.92	19.68	21.67	27.88
10	15.99	18.31	21.16	23.21	29.59
11	17.28	19.68	22.62	24.72	31.26
12	18.55	21.03	24.05	26.22	32.91
13	19.81	22.36	25.47	27.69	34.53
14	21.06	23.68	26.87	29.14	36.12
15	22.31	25.00	28.26	30.58	37.70
16	23.54	26.30	29.63	32.00	39.25
17	24.77	27.59	31.00	33.41	40.79
18	25.99	28.87	32.35	34.81	42.31
19	27.20	30.14	33.69	36.19	43.82
20	28.41	31.41	35.02	37.57	45.32
21	29.62	32.67	36.34	38.93	46.80
22	30.81	33.92	37.66	40.29	48.27
23	32.01	35.17	38.97	41.64	49.73
24	33.20	36.42	40.27	42.98	51.18
25	34.38	37.65	41.57	44.31	52.62
26	35.56	38.89	42.86	45.64	54.05
27	36.74	40.11	44.14	46.96	55.48
28	37.92	41.34	45.42	48.28	56.89
29	39.09	42.56	46.69	49.59	58.30
30	40.26	43.77	47.96	50.89	59.70

From Siegel S (1956). *Nonparametric statistics for the behavioral sciences.* New York: McGraw-Hill Book Co Inc.

Appendix E The *t* distribution

df	Alpha level (directional)					
	.10	.05	.025	.01	.005	.0005
	Alpha level (nondirectional)					
	.20	.10	.05	.02	.01	.001
1	3.078	6.314	12.706	31.821	63.657	636.619
2	1.886	2.920	4.303	6.965	9.925	31.598
3	1.638	2.353	3.182	4.541	5.841	12.924
4	1.533	2.132	2.776	3.747	4.604	8.610
5	1.476	2.015	2.571	3.365	4.032	6.869
6	1.440	1.943	2.447	3.143	3.707	5.959
7	1.415	1.895	2.365	2.998	3.499	5.408
8	1.397	1.860	2.306	2.896	3.355	5.041
9	1.383	1.833	2.262	2.821	3.250	4.781
10	1.372	1.812	2.228	2.764	3.169	4.587
11	1.363	1.796	2.201	2.718	3.106	4.437
12	1.356	1.782	2.179	2.681	3.055	4.318
13	1.350	1.771	2.160	2.650	3.012	4.221
14	1.345	1.761	2.145	2.624	2.977	4.140
15	1.341	1.753	2.131	2.602	2.947	4.073
16	1.337	1.746	2.120	2.583	2.921	4.015
17	1.333	1.740	2.110	2.567	2.898	3.965
18	1.330	1.734	2.101	2.552	2.878	3.922
19	1.328	1.729	2.093	2.539	2.861	3.883
20	1.325	1.725	2.086	2.528	2.845	3.850
21	1.323	1.721	2.080	2.518	2.831	3.819
22	1.321	1.717	2.074	2.508	2.819	3.792
23	1.319	1.714	2.069	2.500	2.807	3.767
24	1.318	1.711	2.064	2.492	2.797	3.745
25	1.316	1.708	2.060	2.485	2.787	3.725
26	1.315	1.706	2.056	2.479	2.779	3.707
27	1.314	1.703	2.052	2.473	2.771	3.690
28	1.313	1.701	2.048	2.467	2.763	3.674
29	1.311	1.699	2.045	2.462	2.756	3.659
30	1.310	1.697	2.042	2.457	2.750	3.646
40	1.303	1.684	2.021	2.423	2.704	3.551
60	1.296	1.671	2.000	2.390	2.660	3.460
120	1.289	1.658	1.980	2.358	2.617	3.373
∞	1.282	1.645	1.960	2.326	2.576	3.291

From Fisher RA and Yates F (1978). *Statistical tables for biological, agricultural and medical research.* London: Longman Group Ltd (previously published by Oliver & Boyd Ltd, Edinburgh). By permission of the authors and publishers.

Appendix F Tables of critical values of U in the Mann-Whitney test

Table F-1 Probabilities associated with values as small as observed values of U in the Mann-Whitney test ($n_2 < 9$)

$n_2 = 3$

U \ n_1	1	2	3
0	.250	.100	.050
1	.500	.200	.100
2	.750	.400	.200
3		.600	.350
4			.500
5			.650

$n_2 = 4$

U \ n_1	1	2	3	4
0	.200	.067	.028	.014
1	.400	.133	.057	.029
2	.600	.267	.114	.057
3		.400	.200	.100
4		.600	.314	.171
5			.429	.243
6			.571	.343
7				.443
8				.557

From Siegel S (1956). *Nonparametric statistics for the behavioral sciences.* New York: McGraw-Hill Book Co Inc.
Table probabilities are one tailed. For two-tailed probabilities, double the value in the table.

$n_2 = 5$

$U \backslash n_1$	1	2	3	4	5
0	.167	.047	.018	.008	.004
1	.333	.095	.036	.016	.008
2	.500	.190	.071	.032	.016
3	.667	.286	.125	.056	.028
4		.429	.196	.095	.048
5		.571	.286	.143	.075
6			.393	.206	.111
7			.500	.278	.155
8			.607	.365	.210
9				.452	.274
10				.548	.345
11					.421
12					.500
13					.579

$n_2 = 6$

$U \backslash n_1$	1	2	3	4	5	6
0	.143	.036	.012	.005	.002	.001
1	.286	.071	.024	.010	.004	.002
2	.428	.143	.048	.019	.009	.004
3	.571	.214	.083	.033	.015	.008
4		.321	.131	.057	.026	.013
5		.429	.190	.086	.041	.021
6		.571	.274	.129	.063	.032
7			.357	.176	.089	.047
8			.452	.238	.123	.066
9			.548	.305	.165	.090
10				.381	.214	.120
11				.457	.268	.155
12				.545	.331	.197
13					.396	.242
14					.465	.294
15					.535	.350
16						.409
17						.469
18						.531

$n_2 = 7$

U / n_1	1	2	3	4	5	6	7
0	.125	.028	.008	.003	.001	.001	.000
1	.250	.056	.017	.006	.003	.001	.001
2	.375	.111	.033	.012	.005	.002	.001
3	.500	.167	.058	.021	.009	.004	.002
4	.625	.250	.092	.036	.015	.007	.003
5		.333	.133	.055	.024	.011	.006
6		.444	.192	.082	.037	.017	.009
7		.556	.258	.115	.053	.026	.013
8			.333	.158	.074	.037	.019
9			.417	.206	.101	.051	.027
10			.500	.264	.134	.069	.036
11			.583	.324	.172	.090	.049
12				.394	.216	.117	.064
13				.464	.265	.147	.082
14				.538	.319	.183	.104
15					.378	.223	.130
16					.438	.267	.159
17					.500	.314	.191
18					.562	.365	.228
19						.418	.267
20						.473	.310
21						.527	.355
22							.402
23							.451
24							.500
25							.549

$n_2 = 8$

U \ n_1	1	2	3	4	5	6	7	8	t	Normal
0	.111	.022	.006	.002	.001	.000	.000	.000	3.308	.001
1	.222	.044	.012	.004	.002	.001	.000	.000	3.203	.001
2	.333	.089	.024	.008	.003	.001	.001	.000	3.098	.001
3	.444	.133	.042	.014	.005	.002	.001	.001	2.993	.001
4	.556	.200	.067	.024	.009	.004	.002	.001	2.888	.002
5		.267	.097	.036	.015	.006	.003	.001	2.783	.003
6		.356	.139	.055	.023	.010	.005	.002	2.678	.004
7		.444	.188	.077	.033	.015	.007	.003	2.573	.005
8		.556	.248	.107	.047	.021	.010	.005	2.468	.007
9			.315	.141	.064	.030	.014	.007	2.363	.009
10			.387	.184	.085	.041	.020	.010	2.258	.012
11			.461	.230	.111	.054	.027	.014	2.153	.016
12			.539	.285	.142	.071	.036	.019	2.048	.020
13				.341	.177	.091	.047	.025	1.943	.026
14				.404	.217	.114	.060	.032	1.838	.033
15				.467	.262	.141	.076	.041	1.733	.041
16				.533	.311	.172	.095	.052	1.628	.052
17					.362	.207	.116	.065	1.523	.064
18					.416	.245	.140	.080	1.418	.078
19					.472	.286	.168	.097	1.313	.094
20					.528	.331	.198	.117	1.208	.113
21						.377	.232	.139	1.102	.135
22						.426	.268	.164	.998	.159
23						.475	.306	.191	.893	.185
24						.525	.347	.221	.788	.215
25							.389	.253	.683	.247
26							.433	.287	.578	.282
27							.478	.323	.473	.318
28							.522	.360	.368	.356
29								.399	.263	.396
30								.439	.158	.437
31								.480	.052	.481
32								.520		

Table F-2 Critical values of the U statistic of the Mann-Whitney test ($n_2 \geq 9$)

α = .002 (two-tailed) and .001 (one-tailed)

n_1 \ n_2	9	10	11	12	13	14	15	16	17	18	19	20
1												
2												
3									0	0	0	0
4		0	0	0	1	1	1	2	2	3	3	3
5	1	1	2	2	3	3	4	5	5	6	7	7
6	2	3	4	4	5	6	7	8	9	10	11	12
7	3	5	6	7	8	9	10	11	13	14	15	16
8	5	6	8	9	11	12	14	15	17	18	20	21
9	7	8	10	12	14	15	17	19	21	23	25	26
10	8	10	12	14	17	19	21	23	25	27	29	32
11	10	12	15	17	20	22	24	27	29	32	34	37
12	12	14	17	20	23	25	28	31	34	37	40	42
13	14	17	20	23	26	29	32	35	38	42	45	48
14	15	19	22	25	29	32	36	39	43	46	50	54
15	17	21	24	28	32	36	40	43	47	51	55	59
16	19	23	27	31	35	39	43	48	52	56	60	65
17	21	25	29	34	38	43	47	52	57	61	66	70
18	23	27	32	37	42	46	51	56	61	66	71	76
19	25	29	34	40	45	50	55	60	66	71	77	82
20	26	32	37	42	48	54	59	65	70	76	82	88

$\alpha = .02$ (two-tailed) and .01 (one-tailed)

n₁ \ n₂	9	10	11	12	13	14	15	16	17	18	19	20
1												
2					0	0	0	0	0	0	1	1
3	1	1	1	2	2	2	3	3	4	4	4	5
4	3	3	4	5	5	6	7	7	8	9	9	10
5	5	6	7	8	9	10	11	12	13	14	15	16
6	7	8	9	11	12	13	15	16	18	19	20	22
7	9	11	12	14	16	17	19	21	23	24	26	28
8	11	13	15	17	20	22	24	26	28	30	32	34
9	14	16	18	21	23	26	28	31	33	36	38	40
10	16	19	22	24	27	30	33	36	38	41	44	47
11	18	22	25	28	31	34	37	41	44	47	50	53
12	21	24	28	31	35	38	42	46	49	53	56	60
13	23	27	31	35	39	43	47	51	55	59	63	67
14	26	30	34	38	43	47	51	56	60	65	69	73
15	28	33	37	42	47	51	56	61	66	70	75	80
16	31	36	41	46	51	56	61	66	71	76	82	87
17	33	38	44	49	55	60	66	71	77	82	88	93
18	36	41	47	53	59	65	70	76	82	88	94	100
19	38	44	50	56	63	69	75	82	88	94	101	107
20	40	47	53	60	67	73	80	87	93	100	107	114

α = .05 (two-tailed) and .025 (one-tailed)

n_1 \ n_2	9	10	11	12	13	14	15	16	17	18	19	20
1												
2	0	0	0	1	1	1	1	1	2	2	2	2
3	2	3	3	4	4	5	5	6	6	7	7	8
4	4	5	6	7	8	9	10	11	11	12	13	13
5	7	8	9	11	12	13	14	15	17	18	19	20
6	10	11	13	14	16	17	19	21	22	24	25	27
7	12	14	16	18	20	22	24	26	28	30	32	34
8	15	17	19	22	24	26	29	31	34	36	38	41
9	17	20	23	26	28	31	34	37	39	42	45	48
10	20	23	26	29	33	36	39	42	45	48	52	55
11	23	26	30	33	37	40	44	47	51	55	58	62
12	26	29	33	37	41	45	49	53	57	61	65	69
13	28	33	37	41	45	50	54	59	63	67	72	76
14	31	36	40	45	50	55	59	64	67	74	78	83
15	34	39	44	49	54	59	64	70	75	80	85	90
16	37	42	47	53	59	64	70	75	81	86	92	98
17	39	45	51	57	63	67	75	81	87	93	99	105
18	42	48	55	61	67	74	80	86	93	99	106	112
19	45	52	58	65	72	78	85	92	99	106	113	119
20	48	55	62	69	76	83	90	98	105	112	119	127

α = .10 (two-tailed) and .05 (one-tailed)

n_1 \ n_2	9	10	11	12	13	14	15	16	17	18	19	20
1											0	0
2	1	1	1	2	2	2	3	3	3	4	4	4
3	3	4	5	5	6	7	7	8	9	9	10	11
4	6	7	8	9	10	11	12	14	15	16	17	18
5	9	11	12	13	15	16	18	19	20	22	23	25
6	12	14	16	17	19	21	23	25	26	28	30	32
7	15	17	19	21	24	26	28	30	33	35	37	39
8	18	20	23	26	28	31	33	36	39	41	44	47
9	21	24	27	30	33	36	39	42	45	48	51	54
10	24	27	31	34	37	41	44	48	51	55	58	62
11	27	31	34	38	42	46	50	54	57	61	65	69
12	30	34	38	42	47	51	55	60	64	68	72	77
13	33	37	42	47	51	56	61	65	70	75	80	84
14	36	41	46	51	56	61	66	71	77	82	87	92
15	39	44	50	55	61	66	72	77	83	88	94	100
16	42	48	54	60	65	71	77	83	89	95	101	107
17	45	51	57	64	70	77	83	89	96	102	109	115
18	48	55	61	68	75	82	88	95	102	109	116	123
19	51	58	65	72	80	87	94	101	109	116	123	130
20	54	62	69	77	84	92	100	107	115	123	130	138

Appendix G   Probabilities associated with values as small as observed values of *x* in the binomial test

N \ x	0	1	2	3	4	5	6	7	8	9	10	11	12	13	14	15
5	031	188	500	812	969	*										
6	016	109	344	656	891	984	*									
7	008	062	227	500	773	938	992	*								
8	004	035	145	363	637	855	965	996	*							
9	002	020	090	254	500	746	910	980	998	*						
10	001	011	055	172	377	623	828	945	989	999	*					
11		006	033	113	274	500	726	887	967	994	*	*				
12		003	019	073	194	387	613	806	927	981	997	*	*			
13		002	011	046	133	291	500	709	867	954	989	998	*	*		
14		001	006	029	090	212	395	605	788	910	971	994	999	*	*	
15			004	018	059	151	304	500	696	849	941	982	996	*	*	*
16			002	011	038	105	227	402	598	773	895	962	989	998	*	*
17			001	006	025	072	166	315	500	685	834	928	975	994	999	*
18			001	004	015	048	119	240	407	593	760	881	952	985	996	999
19				002	010	032	084	180	324	500	676	820	916	968	990	998
20				001	006	021	058	132	252	412	588	748	868	942	979	994
21				001	004	013	039	095	192	332	500	668	808	905	961	987
22					002	008	026	067	143	262	416	584	738	857	933	974
23					001	005	017	047	105	202	339	500	661	798	895	953
24					001	003	011	032	076	154	271	419	581	729	846	924
25						002	007	022	054	115	212	345	500	655	788	885

Adapted from Walker H and Lev J (1953). *Statistical inference.* New York: Holt, Rinehart & Winston. In Siegel S (1956). *Nonparametric statistics for the behavioral sciences.* New York: McGraw-Hill Book Co Inc.

Given in the body of this table are one-tailed probabilities under H_o for the binomial test when $P = Q = \frac{1}{2}$. To save space, decimal points are omitted in the p's.

*1.0 or approximately 1.0.

Appendix H   Percentage points of the F distribution

Degrees of freedom; $\alpha = .05$

v_2 \ v_1	1	2	3	4	5	6	7	8	9
1	161.4	199.5	215.7	224.6	230.2	234.0	236.8	238.9	240.5
2	18.51	19.00	19.16	19.25	19.30	19.33	19.35	19.37	19.38
3	10.13	9.55	9.28	9.12	9.01	8.94	8.89	8.85	8.81
4	7.71	6.94	6.59	6.39	6.26	6.16	6.09	6.04	6.00
5	6.61	5.79	5.41	5.19	5.05	4.95	4.88	4.82	4.77
6	5.99	5.14	4.76	4.53	4.39	4.28	4.21	4.15	4.10
7	5.59	4.74	4.35	4.12	3.97	3.87	3.79	3.73	3.68
8	5.32	4.46	4.07	3.84	3.69	3.58	3.50	3.44	3.39
9	5.12	4.26	3.86	3.63	3.48	3.37	3.29	3.23	3.18
10	4.96	4.10	3.71	3.48	3.33	3.22	3.14	3.07	3.02
11	4.84	3.98	3.59	3.36	3.20	3.09	3.01	2.95	2.90
12	4.75	3.89	3.49	3.26	3.11	3.00	2.91	2.85	2.80
13	4.67	3.81	3.41	3.18	3.03	2.92	2.83	2.77	2.71
14	4.60	3.74	3.34	3.11	2.96	2.85	2.76	2.70	2.65
15	4.54	3.68	3.29	3.06	2.90	2.79	2.71	2.64	2.59
16	4.49	3.63	3.24	3.01	2.85	2.74	2.66	2.59	2.54
17	4.45	3.59	3.20	2.96	2.81	2.70	2.61	2.55	2.49
18	4.41	3.55	3.16	2.93	2.77	2.66	2.58	2.51	2.46
19	4.38	3.52	3.13	2.90	2.74	2.63	2.54	2.48	2.42
20	4.35	3.49	3.10	2.87	2.71	2.60	2.51	2.45	2.39
21	4.32	3.47	3.07	2.84	2.68	2.57	2.49	2.42	2.37
22	4.30	3.44	3.05	2.82	2.66	2.55	2.46	2.40	2.34
23	4.28	3.42	3.03	2.80	2.64	2.53	2.44	2.37	2.32
24	4.26	3.40	3.01	2.78	2.62	2.51	2.42	2.36	2.30
25	4.24	3.39	2.99	2.76	2.60	2.49	2.40	2.34	2.28
26	4.23	3.37	2.98	2.74	2.59	2.47	2.39	2.32	2.27
27	4.21	3.35	2.96	2.73	2.57	2.46	2.37	2.31	2.25
28	4.20	3.34	2.95	2.71	2.56	2.45	2.36	2.29	2.24
29	4.18	3.33	2.93	2.70	2.55	2.43	2.35	2.28	2.22
30	4.17	3.32	2.92	2.69	2.53	2.42	2.33	2.27	2.21
40	4.08	3.23	2.84	2.61	2.45	2.34	2.25	2.18	2.12
60	4.00	3.15	2.76	2.53	2.37	2.25	2.17	2.10	2.04
120	3.92	3.07	2.68	2.45	2.29	2.17	2.09	2.02	1.96
$\propto$	3.84	3.00	2.60	2.37	2.21	2.10	2.01	1.94	1.88

From Merrington M and Thompson CM (1943). *Biometrika* 33:73-78.

10	12	15	20	24	30	40	60	120	∝	v_1 / v_2
241.9	243.9	245.9	248.0	249.1	250.1	251.1	252.2	253.3	254.3	1
19.40	19.41	19.43	19.45	19.45	19.46	19.47	19.48	19.49	19.50	2
8.79	8.74	8.70	8.66	8.64	8.62	8.59	8.57	8.55	8.53	3
5.96	5.91	5.86	5.80	5.77	5.75	5.72	5.69	5.66	5.63	4
4.74	4.68	4.62	4.56	4.53	4.50	4.46	4.43	4.40	4.36	5
4.06	4.00	3.94	3.87	3.84	3.81	3.77	3.74	3.70	3.67	6
3.64	3.57	3.51	3.44	3.41	3.38	3.34	3.30	3.27	3.23	7
3.35	3.28	3.22	3.15	3.12	3.08	3.04	3.01	2.97	2.93	8
3.14	3.07	3.01	2.94	2.90	2.86	2.83	2.79	2.75	2.71	9
2.98	2.91	2.85	2.77	2.74	2.70	2.66	2.62	2.58	2.54	10
2.85	2.79	2.72	2.65	2.61	2.57	2.53	2.49	2.45	2.40	11
2.75	2.69	2.62	2.54	2.51	2.47	2.43	2.38	2.34	2.30	12
2.67	2.60	2.53	2.46	2.42	2.38	2.34	2.30	2.25	2.21	13
2.60	2.53	2.46	2.39	2.35	2.31	2.27	2.22	2.18	2.13	14
2.54	2.48	2.40	2.33	2.29	2.25	2.20	2.16	2.11	2.07	15
2.49	2.42	2.35	2.28	2.24	2.19	2.15	2.11	2.06	2.01	16
2.45	2.38	2.31	2.23	2.19	2.15	2.10	2.06	2.01	1.96	17
2.41	2.34	2.27	2.19	2.15	2.11	2.06	2.02	1.97	1.92	18
2.38	2.31	2.23	2.16	2.11	2.07	2.03	1.98	1.93	1.88	19
2.35	2.28	2.20	2.12	2.08	2.04	1.99	1.95	1.90	1.84	20
2.32	2.25	2.18	2.10	2.05	2.01	1.96	1.92	1.87	1.81	21
2.30	2.23	2.15	2.07	2.03	1.98	1.94	1.89	1.84	1.78	22
2.27	2.20	2.13	2.05	2.01	1.96	1.91	1.86	1.81	1.76	23
2.25	2.18	2.11	2.03	1.98	1.94	1.89	1.84	1.79	1.73	24
2.24	2.16	2.09	2.01	1.96	1.92	1.87	1.82	1.77	1.71	25
2.22	2.15	2.07	1.99	1.95	1.90	1.85	1.80	1.75	1.69	26
2.20	2.13	2.06	1.97	1.93	1.88	1.84	1.79	1.73	1.67	27
2.19	2.12	2.04	1.96	1.91	1.87	1.82	1.77	1.71	1.65	28
2.18	2.10	2.03	1.94	1.90	1.85	1.81	1.75	1.70	1.64	29
2.16	2.09	2.01	1.93	1.89	1.84	1.79	1.74	1.68	1.62	30
2.08	2.00	1.92	1.84	1.79	1.74	1.69	1.64	1.58	1.51	40
1.99	1.92	1.84	1.75	1.70	1.65	1.59	1.53	1.47	1.39	60
1.91	1.83	1.75	1.66	1.61	1.55	1.50	1.43	1.35	1.25	120
1.83	1.75	1.67	1.57	1.52	1.46	1.39	1.32	1.22	1.00	∝

Degrees of freedom; $\alpha = .01$

v_2 \ v_1	1	2	3	4	5	6	7	8	9
1	4052	4999.5	5403	5625	5764	5859	5928	5982	6022
2	98.50	99.00	99.17	99.25	99.30	99.33	99.36	99.37	99.39
3	34.12	30.82	29.46	28.71	28.24	27.91	27.67	27.49	27.35
4	21.20	18.00	16.69	15.98	15.52	15.21	14.98	14.80	14.66
5	16.26	13.27	12.06	11.39	10.97	10.67	10.46	10.29	10.16
6	13.75	10.92	9.78	9.15	8.75	8.47	8.26	8.10	7.98
7	12.25	9.55	8.45	7.85	7.46	7.19	6.99	6.84	6.72
8	11.26	8.65	7.59	7.01	6.63	6.37	6.18	6.03	5.91
9	10.56	8.02	6.99	6.42	6.06	5.80	5.61	5.47	5.35
10	10.04	7.56	6.55	5.99	5.64	5.39	5.20	5.06	4.94
11	9.65	7.21	6.22	5.67	5.32	5.07	4.89	4.74	4.63
12	9.33	6.93	5.95	5.41	5.06	4.82	4.64	4.50	4.39
13	9.07	6.70	5.74	5.21	4.86	4.62	4.44	4.30	4.19
14	8.86	6.51	5.56	5.04	4.69	4.46	4.28	4.14	4.03
15	8.68	6.36	5.42	4.89	4.56	4.32	4.14	4.00	3.89
16	8.53	6.23	5.29	4.77	4.44	4.20	4.03	3.89	3.78
17	8.40	6.11	5.18	4.67	4.34	4.10	3.93	3.79	3.68
18	8.29	6.01	5.09	4.58	4.25	4.01	3.84	3.71	3.60
19	8.18	5.93	5.01	4.50	4.17	3.94	3.77	3.63	3.52
20	8.10	5.85	4.94	4.43	4.10	3.87	3.70	3.56	3.46
21	8.02	5.78	4.87	4.37	4.04	3.81	3.64	3.51	3.40
22	7.95	5.72	4.82	4.31	3.99	3.76	3.59	3.45	3.35
23	7.88	5.66	4.76	4.26	3.94	3.71	3.54	3.41	3.30
24	7.82	5.61	4.72	4.22	3.90	3.67	3.50	3.36	3.26
25	7.77	5.57	4.68	4.18	3.85	3.63	3.46	3.32	3.22
26	7.72	5.53	4.64	4.14	3.82	3.59	3.42	3.29	3.18
27	7.68	5.49	4.60	4.11	3.78	3.56	3.39	3.26	3.15
28	7.64	5.45	4.57	4.07	3.75	3.53	3.36	3.23	3.12
29	7.60	5.42	4.54	4.04	3.73	3.50	3.33	3.20	3.09
30	7.56	5.39	4.51	4.02	3.70	3.47	3.30	3.17	3.07
40	7.31	5.18	4.31	3.83	3.51	3.29	3.12	2.99	2.89
60	7.08	4.98	4.13	3.65	3.34	3.12	2.95	2.82	2.72
120	6.85	4.79	3.95	3.48	3.17	2.96	2.79	2.66	2.56
∞	6.63	4.61	3.78	3.32	3.02	2.80	2.64	2.51	2.41

10	12	15	20	24	30	40	60	120	∝	v_1 / v_2
6056	6106	6157	6209	6235	6261	6287	6313	6339	6366	1
99.40	99.42	99.43	99.45	99.46	99.47	99.47	99.48	99.49	99.50	2
27.23	27.05	26.87	26.69	26.60	26.50	26.41	26.32	26.22	26.13	3
14.55	14.37	14.20	14.02	13.93	13.84	13.75	13.65	13.56	13.46	4
10.05	9.89	9.72	9.55	9.47	9.38	9.29	9.20	9.11	9.02	5
7.87	7.72	7.56	7.40	7.31	7.23	7.14	7.06	6.97	6.88	6
6.62	6.47	6.31	6.16	6.07	5.99	5.91	5.82	5.74	5.65	7
5.81	5.67	5.52	5.36	5.28	5.20	5.12	5.03	4.95	4.86	8
5.26	5.11	4.96	4.81	4.73	4.65	4.57	4.48	4.40	4.31	9
4.85	4.71	4.56	4.41	4.33	4.25	4.17	4.08	4.00	3.91	10
4.54	4.40	4.25	4.10	4.02	3.94	3.86	3.78	3.69	3.60	11
4.30	4.16	4.01	3.86	3.78	3.70	3.62	3.54	3.45	3.36	12
4.10	3.96	3.82	3.66	3.59	3.51	3.43	3.34	3.25	3.17	13
3.94	3.80	3.66	3.51	3.43	3.35	3.27	3.18	3.09	3.00	14
3.80	3.67	3.52	3.37	3.29	3.21	3.13	3.05	2.96	2.87	15
3.69	3.55	3.41	3.26	3.18	3.10	3.02	2.93	2.84	2.75	16
3.59	3.46	3.31	3.16	3.08	3.00	2.92	2.83	2.75	2.65	17
3.51	3.37	3.23	3.08	3.00	2.92	2.84	2.75	2.66	2.57	18
3.43	3.30	3.15	3.00	2.92	2.84	2.76	2.67	2.58	2.49	19
3.37	3.23	3.09	2.94	2.86	2.78	2.69	2.61	2.52	2.42	20
3.31	3.17	3.03	2.88	2.80	2.72	2.64	2.55	2.46	2.36	21
3.26	3.12	2.98	2.83	2.75	2.67	2.58	2.50	2.40	2.31	22
3.21	3.07	2.93	2.78	2.70	2.62	2.54	2.45	2.35	2.26	23
3.17	3.03	2.89	2.74	2.66	2.58	2.49	2.40	2.31	2.21	24
3.13	2.99	2.85	2.70	2.62	2.54	2.45	2.36	2.27	2.17	25
3.09	2.96	2.81	2.66	2.58	2.50	2.42	2.33	2.23	2.13	26
3.06	2.93	2.78	2.63	2.55	2.47	2.38	2.29	2.20	2.10	27
3.03	2.90	2.75	2.60	2.52	2.44	2.35	2.26	2.17	2.06	28
3.00	2.87	2.73	2.57	2.49	2.41	2.33	2.23	2.14	2.03	29
2.98	2.84	2.70	2.55	2.47	2.39	2.30	2.21	2.11	2.01	30
2.80	2.66	2.52	2.37	2.29	2.20	2.11	2.02	1.92	1.80	40
2.63	2.50	2.35	2.20	2.12	2.03	1.94	1.84	1.73	1.60	60
2.47	2.34	2.19	2.03	1.95	1.86	1.76	1.66	1.53	1.38	120
2.32	2.18	2.04	1.88	1.79	1.70	1.59	1.47	1.32	1.00	∝

Appendix I Probabilities associated with values as large as observed values of H in the Kruskal-Wallis one-way analysis of variance by ranks test

Sample sizes					Sample sizes				
n_1	n_2	n_3	H	p	n_1	n_2	n_3	H	p
2	1	1	2.7000	.500	4	3	2	6.4444	.008
2	2	1	3.6000	.200				6.3000	.011
2	2	2	4.5714	.067				5.4444	.046
			3.7143	.200				5.4000	.051
3	1	1	3.2000	.300				4.5111	.098
								4.4444	.102
3	2	1	4.2857	.100	4	3	3	6.7455	.010
			3.8571	.133				6.7091	.013
3	2	2	5.3572	.029				5.7909	.046
			4.7143	.048				5.7273	.050
			4.5000	.067				4.7091	.092
			4.4643	.105				4.7000	.101
3	3	1	5.1429	.043	4	4	1	6.6667	.010
			4.5714	.100				6.1667	.022
			4.0000	.129				4.9667	.048
3	3	2	6.2500	.011				4.8667	.054
			5.3611	.032				4.1667	.082
			5.1389	.061				4.0667	.102
			4.5556	.100	4	4	2	7.0364	.006
			4.2500	.121				6.8727	.011
3	3	3	7.2000	.004				5.4545	.046
			6.4889	.011				5.2364	.052
			5.6889	.029				4.5545	.098
			5.6000	.050				4.4455	.103
			5.0667	.086	4	4	3	7.1439	.010
			4.6222	.100				7.1364	.011
4	1	1	3.5714	.200				5.5985	.049
4	2	1	4.8214	.057				5.5758	.051
			4.5000	.076				4.5455	.099
			4.0179	.114				4.4773	.102
4	2	2	6.0000	.014	4	4	4	7.6538	.008
			5.3333	.033				7.5385	.011
			5.1250	.052				5.6923	.049
			4.4583	.100				5.6538	.054
			4.1667	.105				4.6539	.097
4	3	1	5.8333	.021				4.5001	.104
			5.2083	.050	5	1	1	3.8571	.143
			5.0000	.057	5	2	1	5.2500	.036
			4.0556	.093				5.0000	.048
			3.8889	.129				4.4500	.071
								4.2000	.095
								4.0500	.119

Sample sizes					Sample sizes				
n_1	n_2	n_3	*H*	*p*	n_1	n_2	n_3	*H*	*p*
5		2	6.5333	.008				5.6308	.050
			6.1333	.013				4.5487	.099
			5.1600	.034				4.5231	.103
			5.0400	.056	5	4	4	7.7604	.009
			4.3733	.090				7.7440	.011
			4.2933	.122				5.6571	.049
5	3	1	6.4000	.012				5.6176	.050
			4.9600	.048				4.6187	.100
			4.8711	.052				4.5527	.102
			4.0178	.095	5	5	1	7.3091	.009
			3.8400	.123				6.8364	.011
5	3	2	6.9091	.009				5.1273	.046
			6.8218	.010				4.9091	.053
			5.2509	.049				4.1091	.086
			5.1055	.052				4.0364	.105
			4.6509	.091	5	5	2	7.3385	.010
			4.4945	.101				7.2692	.010
5	3	3	7.0788	.009				5.3385	.047
			6.9818	.011				5.2462	.051
			5.6485	.049				4.6231	.097
			5.5152	.051				4.5077	.100
			4.5333	.097	5	5	3	7.5780	.010
			4.4121	.109				7.5429	.010
5	4	1	6.9545	.008				5.7055	.046
			6.8400	.011				5.6264	.051
			4.9855	.044				4.5451	.100
			4.8600	.056				4.5363	.102
			3.9873	.098	5	5	4	7.8229	.010
			3.9600	.102				7.7914	.010
5	4	2	7.2045	.009				5.6657	.049
			7.1182	.010				5.6429	.050
			5.2727	.049				4.5229	.099
			5.2682	.050				4.5200	.101
			4.5409	.098	5	5	5	8.0000	.009
			4.5182	.101				7.9800	.010
5	4	3	7.4449	.010				5.7800	.049
			7.3949	.011				5.6600	.051
			5.6564	.049				4.5600	.100
								4.5000	.102

From Siegel S (1956). *Nonparametric statistics for the behavioral sciences.* New York: McGraw-Hill Book Co Inc.

Index